Modern Practical Neurology

*An Introduction to
Diagnosis and Management of
Common Neurologic Disorders*

Second Edition

Modern Practical Neurology

An Introduction to Diagnosis and Management of Common Neurologic Disorders

Second Edition

Peritz Scheinberg, M.D.

Professor and Chairman
Department of Neurology
University of Miami School of Medicine
Miami, Florida

Raven Press ▪ New York

**Raven Press, 1140 Avenue of the Americas, New York,
New York 10036**

Great care has been taken to maintain the accuracy of the information
contained in the volume. However, Raven Press cannot be held responsible
for errors or for any consequences arising from the use of the information
contained herein.

Library of Congress Cataloging in Publication Data

Scheinberg, Peritz.
   Modern practical neurology.

   Includes bibliographical references and index.
   1. Nervous system—Diseases.   I. Title.
RC346.S345   1981   616.8   80-28008
ISBN 0-89004-521-6

Preface

The second edition of *Modern Practical Neurology* has been completely revised and details added to make it more responsive to the needs of medical students, house officers, and physicians who undertake to manage patients with neurological disorders. Its format is different from most standard texts of neurology in that historical, neuroanatomical, neurophysiologic, and neuropathological descriptions are not extensive but are limited to what is required to clarify the mechanisms of the disorder being described. Although the organization of the book is disease-oriented, a special effort has been made to explain symptoms and signs in the context of the mechanism of their causation.

Many medical students and physicians regard clinical neurology as a specialty concerned with the differential diagnosis of complex, degenerative disorders for which there is no useful treatment. It is true that many neurologic diseases, even some common ones, cannot be successfully treated, but the same problem exists in most of medicine, with the physician offering amelioration rather than cure. It is also true—and in this regard the public relations of neurology have not been good—that neurologists have a great deal to offer the majority of their patients. To that end, one of the major objectives of this book is to emphasize the practical problems of diagnosis and management. Liberal use has been made of computed tomography and other radiographic techniques in discussing diagnosis, and when indicated, specific details of therapy are included.

This volume, then, is less concerned with theories of mechanisms than with a concise review of the diagnosis and management of those neurological disorders most commonly seen in practice. It is not intended to be encyclopedic. Numerous monographs and multiple volume neurology texts are available to the reader who wishes more information. To assist students, residents, and others so interested in a review of pertinent literature, extensive bibliographies have been compiled to accompany each chapter.

The views expressed herein are the construct of personal experience, literature search, and much opinion-seeking from others. The reader should be reminded that, like all single-author texts, these opinions may not be shared by all other authors, authorities, or clinicians.

Peritz Scheinberg, M.D.

Acknowledgments

I am indebted to several colleagues, particularly those in the Divisions of Neuroradiology and Neuropathology of the University of Miami School of Medicine for assistance with the illustrations and to Ms. Judith Parkerson who was responsible for the transcription of the manuscript. Finally, I would like to dedicate this volume to my colleagues, house officers, and students who have contributed greatly to my education and whose stimulation (mutual I hope) continues to be a source of great pleasure, but most of all to the countless patients who have given me the privilege of learning from them.

Contents

1

The Neurologic Examination

The first prerequisite to the proper diagnosis and treatment of the patient with a neurologic disorder is the ability to perform a competent neurologic examination. To the many physicians who recall being intimidated by the vast array of nuclei and tracts that was their introduction to the anatomy of the nervous system, the task of evaluating some abnormality of these structures by a physical examination seems formidable indeed. In addition, some had a rather brief introduction to the neurologic examination during medical school without any subsequent instruction, so that the years have dimmed the original skills and knowledge. Whatever the reason, many physicians who feel perfectly comfortable when examining the heart, lungs, and abdomen feel completely inadequate about their ability to examine the nervous system and are therefore reluctant to deal with neurologic problems at all. Just as it is necessary to learn words to know a language, it is also essential to be able to appraise the nervous system intelligently before undertaking the management of a patient with a neurologic disturbance.

The fact is that the neurologic examination is not complicated. It is an application of rather simple and straightforward principles of the structure and function of the nervous system. The purpose of the neurologic examination is to localize the lesion. This does not preclude the possibility that a person may have neurologic disease in the presence of a normal neurologic examination. Indeed, rather significant central nervous system (CNS) disease may be present despite a normal neurologic examination, and patients with a variety of neurologic complaints (e.g., headaches, dizziness, or pain in an extremity) may be entirely normal to examination. Before a decision can be made about the pathology of a lesion the physician must first localize it by history and examination. This localization is an orderly review of the function of the patient's central and peripheral nervous systems, including the various localizable functions of the cerebral hemispheres, brainstem, medulla, spinal cord, nerve roots, peripheral nerves, and muscles. Although it should be as complete as possible, the examination is not necessarily intricate and should always be modified to suit the situation. Obviously, a comatose patient cannot be examined in the same fashion as can an alert and cooperative patient, but with a little practice it is possible to adjust or modify the examination according to the circumstances and still obtain the data pertinent to the problem.

It goes without saying that a good history is essential to the interpretation of the neurologic examination. Often the experienced clinician can make the appropriate diagnosis from the history and is not often surprised by the findings on examination. A good history allows the examiner to focus in on those aspects of the examination he considers to be most pertinent, thereby enabling him to detect ever more subtle pathology.

Good history-taking is a medical art form that is applicable to all organ systems. It implies the careful dissection of the patient's complaints by questions which spring from an understanding of the symptomatology of various disease states and the effects of pathology on different parts of the nervous system. A good history is never diffuse; it is pointed. The examiner finds out as much as possible about each system, calling on his knowledge of disease to formulate his questions. It is beyond the scope of this work to describe neurologic history-taking in detail, but the principle is always the same. Whether the patient's complaint is pain, weakness, dizziness, or difficulty walking, the examiner finds out enough about that symptom to identify its anatomic origin and obtain a clue as to its pathology. For example, if the patient's complaint is of weakness of an extremity, one must know:

Time of onset
Abrupt or gradual
Progressive, unchanged, or improved
Worse distally or proximally
Affected by activity or exercise
Association with other symptoms which give additional clues as to the location of the lesion, e.g., numbness or paresthesias, sphincter disorders, pain

In most instances the responses gradually fill in the spaces of the puzzle, giving a picture of the responsible pathology and allowing the examiner to approach the examination with greater confidence.

The remainder of the chapter outlines the neurologic examination. Each portion of the examination is treated separately and in some detail. It is important to get into the habit of following a pattern so as to avoid omissions. The following areas are considered:

Mental status	Motor function
Gait and station	Sensation
Head and spine	Reflexes
Cranial nerves	Autonomic and sphincter function

MENTAL STATUS

A great deal is learned about the patient's mental status during the initial interview and history taking, before the formal testing is begun. It is necessary to take note of all of the following during the examination.

State of Consciousness

The state of consciousness may vary from alert to lethargic to stuporous to comatose. Depression of consciousness is a definite indication of organic brain disease, either structural, metabolic, or toxic. Interpretation of the significance of the altered state of consciousness is dependent on the remainder of the examination. A small brainstem lesion may result in coma, but there are practically always accompanying neurologic signs which aid in localizing the lesion. These and other distinguishing features of the evaluation of the comatose patient are discussed in Chapter 11.

Appearance, Behavior, Mood, Affect, Stream of Conversation, and Thought Content

Does the patient appear to be sick, in pain, or restless? Is his behavior appropriate to the occasion and to his complaints? A glaring disparity between the patient's behavior and his symptoms and signs is suggestive of a psychiatric disorder.

Is there evidence of depression or anxiety? Many patients compensate well, so that initial appearances are deceiving. It is therefore necessary to inquire about the symptoms of each, such as:

1. Bouts of gloominess and crying
2. Severe feelings of guilt and worthlessness
3. Reduced interest in surroundings, withdrawal, lack of motivation, early morning insomnia, lack of appetite, constipation
4. Restlessness, inner tension, tremor, irritability, swings of mood

Is the patient's conversation coherent, appropriate, and relevant? Is there evidence of delusions or hallucinations?

Intellectual Functions

Orientation (To Time, Place, and Person)

Disorientation is often associated with other evidence of confusion and may mean diffuse brain disease, intoxication, metabolic disturbance, or simple dementia.

Memory

Memory determines the patient's ability to acquire and retain information. Recent memory is most severely affected in brain disease. Inquiry is made about events of the past few hours or days, and the patient is asked to remember three common objects or names for about 5 min. The examiner may determine that the patient is able to repeat several numbers immediately after they are given but has great difficulty retaining details for more than a few minutes. This represents a defect in the patient's ability to acquire new information, which is the most common abnormality in dementia. Disturbances of memory function may occur from rather localized diseases of the brain (viz., Wernicke-Korsakoff syndrome), in which instance one suspects a lesion of the medial portions of the temporal lobes, the mammillary bodies, and parts of the thalamus, or from diffuse brain disturbances, metabolic or structural.

Calculation

The parameter of calculation may be difficult to evaluate because it is so dependent on prior education and experience, but significant abnormalities suggest a disturbance in the dominant parietal lobe. The patient is asked to subtract sevens serially from 100 or to calculate how much change one would receive from a dollar following purchases of stated amounts. Such questions test the patient's ability to concentrate as well as to perform simple calculations; hence a disorder of attention may also cause difficulty in calculating.

General Information, Insight, and Judgment

The patient's store of general information as well as his insight and judgment are also dependent on his previous experiences, socioeconomic status, and so forth. Subtle alterations in a college professor would not be detectable if he were tested similarly to a poorly educated laborer. The examiner inquires about recent presidents, world or local events, and asks the patient to interpret simple proverbs to determine whether he is excessively literal or capable of deducing meanings. Proverbs frequently used are: "People who live in glass houses should not throw stones." "A bird in the hand is worth two in the bush." "A stitch in time saves nine." Comparisons such as the difference between a lie and a mistake or a baby and a midget are also helpful in evaluating the patient's reasoning capacities.

Language Function

Aside from the intellectual satisfaction of attempting to understand the nature of a patient's language disorder, it is of practical importance to establish if there is any evidence of aphasia for three reasons: (1) It helps in the localization of a lesion to a fairly predictable site in the dominant hemisphere; (2) evaluation of mental status is difficult in an aphasic or partially aphasic (dysphasic) patient; and (3) aphasia decidedly influences the patient's potential for rehabilitation. It is evident that the various mental status functions described above cannot be properly evaluated if the patient cannot understand what is said to him or cannot express himself properly. Aphasic patients are occasionally misdiagnosed as being demented or depressed unless subtle alterations in their ability to understand or communicate are recognized.

Aphasia is an impairment of language function following a lesion in the dominant hemisphere, most frequently in the posterior frontal or temporal lobe, or both. The left cerebral hemisphere is dominant in all right-handed individuals and in about half of sinistrals. Although it is not necessary to be able to classify in detail the various types of aphasia in order to recognize its existence, an understanding of the type of language dysfunction is helpful in lesion localization and in the type of speech therapy to be utilized.

There are many classifications of aphasia, just as there are many schemes for aphasia testing. The classification utilized by the Boston Veterans Administration Aphasia Research Center is a useful one; it classifies aphasias according to whether repetition is disturbed (Table 1.1).

TABLE 1.1. *Classification of aphasia*

Aphasia with abnormal repetition
  Broca's aphasia — *motor, non fluent*
  Wernicke's aphasia *receptive, fluent*
  Conduction aphasia *fluent, paraphasic*
Aphasia with preserved repetition
  Mixed transcortical aphasia
  Transcortical aphasia
  Transcortical sensory aphasia
  Anomic aphasia
Total aphasia
  Global aphasia

Broca's aphasia is the result of a lesion of some type in the dominant (usually left) frontal operculum, the posterior inferior portion of the frontal lobe. There are many names applied to it, viz., motor, executive, and nonfluent. The patient shows a reduced to absent verbal output. Speech is sparse, performed with great effort, and characterized by the use of substantive words with a paucity of prepositions, articles, and modifiers. Articulation is poor, the length of phrases is short, and there is dysprosody. Comprehension is usually good but rarely intact. Repetition of words or phrases is difficult. Dysnomia is almost always present, but this can usually be helped by prompting. Writing is usually severely disturbed as is reading comprehension. Most patients with Broca's aphasia have a right hemiparesis, but small lesions causing aphasia may not produce a motor abnormality.

Wernicke's aphasia is caused by a lesion in the dominant temporal lobe, particularly in the superior–posterior part of the first temporal gyrus. The major abnormality is a severe disturbance of comprehension of spoken and written language along with an inability to repeat words. There is almost always a great deal of verbal output, but it is usually contextually meaningless, replete with substitutions of inexact or inappropriate words for the ones wanted. This substitution is termed paraphasia. Dysnomia is severe and not improved by prompting.

Conduction aphasia is thought to be the result of pathology in the white matter fasciculus which connects Broca's and Wernicke's areas. The patients have fluent paraphasic speech, fairly good comprehension, but severe difficulty with repetition. They can comprehend what they read but cannot read aloud because of paraphasic contamination. Writing is affected by insertion of inappropriate letters or reversal of words or letters, and dysnomia is common. The dysnomia is characterized by the use of incorrect phonemes so that the word produced may be unrecognizable to the listener (neologism).

The *transcortical aphasias* are characterized by either nonfluent (transcortical motor) or fluent (transcortical sensory) aphasia with preservation of repetition. They often exhibit *echolalia*, a tendency to repeat what the examiner has said, and may be able to complete overlearned phrases. The pathology of these lesions is not precisely established. In transcortical motor aphasia the pathologic site is usually anterior or superior to Broca's area. These aphasias have been described as an isolation or disconnection of the primary speech areas from other parts of the cortex.

Anomic aphasia, or variations thereof, may occur from a lesion in almost any part of the dominant hemisphere, particularly in the general region of the language centers. The patient manifests difficulty in finding the precise word with which to express himself and often substitutes a less appropriate one.

Global aphasia is said to exist when language loss is nearly complete. There is poor verbal output and comprehension as well as repetition. The pathology is usually widespread, involving Broca's and Wernicke's areas and often much of the brain between them.

Aphasia can be diagnosed with little difficulty by the trained observer, but detailed aphasia testing requires considerable time and often a great deal of patience on the part of the examiner. The Porch Index of Communicative Ability (PICA) is a popular, relatively brief (1 hr) test for aphasia which can be administered fairly easily, but it requires considerable experience for interpretation and scoring. Most clinicians rely on straightforward bedside observations performed as part of a routine neurologic examination to obtain a perspective of the patient's language disability and the presumed location of the responsible pathology.

Reading

Although reading ability may properly be considered a part of language function, its loss may occur without aphasia. Acquired dyslexia (i.e., impairment of reading function that occurs in a previously literate adult) usually denotes a lesion of the dominant parietal lobe and is often accompanied by right homonymous hemianopsia. Primary dyslexia (i.e., difficulty in learning to read) is a more complex neurologic problem and is of little value as a sign of cerebral localization.

Praxis

Praxis is a term used to describe a variety of skilled, learned (noninstinctual) motor acts, e.g., drawing, copying figures, ability to use a simple tool or pencil, putting on one's clothes, imitating other's movements. Apraxia means loss or impairment of such functions, and it may be caused by lesions in either parietal lobe and occasionally in the frontal lobes as well. This is tested for by having the patient light a cigarette, use a screwdriver, perform a military salute, or use a comb properly.

General Observations

In addition to the above functions evaluated in a mental status examination, there are a number of other clues to the location of the patient's lesion that can be obtained from simple observation or questioning. Patients with nondominant parietal lobe lesions (usually right) may actually deny they are ill even though the opposite limbs are paralyzed (anosognosia). They may even deny that the paralyzed body parts belong to them (asomatognosia). Another clue to nondominant hemisphere disease is *motor impersistence*, characterized by inability of the patient to sustain a simple motor act (e.g., keeping his eyes closed or an arm outstretched) even though no actual motor weakness is present. Further evidence of nondominant parietal lobe disease can be determined by having the patient copy a few simple figures or draw the face of a clock with the hands of the clock pointing to a designated time. Patients with such lesions cannot copy figures or objects accurately, and they often crowd all the figures on the clock into the right half of the face (Fig. 1.1).

Dressing apraxia also occurs in nondominant parietal lobe lesions. The patient has difficulty putting on his shirt or trousers, not seeming to be able to identify which extremity goes into which sleeve or pant leg.

GAIT AND STATION

A reasonably practiced and observant physician can learn a great deal about the localization of a patient's neurologic disorder by watching him walk. Indeed, there is probably no single performance in the neurologic examina-

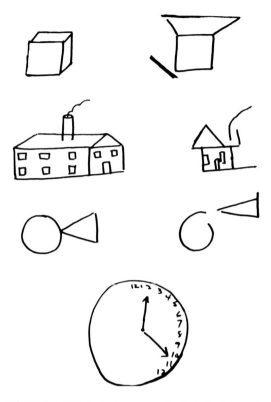

FIG. 1.1. Drawing and copying defects that occur particularly in right parietal lobe lesions but which may also occur in diffuse cortical disease. The patient has attempted to copy, on the right, figures drawn by the examiner on the left. He was also asked to draw the face of a clock with the hands pointing to 10 min after 2 o'clock. The crowding of the clock numbers to one side of the face is particularly characteristic of nondominant parietal lobe lesions. The distortions of the figures drawn by the patient are evident and denote a disorder of spatial perception.

tion so revealing as the observation of gait and station. The observer watches the patient carefully first during normal walking, observing the way in which he moves his trunk, legs, and arms, noting the rhythm of the patient's movements, observing whether there is decreased or absent arm swing (associated movements) and whether the trunk is rigid or moves naturally, checking for foot drop and the ability to turn sharply and to start and stop abruptly and smoothly. A widened base in walking means ataxia even before gross stumbling or staggering occur. The patient should be made to walk on his toes and then his heels to accentuate mild weakness of dorsiflexion or plantar flexion of the feet. Disturbances of vestibular or cerebellar function can be accentuated by tandem walking, heel to toe in a straight line, and can cause the patient to step out of the pattern or stagger to one side. Proprioceptive abnormalities (decrease in joint sensibility or position sense) are suspected if the patient complains of difficulty walking in the dark, and if the gait is characterized by slapping of the feet, exaggerated lifting of the feet, or ataxia.

The posture of the head, arms, and trunk are important in the evaluation of gait, as they may be affected in extrapyramidal or cerebellar disorders as well as in weakness of the extremities. Patients with early parkinsonism walk with few associated arm movements and turn in a characteristically rigid fashion, like a toy soldier. As the disease progresses, these patients may demonstrate festination, wherein the steps are increasingly small and rapid, until they are actually running. Certain dementias (particularly normal-pressure hydrocephalus) and frontal lobe lesions may be accompanied by difficulty in initiating coordinated walking movements, retropulsion (falling backward), and a strange awkwardness of gait. Although this is frequently termed gait apraxia, there is doubt that this meets the requirements for such a definition.

The Romberg test is designed to detect abnormalities in proprioceptive function. The patient is asked to stand with feet together. If the patient sways excessively, falls, or cannot maintain that posture with open eyes, a cerebellar lesion must be suspected. A positive Romberg test is present if the patient has difficulty maintaining that posture with closed eyes; this should be confirmed by the sensory examination of the lower extremities, which should indicate impairment of position, vibration sensibility, or both.

HEAD AND SPINE

Examination of the head and spine requires little additional time and may pay huge dividends, particularly if one is examining a comatose patient, wherein the examiner must look carefully for any signs of head injury (e.g., abrasions or lacerations) or Battle's sign (ecchymoses over the mastoid region), which frequently accompanies basilar skull fracture. Abnormalities in head size or configuration may be helpful in diagnosis, particularly in children. Similarly, scoliosis or unusual spine configurations should be noted, for they may point to an underlying neurologic problem. Scoliosis is particularly common in muscular dystrophy, certain types of cerebellar system diseases, and slow-growing spinal cord tumors, e.g., astrocytoma. Spine tenderness may indicate underlying bone disease (e.g., tumor or infection), and flexibility of the spine is important when the patient complains of neck, low back, or extremity pain. If there is any suspicion of meningitis or subarachnoid hemorrhage, one must look for neck rigidity, pain on flexion of the neck, and a positive Kernig or Brudzinski sign. When examining a patient with complaints of low back or lower extremity pain, a useful trick is to have the patient bend forward as far as possible without bending the knees, at which time percussion or finger pressure over the sciatic notch (the upper–outer quadrant of the gluteus muscle) may provoke local or radiating pain if the patient's problem is caused by compression of one of the roots of the sciatic nerve, as by a herniated disc.

CRANIAL NERVES

The cranial nerves are usually examined in sequence. Appreciation of normal or abnormal function is dependent on a few neuroanatomic principles.

Olfactory

It is helpful to test for appreciation, but not necessarily identification, of aromatic, nonirritating odors (e.g., coffee, peppermint, cloves). Most of the time it is sufficient to know if the patient can taste food flavors, for this faculty is dependent on intact olfaction. Olfaction should be evaluated in any patient suspected of having frontal lobe disease (viz., dementia, personality change, or unexplained gait disorders) because of the possibility of a tumor on the orbital surface of the frontal lobes in such an instance. Other causes for anosmia include local nasal or nasopharyngeal disease, head trauma with injury to the olfactory bulbs, psychogenic disturbance, and pernicious anemia.

Optic

Tests for visual function include evaluation of visual acuity and fields of vision. A Snellen eye chart or a J. G. Rosenbaum Pocket Vision Screener, which is inexpensive and commercially available, may be used. The card is held in good light, and best corrected visual acuity is measured in each eye, allowing the patient to hold the card at the most comfortable distance. If the patient's best corrected visual acuity is faulty, it means that there is a defect in the macula or the optic nerve, provided there is no abnormality in the ocular media (lens, vitreous, etc.). Such a finding always demands explanation, which should be sought from an ophthalmologist if it is not apparent to the examiner.

A person's visual fields include all that he can see when he fixes his gaze on one target. The examination should therefore include the area around the fixation points of both eyes as well as the periphery. Defects in the visual fields may be caused by lesions of the retina, optic nerve, chiasm, optic tracts, and optic radiations. The abnormalities caused by lesions in each of these areas are fairly stereotyped, so that the location of the lesion can usually be predicted from the pattern of the field deficit. Lesions of the optic nerve cause central scotomas or complete blindness in the affected eye. The field deficit caused by lesions of the optic chiasm depends on the portion of the chiasm involved, but the usual and "characteristic" chiasmatic deficit is bitemporal hemianopsia, caused by interruption of the crossing fibers in the center of the chiasm by a pituitary or other perichiasmal tumor. Lesions involving the visual pathways posterior to the chiasm, namely the optic tract, lateral geniculate body, optic radiations, or visual cortex cause *homonymous hemianop-*

sia, (i.e., a visual defect in corresponding or homonymous half-fields of both eyes). The congruity of the visual field defect refers to the similarity of size and shape of the paired defects. The congruity of the defect may give a clue as to its location. A complete anatomical lesion will cause a complete homonymous field defect, which, therefore, gives little clue as to the anatomical location of the lesion. Optic tract lesions are rarely complete and the resultant hemianopsia is therefore rarely congruous. Lesions of the anterior temporal lobe may characteristically cause a superior quadrantanopsia which is incongruous, because of the anatomical disposition of Meyer's loop. More posteriorly the fibers in the geniculocalcarine radiations become increasingly contiguous so that lesions are somewhat likelier to cause congruous field defects or complete homonymous hemianopsias. The absence of any other neurologic deficit in the presence of a congruous field defect or complete hemianopsia points to the occipital lobe as the location of the lesion. Macular sparing is said to be characteristic of occipital lobe lesions, presumably due to a double blood supply to the area of macular representation in the cortex. In some instances macular sparing may be an artifact of poor ocular fixation during the testing.

There are several methods of examining the visual fields quickly and accurately by confrontation. All depend upon the patient's ability to fixate vision reasonably well upon one object (examiner's nose). The four quadrants of vision of each eye should be tested.

One way is to compare the patient's fields with those of the examiner by using a small object, remembering that the fields include the central 30° of vision as well as the periphery. Other methods include asking the patient to compare the appearance of the examiner's hands when they are held up simultaneously, on either side of the vertical meridian of each eye. One hand will appear darker or less clear than the other if there is a defect in that field of vision. In this way the nasal and temporal fields of the patient's eye can be compared to each other. Another similar method is to use a red object rather than one's hand as the target. The red color will appear brighter in a normal than in a defective field.

There are other even simpler methods which must occasionally be resorted to, depending upon the patient's state of awareness or cooperation. On occasion the examiner must rely on the patient's blinking or flinching to a threatening hand movement aimed at his face from each field of vision. Persistence and resourcefulness are important assets when adapting the testing procedure to the patient's capabilities.

Ophthalmoscopic examination should be performed in every patient. One must examine for the state of the optic disc, the adjacent retina, the arterioles and venules, and, if possible, the macula. The optic disc is examined to determine if there is any evidence of papilledema or atrophy. Recognition of early papilledema may be difficult, but there are several helpful criteria:

1. *Color of the disc.* The swollen disc usually has a congested appearance, being darker or pinker than normal.

2. *Margins of the disc.* There may be blurring of the disc margins, which are normally distinct.

3. *Venular size.* In early papilledema, the retinal venules are engorged and increased in diameter.

4. *Venular pulsations.* Pulsation of the venules on the disc are usually seen in the normal eye, but absence of pulsations is not necessarily pathologic. If venular pulsations are present, it is highly unlikely that there is papilledema, regardless of other findings.

5. *Physiologic cup.* Contrary to popular conception, the physiologic cup does not usually disappear in early papilledema. Its absence suggests pseudopapilledema, a congenital anomaly of the disc.

6. *Retinal hemorrhages.* The finding of small splinter hemorrhages adjacent to the disc is strongly confirmatory of papilledema in suspected cases, but their presence is not necessary to make the diagnosis.

Sometimes even experts cannot be certain whether a disc is swollen, in which instance the clinical setting must be considered. Careful evaluation of the above points, however, usually allows the examiner to determine if papilledema is present.

Optic atrophy is characterized by pallor of the disc and distinctness of the disc margin. Early optic atrophy can be detected by counting the arterioles that traverse the disc margin. There should be 10 or more such arterioles, whereas in early optic atrophy the number is reduced to six or seven. Optic atrophy is almost always accompanied by a diminution of vision in the affected eye and may be the result of a prior episode of retrobulbar optic neuritis or retinal occlusive vascular disease, or it may be the end result of papilledema. In any case, the cause should be determined.

Oculomotor, Trochlear, and Abducens Nerves

This part of the examination concerns itself with pupillary function, extra-ocular movements, and the appearance and motility of the eye-lids. The major interest in the pupils is in their reactivity to light, although symmetry is sometimes diagnostically important and should be evaluated. The patient should fix his gaze on a distant object in a dimly-lighted room while both pupils are simultaneously indirectly illuminated by a dim light from below. Pupillary size in this mid-dilated state should be estimated or measured in millimeters and equality and regularity noted. Pupillary inequality is an important finding and requires an explanation; it should not simply be observed and then ignored. Unilateral pupillary dilatation may denote an early 3rd nerve lesion, even if eye movements are intact. As is described in detail in Chapter 11, changes in pupillary size are of critical importance in the evaluation of a stuporous or comatose patient. A dilated, poorly reactive pupil in such a setting may indicate compression of the 3rd nerve by transtentorial herniation of the medial portion of the temporal lobe due to a mass lesion. An abnormally small pupil on one side suggests Horner's syndrome, which may be caused by any lesion which affects the sympathetic fibers to the pupil. It is usually accompanied by narrowing of the palpebral fissure and homolateral anhidrosis of the face. Horner's syndrome may be caused by a lesion of the medulla, cervical cord, or cervical sympathetic chain. The anisocoria of Horner's syndrome is much more evident in dim light because of failure of pupillary dilatation on the involved side. Contrary to popular conception unilateral visual field or acuity defects do not cause anisocoria because unilateral afferent visual stimulation causes bilateral equal pupillary stimulation.

Reaction to light should preferably be tested in a dimly lighted room, using a bright light. The rate and extent of constriction of the pupils is noted by direct stimulation of each separately. If a pupil reacts poorly to direct stimulation, the consensual reaction should be observed by shining the light on the other pupil. If the consensual response is greater than the direct response, it signifies a defect in the afferent visual arc, usually the optic nerve, as occurs in optic neuritis. Visual acuity is usually found to be defective in the eye with the diminished direct response to light, although the pupillary defect may persist after complete recovery of visual acuity following an episode of optic neuritis. In the presence of a unilateral visual arc defect both pupils respond slowly and incompletely when the affected eye is light-stimulated, but normally when light is shone into the good eye. This difference or alteration in pupillary reactions may be emphasized by the swinging flashlight test, in which the light is swung back and forth from one eye to the other. This is sometimes called the Marcus Gunn phenomenon and is dependent upon bilateral innervation of each Edinger-Westphal nucleus from the pre-tectal nuclear complex which receives the afferent light signals.

Poorly reactive pupils must be examined for the near reflex by having the patient fixate vision first upon a distant object and then upon his own finger held immediately in front of his nose. If the pupillary reaction to light is appreciably slower and less complete than it is to near vision, and one or both pupils are miotic, the diagnosis of central nervous system lues must be considered. Bilateral poorly reactive dilated pupils may be caused by anticholinergic drugs; unilateral pupillary fixation and dilatation in the absence of other pathology suggests local application of a mydriatic, either accidentally or factitiously.

Horner's syndrome may indicate the presence of serious pathology involving the oculo-sympathetic system and these patients require careful evaluation. The clarification of sympathetic paralysis of the pupil can usually be accomplished by 4% cocaine drops in each eye. The normal pupil dilates, whereas the Horner's pupil will not.

Extraocular movements are mediated through the action of the 3rd, 4th, and 6th cranial nerves. The 6th nerve (abducens) innervates the lateral rectus muscle, the sole function of which is to abduct the eye. Lesions of the 6th nerve cause double vision, and examination indicates that the eye cannot be abducted (turned laterally). The 4th nerve innervates the superior oblique muscle, and the 3rd nerve innervates all the other extraocular muscles, including the levator palpebrae superioris. An acute lesion of one of these nerves or one of the muscles innervated by them usually produces diplopia, which is corrected by covering one eye. Diplopia is often absent in longstanding extraocular lesions because the patient has learned to suppress the extra image. Because each of the extraocular muscles has a special function according to the position of the eye, it is best to follow a simple pattern in this examination, as indicated in Fig. 1.2.

The patient's eyes follow a light or target. When the target is moved to the patient's right, one is testing the right lateral rectus (6th nerve) and the left medial rectus (3rd nerve). In that position (eyes turned to the right), the patient is asked to follow the target up and then down. This tests the right superior rectus (3rd nerve) and left inferior oblique (3rd nerve) on up gaze and the right inferior rectus (3rd nerve) and left superior oblique (4th nerve) on down gaze. The patient then follows the target to the left and the movements are repeated. This simple and rapid format permits all extraocular muscles to be tested, and the observer can determine if there is a defect. The observer will also thus be able to detect a disturbance in conjugate gaze (ability to move eyes together), which denotes a CNS lesion.

Aside from evaluation of the individual extraocular muscles the above testing procedure also gives a great deal of information about conjugate eye movements, that is, the ability to move the eyes simultaneously in the same vertical or horizontal direction. Rapid versional movements are called saccades; whereas tracking movements, as in visual pursuit, are called pursuit

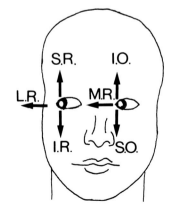

FIG. 1.2. Examination of extraocular movements. LR = lateral rectus. IR = inferior rectus. SR = superior rectus. MR = medical rectus. IO = inferior oblique. SO = superior oblique.

movements. Lesions of the frontal lobe cause impairment of conjugate gaze to the opposite side and pontine lesions impair conjugate movements toward the side of the lesion. Vertical upward conjugate movements are physiologically reduced with age and are also impaired by bilateral pretectal lesions (pineal tumor). Vertical downward conjugate movement defects are rare and appear to be caused by lesions dorsal and medial to the red nuclei. The cause of conjugate movement disorders is always some type of lesion of the central nervous system. Because synchronous eye movement, even though impaired, is retained, diplopia is not a symptom.

Opticokinetic nystagmus (OKN) is a physiologic phenomenon which occurs when a series of vertical bars is moved horizontally in front of the eyes. The eyes follow the bars slowly to the side of the movement direction and then snap back to follow the succeeding bar. Failure or impairment of OKN in one direction of target movement denotes a lesion in the cerebral hemisphere on the side toward which the target was moving. OKN defects often occur with hemianopsias and are most prominent in lesions of the parietal lobes. OKN testing may be of great value in determining whether sight is present in malingering or hysterical patients.

Patients with extraocular motor defects often complain of diplopia, the mechanism of which will frequently be elucidated by the plan of extraocular motor testing described above. The objective of diplopia testing is to determine which extraocular muscle(s) is weak, and history taking is designed to elucidate the pathology (myasthenia gravis, trauma, aneurysm, diabetes, multiple sclerosis, thyroid disease, etc.). If the ocular mechanism responsible for the diplopia cannot be discovered by the examination procedure previously described, it becomes necessary to undertake special testing with lenses or Maddox rod; details of these examinations are beyond the scope of this book.

A great deal can be learned by careful examination of the position and motility of the eye-lids, which are innervated by the 3rd nerve. Aside from ptosis, which may signify 3rd nerve palsy, a congenital lesion, myasthenia, thyroid disease, facial trauma, Horner's syndrome, or a variety of other less common entities, the examiner must also inspect for lid retraction, which may suggest thyroid disease, lesions of the posterior 3rd ventricle, myasthenia gravis, or infantile hydrocephalus.

When testing eye movements, the presence or absence of nystagmus is noted. It is not within the province of this book to discuss in detail either the mechanisms of nystagmus or the different varieties and their pathologic significance, but because nystagmus is such an important diagnostic finding some clarification and embellishment are required here.

Nystagmus is a to and fro ocular oscillation in which the two phases have approximately similar amplitudes. Convention has decreed that nystagmus be characterized as either *pendular* in which the to and fro movements are about equal in intensity (amplitude frequency) and *jerk*, in which there is a slow phase away from an object of fixation and a fast (saccadic) return phase. Convention also requires that *the direction of the fast component defines the direction of the nystagmus*. With these semantic considerations it becomes possible for clinicians to communicate their findings accurately and consistently to each other, and it has been established that certain kinds of nystagmus are associated with lesions in specific anatomic regions. It should be emphasized that these correlations, although clinically useful, are nevertheless empiric and the precise explanation of the physiologic mechanisms responsible for these eye movements is far from complete.

Pendular nystagmus is almost always congenital; rarely it may occur secondary to brainstem or cerebellar disease.

The commonest causes of horizontal jerk nystagmus are:

1. Gaze-evoked nystagmus (GEN) which is elicited by attempted maintenance of an eccentric eye position. A few beats of GEN is normal, whereas sustained GEN may be pathological. Probably the most frequent causes of bidirectional GEN are sedatives or anticonvulsants. Unilateral GEN is always pathological and suggests vestibular system disease.

2. Vestibular nystagmus. The fast component beats away from the diseased end organ. It may be present in primary position of gaze or gaze-evoked and is usually worse with ocular deviation in a specific direction. The nystagmus of peripheral vestibular pathology is often rotatory and horizontal whereas lesions of the retrocochlear vestibular anatomy may cause purely horizontal nystagmus. Pure vertical or pure rotatory nystagmus is never of peripheral origin but rather suggest a central lesion.

A large number of special nystagmus types have been identified. In most instances these will be described in this book in the discussion of the diseases which produce them. A few are mentioned briefly here:

1. *Downbeat nystagmus*. Nystagmus in primary position of gaze beating downward. This is seen mainly in lesions of the cranio-cervical junction.

2. *Rotary nystagmus*. Pure rotary nystagmus points to a lesion in the diencephalon. *See-saw nystagmus* is a variant.

3. *Dissociated nystagmus* is asymmetrical in the two eyes in either amplitude or duration. It is seen most commonly in the presence of inter-nuclear ophthalmoplegia.

Four other unusual forms of eye movement should be mentioned because they may be observed during the ocular examination:

1. *Ocular dysmetria* is a common eye sign in cerebellar disease. The patient's eyes overshoot the fixation point when he is asked to gaze back and forth between two objects. Re-fixation saccades are evident and give the visual impression of dysmetria.

2. *Ocular bobbing* is observed as fast downward jerks of both eyes with a slow return to mid-position, occurring in patients with severe pontine lesions, usually hemorrhage.

3. *Ocular myoclonus* is a continuous horizontal or vertical ocular oscillation with a frequency of 2 to 5 per second. It usually occurs in conjunction with palatal myoclonus and the pathology is in the central tegmental tract.

4. *Opsoclonus* consists of rapid, chaotic, repetitive, conjugate eye movements in all directions, persisting during sleep. It may be seen in post-infectious encephalopathy or, together with cerebellar ataxia, as a sign of neuroblastoma.

Trigeminal Nerve

The trigeminal nerve has a sensory and motor component. The sensory portion is divided into three distinct peripheral nerves: (1) ophthalmic branch: sensation to forehead and anterior 2 to 3 inches of the scalp; (2) maxillary division: sensation from the maxillary region; (3) mandibular division: mandibular area, lower lip, chin, down to mandibular line (Fig. 1.3).

The examiner tests each division separately with a pin and compares the two sides. The corneal reflex is tested by touching the cornea lightly with a wisp of cotton. The efferent arc of the corneal reflex is the 7th nerve.

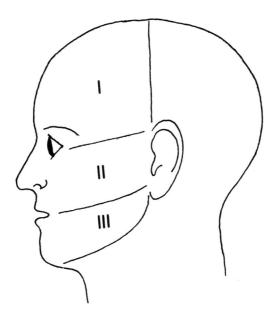

FIG. 1.3. Distribution of the three sensory divisions of the 5th cranial nerve.

The muscles of mastication are innervated by the motor division of the trigeminal nerve. The examiner palpates the bulk and symmetry of the masseter and temporal muscles while the patient clenches his teeth. When the jaw is opened it deviates toward the side of the weak pterygoid muscle. Pterygoid weakness can also be assessed by asking the patient to move the jaw horizontally. Weakness of the right pterygoid causes weak movement toward the left and vice-versa.

The muscles innervated by the trigeminal nerve must be examined with particular care in a patient complaining of facial pain, for motor 5th nerve involvement may occur early in lesions involving the skull base, e.g., nasopharyngeal carcinoma.

Facial Nerve

The motor division of the 7th cranial nerve innervates the mimetic muscles of the face, the frontalis, orbicularis oculi and oris, and platysma. One looks for symmetry of function during spontaneous movement, at rest, and on command to close eyes, grimace, and wrinkle the forehead. The examiner must look for minor degrees of dysfunction. Note that when a lesion is present in the CNS pathways above the level of the 7th nerve nucleus in the pons, there is relative sparing of involvement of eye closure and forehead wrinkling. Peripheral 7th nerve lesions (e.g., Bell's palsy) cause weakness of all homolateral facial muscles. Testing for taste on the anterior two-thirds of the tongue may be useful in peripheral 7th nerve lesions to detect whether the nerve is involved proximal or distal to the entry of the chorda tympani (taste).

Subtle twitching of the orbicularis oculi muscles is not uncommon when a patient is fatigued or under emotional stress, but other involuntary facial movements may be a cause for concern. These include facial hemispasm and facial myokymia. Facial hemispasm usually begins with infrequent involuntary unilateral facial contractions lasting for a few seconds. These may increase in frequency, severity, and duration, causing discomfort and embarrassment. The etiology is not often established, although it is believed that the spasm may be caused by a lesion involving the 7th nerve, either a tumor or compression by a sclerotic or aberrant artery. Certainly such pathology should be sought in these patients. Facial myokymia is characterized by discrete vermicular movements of facial muscles and is usually associated with a serious brainstem lesion, either multiple sclerosis or tumor.

Auditory and Vestibular Nerves

There may be significant reduction in hearing without the patient's knowledge. Evaluation of hearing is particularly important if an 8th nerve tumor or other posterior fossa tumor is suspected. Gross testing can be accomplished by asking the patient to compare the tick of a watch or a tuning fork (256 vibrations per second) in each ear and with a normal control (the examiner).

The Weber test is designed to give rough information about the location of the lesion responsible for hearing loss. If hearing loss in one ear is caused by middle ear disease (conduction), a tuning fork placed against the middle of the forehead is heard better in the deaf ear, whereas if the hearing loss is secondary to nerve disease it is heard better in the opposite ear. If the Weber lateralizes to one ear, the examiner must then decide if the cause is middle ear disease in the lateralized ear or nerve disease of the opposite ear. In fact, if air conduction (tuning fork held adjacent to ear) is reduced on the side to which the Weber lateralizes, the examiner can conclude that the problem is middle ear deafness on that side. Traditionally if the Weber test lateralizes, the Rinne test may be used to clarify whether nerve or conduction deafness is present. The vibrating tuning fork is placed first on the mastoid and then adjacent to the auricle. The patient with normal hearing or mild nerve deafness will hear it better in the latter position, that is, air conduction will be louder than bone conduction, whereas in middle ear disease (conductive deafness) the tuning fork will be louder when held on the bone. *Audiometry is essential to any situation in which hearing evaluation or characterization of hearing deficit is important to the diagnosis.*

The distinction between conduction and nerve deafness is of the greatest importance in evaluation of hearing disturbances, as is the finer distinction between cochlear and retrocochlear lesions. These distinctions and their evaluation will be discussed in greater detail in Chapter 6.

Precise evaluation of vestibular function is difficult. Lesions of the 8th nerve may cause vertigo or a feeling of disequilibrium; and these may be reflected in gait or by the presence of nystagmus. The examiner may turn the patient's head and neck sharply to either side to attempt to induce vertigo or have the patient lie supine with his head about 45° below the horizontal and then turn his head sharply to either side in an effort to induce vertigo and/or nystagmus. Ice water caloric testing is usually reserved for evaluation of the comatose patient (Chapter 11) or to determine if there is unilateral reduction of vestibular function in a patient suspected of having an 8th nerve tumor.

Bulbar Functions

Bulbar functions are the combined function of the 9th, 10th, and 12th nerves. The 9th and 10th nerves (glossopharyngeal and vagus) actually constitute one nuclear complex in the medulla, so that function of both is tested together. These two nerves supply, among other things, motor and sensory function to the palate and larynx and, therefore, their disease or injury cause dysphagia (difficulty in swallowing) associated usually with pooling of saliva in the mouth and pharynx and drooling. Swallowing of liquids is accompanied by nasal regurgitation or aspiration and the patient may be unable to swallow a bolus of solid food without choking. Speech is usually nasal in quality, the tone being induced by inability to close off the nasopharynx from the oropharynx during speech. Hoarseness suggests laryngeal paralysis or weakness. Unilateral vocal cord paralysis makes it difficult for the patient to say "e" because the cords cannot be properly approximated.

On examination one looks for symmetrical elevation of the palate. Drawing up of the palate on one side with deviation of the uvula to that side denotes weakness of the opposite palate (9th and 10th nerves). The gag reflex is done to test both sensation (9th nerve) and motor function (10th nerve). The back of the throat is touched with an applicator stick and the resultant gag response and palatal elevation are noted. Unilateral loss of the gag reflex is always abnormal. It must be determined if the loss of the reflex is due to impaired sensation or motor function. Bilateral decrease or absence of the gag reflex may be found in certain normal subjects.

It is difficult to test taste on the posterior third of the tongue (9th nerve) and this is rarely required in order to establish the presence or absence of a lesion.

The tongue is first examined unprotruded, looking for asymmetry, muscle twitching (fasciculations), or atrophy. The tongue always protrudes toward the side of the weakness, whether the lesion is supranuclear or peripheral. Wasting or fasciculations denote disease of the hypoglossal nucleus (amyotrophic lateral sclerosis or syringobulbia) or of the hypoglossal nerve itself. Tremor and involuntary movements of the protruded tongue are common in certain movement disorders and dyskinesias produced by drugs.

Dysarthria may occur in the absence of weakness of the bulbar muscles, but may indicate lack of normal coordination of diaphragm, intercostal muscles, larynx, pharynx, tongue and lips. Excellent examples of this type of problem include cerebral palsy, particularly the athetoid type, dystonia of any sort, multiple sclerosis, drug or alcohol intoxication, Parkinson's syndrome, and other movement disorders and cerebellar system lesions.

Spinal Accessory Nerve

The 11th cranial nerve innervates the sternocleidomastoid and upper one-third of the trapezius muscles. It should be tested for by shoulder elevation, head turning, head flexion, and extension. Recall that the right sternomastoid turns the head to the left. Careful examination of these muscle functions is indicated if a lesion is suspected in the region of the foramen magnum (cervical medullary junction). Tumors or congenital anomalies (Arnold-Chiari syndrome) may affect the various branches of the 11th nerve and thereby offer an important clue to diagnosis.

MOTOR FUNCTION

A complete and detailed examination for motor function requires considerable time and practice as well as knowledge of the innervation and action of each individual muscle. Fortunately, such a detailed examination is not necessary for the great majority of patients. Lesions of the CNS produce weakness or alteration in function of groups of muscles, and ordinarily that is all that is necessary to test. If the problem is to localize a specific peripheral nerve or nerve root lesion by muscle testing, individual muscle testing is required. The interested reader is referred to the many complete tests of neurologic diagnoses and particularly to the paper bound *Aids to the Investigation of Peripheral Nerve Injuries*, published by Her Majesty's Stationery Office. The motor examination is much more than an appraisal of muscle strength; rather it tests all aspects of motor function. The following pattern is suggested:

1. *Inspect* the muscles and extremities carefully looking for symmetry, atrophy, hypertrophy, and adventitious movements. Disuse muscle atrophy (e.g., immobilization of a limb for treatment of fracture) is diffuse involving all affected muscles, whereas atrophy secondary to lower motor neuron disease may involve one or two muscle groups only and is often irregular in distribution. The clinical distinction is not always simple. Adventitious movements give a great deal of information as to the localization and type of pathology.

Fasciculations. These are irregularly occurring twitches under the skin, frequently accentuated after activity. Fine fasciculations indicate lower motor neuron disease. They must be distinguished from myokymia, which usually appears as twitching of the orbicularis oculi after stress or excessive physical activity.

Spasm. Spasm of the extremities, particularly the lower extremities, is usually characterized by brief episodes of extensor rigidity and almost invariably means progressive spinal cord disease. It is a sign of upper motor neuron disease.

Myoclonus. Myoclonus is a jerking of a limb or muscle (or group of muscles) and is seen in lesions in a number of anatomic locations. It occurs most commonly in the course of severe metabolic encephalopathies and in certain progressive diseases of the CNS, e.g., myoclonus epilepsy, subacute sclerosing panencephalitis (measles), and Jakob-Creutzfeldt syndrome. The last two entities are considered slow-virus invasions of the CNS.

Tremor. A disorder of postural adjustment of the extremities, tremor at rest, is seen characteristically in Parkinson's syndrome, in which the tremor is usually rhythmic and characterized by a pill-rolling movement of the fingers. Benign familial tremor is more evident when the extremities are used, and so-called cerebellar tremor, or intention tremor, is actually a form of dysmetria, i.e., an inability to coordinate agonist and antagonist muscle groups so that the extremity over- and underreaches and cannot fixate properly. Action tremor is the term applied to tremor that occurs primarily or is aggravated by placing the extremities in certain postures, e.g., the tremor of hyperthyroidism, which is accentuated when the hands and arms are extended in front of the body. The postural tremor differs, therefore, from a resting tremor or intention tremor.

Chorea. Chorea is characterized by quick, inappropriate thrusting movements of the extremities, head, neck, or trunk, so that the patient may drop objects repeatedly. It is presumably caused by a lesion of putamen and caudate, and is seen during childhood as Sydenham's chorea and in adults in Huntington's disease.

Athetosis and other tonic movements. Athetosis is a writhing, nondeforming movement of the extremities, head, neck, tongue, cranial musculature, and trunk which occurs almost invariably as a consequence of neonatal

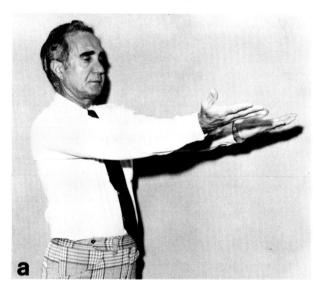

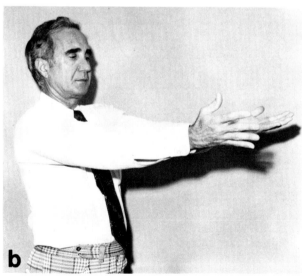

FIG. 1.4. The pronator-drift test for mild arm weakness. **a:** Arms are extended in a supinated position. **b:** Partial pronation occurs before the right arm drifts downward.

hypoxia and is usually classified as a form of "cerebral palsy." *Torsion dystonia* is an exaggeration of athetosis that appears during early adolescence or adulthood. It may begin with sustained posturing of an extremity but eventually involves practically all muscle groups and produces severe deformity. *Dystonic movements* are not uncommon signs of intoxication by certain drugs (phenothiazines, L-DOPA). When the dystonic movements involve mainly the tongue and mouth, they are called *buccal-lingual dyskinesia*.

Hemiballismus is a rare movement disorder characterized by throwing movements of the extremities on one side. It is thought to be secondary to infarction to the subthalamic nucleus of Luys.

Spasmodic torticollis is a rare disorder related to the dystonias in which the patient's head and neck are spasmodically twisted to one side or bent backward. The anatomic basis is not known.

Habit spasms are seen in children. They are called *tics* and are probably psychogenic in origin. These are characterized by compulsive movements of the face, eye-blinking, etc.

2. *Test for power and fatigability.* As indicated above, the extent of this examination is determined by the need. In an examination to exclude brain disease, gross strength of extremities is compared bilaterally. The patient holds his arms out in front of him, fingers and thumb extended, with the hands supinated and the eyes closed. Inability to maintain this posture on one side may be the only clue to weakness (Fig. 1.4). If detailed muscle testing is required, the examiner proceeds from the proximal portions of the extremities distally, following the segmental innervation of the muscles. *As a general rule,*

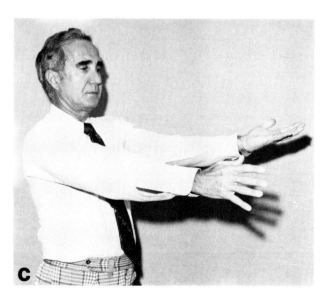

FIG. 1.4. c: Increased pronation as the weak right arm begins a downward drift.

it is worthwhile to remember that symmetrical weakness of the proximal muscles suggests myopathy, whereas distal weakness usually denotes neuropathy. Excessive muscle fatigability may occur even if the initial effort is of normal strength. This is seen in myasthenia gravis and in the myasthenic syndrome.

Although a detailed description of individual muscle testing is beyond the scope of this book, it is important for the serious examiner to know how to test the function of the major muscles or muscle groups and to have access to a chart which describes the innervation of the muscles. Muscle strength can be quantitated reasonably well using a simple scale; this can be useful when assaying worsening or recovery of the weakness. The scale is in terms of strength:

5 = Normal
4 = Overcome by resistance
3 = Can move against gravity only
2 = Can move only if gravity is eliminated
1 = Only a trace of contraction *(no movement across joint)*
0 = No muscular contraction

Since all muscles are innervated by more than a single nerve root, no simple correlation can be made. The following is one that may be used for rapid screening:

Trapezius	C_{3-4}	Iliopsoas	$L_{1,2,3}$
Supra- and infraspinatus	C_{5-6}	Quadriceps	$L_{2,3,4}$
Deltoid	C_{5-6}	Hamstrings	L_5,S_1
Biceps	C_{5-6}	Gastrocnemius	S_1,S_2
Triceps	C_{7-8}	Anterior tibial (dorsiflexes	
Wrist and finger extensors	C_{7-8}	ankle)	$L_{4,5}$
Wrist and finger flexors	C_8-D_1	Extensor digitorum longus	L_5,S_1
Interossei	C_8-D_1	Small muscles of foot	$S_{1,2}$

3. *Test the resistance to rapidly repeated passive stretch* to detect the presence of rigidity (basal ganglia disease), spasticity (corticospinal tract disease) or hypotonia (cerebellar disease). I acknowledge that the clinical and physiologic differentiation between rigidity and spasticity may be hazy. The terms are used here in their most clinically accepted sense. The rigidity of parkinsonism is typical in its characterization as cogwheel type, for that is how it feels, whereas the spasticity of upper motor neuron lesions (as in spastic hemiplegia) is a feeling of resistance followed by sudden release of resistance (clasp knife). Patients with severe bilateral frontal lobe disease may exhibit increased resistance with increasing efforts by the examiner to flex or extend an extremity. This is sometimes called *Gegenhalten* or paratonia and usually is an indication of severe and widespread brain disease.

4. *Accuracy and coordination* are cerebellar and cortical functions. They are tested by (1) having the patient touch his or her nose or the examiner's finger in rapid succession with one finger of each hand; (2) the heel-to-shin test familiar to all physicians; (3) asking the patient to clench his fists and rotate one arm rapidly around the other; or (4) rapid alternating movements, sometimes called diadochokinesis. Rapid accurate finger movements may also be used to test for coordination.

5. *Testing for learned acts* was already described under *Praxis, Mental Status*, above. This can be evaluated only if there is no primary motor dysfunction, e.g., weakness or incoordination. The patient is asked to use common tools, copy simple geometric designs, and fill in the face of a clock. Anatomic localization of apraxias may be difficult unless other signs are also present.

SENSATION

An examination for sensation requires the cooperation of the patient. About all that can be determined in stuporous or poorly cooperative patients is whether the patient is able to perceive pinprick at various sites, and this is done by judging the patient's response (withdrawal, etc.) to the painful stimulus. As in the muscle function evaluation, the goal of the examination should be kept in mind when testing sensation. Clearly, it is of the greatest importance to test all modalities carefully if a peripheral neuropathy or a nerve root or spinal cord lesion is suspected. In the last, the sensory level may be the most important single clinical finding. Similarly, the physician must keep in mind a simple dermatome scheme or else he will be unable to distinguish neuropathies from radiculopathies. An acceptable sensory segmental dermatome scheme is shown in Fig. 1.5. Moreover, the types of sensory abnormalities that occur with spinal cord lesions can be appreciated only if the anatomy of the spinal cord is recalled. Pinprick (pain) must always be tested. It is best to examine both sides simultaneously for comparison and to check key dermatomes beginning distally (sacraldermatomes), and then moving proximally up the lower extremities, trunk, upper extremities, and neck. Delay in response to the stimulus usually means prolonged nerve conduction time, an almost certain indication of peripheral neuropathy, as does hyperpathia or hyperesthesia. If a spinal cord lesion is suspected, check carefully for a "level" at which the quality of the pinprick sensation seems to change, starting at the bottom and moving upward.

Position sensibility is tested by the patient's ability to detect slight movements of the fingers or toes. The simplest way to detect early changes is to grasp a big toe between two fingers and ask the patient when and in what direction the movement is perceived. Disturbances are characterized by the necessity to move the digit up or down several degrees before any movement

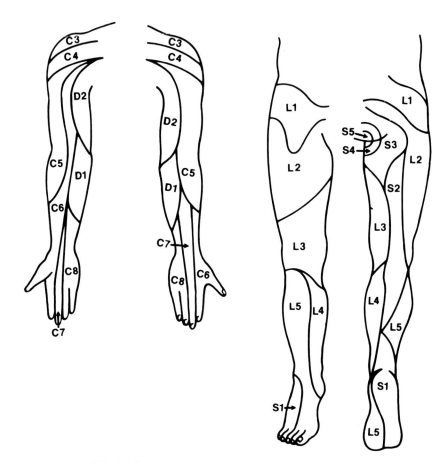

FIG. 1.5. Dermatome pattern in upper and lower extremities.

is detected by the patient. With severe lesions, the abnormality is obvious if any attempt is made to test it.

Vibration sense is tested with a 128-vps tuning fork, beginning distally. If distal vibration sense is intact, there is little need to proceed up the extremity. Moderate (not maximum) intensity vibration should be used if early lesions are to be detected. Vibration sensitivity is normally impaired in the toes and feet of elderly people.

Touch and temperature discrimination require testing only if the examiner wishes to confirm another finding or if the problem is obscure and every possible clue must be obtained.

The rule of thumb is that generalized peripheral neuropathies produce distal (stocking-glove) type impairment of all or most sensory modalities, although one (e.g., vibration in diabetes mellitus) may be involved much more than others. Nerve root lesions may produce restricted sensory loss, but then always in a dermatomal pattern. Spinal cord disease may cause loss of all sensory modalities below a certain level, or it may result in impairment of specific modalities (as in vitamin B_{12} deficiency in which only the dorsal sensory columns are involved) or a dissociated and suspended loss of pain and temperature (as in syringomyelia).

Higher orders of sensation are sometimes impaired in disease of the parietal lobes. The most common form of this is called *astereognosis*, in which the patient is unable to recognize by touch an object placed in his hand, even if primary sensations are intact. The anatomic significance of defects in two-point discrimination, figure writing, and object weight discrimination is still debated. Generally these represent cortical dysfunction.

REFLEXES

The stretch reflexes are easily tested and are graded from 0 to 4+, 0 indicating an absence of reflexes and therefore pathology, and 4+ indicating pathologically hyperactive reflexes. The normal variation ranges from 1+ to 3+, 2+ being average. Not only are the stretch reflexes scaled in this fashion, they are also compared from side to side and in different parts of the same limb. The stretch reflexes routinely tested and their segmental levels are as follows:

Biceps C_{5-6}	Adductor of thigh L_{2-3}
Triceps C_{6-7}	Knee L_{3-4}
Brachioradialis C_{6-7-8}	Ankle S_{1-2}

The plantar response is always evaluated. A semisharp instrument (key) is stroked upward along the lateral margin of the foot. The classic Babinski reflex is extension of the great toe and fanning of the other toes, but modifications of this are important to note. It is relevant to note a difference in the nature of the response between the two sides, for absence of any response to plantar stimulus in the presence of a strong normal flexor response on the opposite foot may well indicate pathology. Of course, it is important to distinguish withdrawal from a pathologic extension response.

Several other reflexes may be useful when evaluating specific problems. Some of these may be grouped together and called "cortical release signs," so designated because they usually appear in patients with severe bihemispheric (frontal lobe) disease.

The snout reflex is elicited by placing a finger vertically over the patient's lips and gently tapping it with a reflex hammer; a positive response is a puckering movement of the lips. The sucking or rooting reflex is elicited by lightly stimulating the corners of the patient's mouth with a finger or tongue blade. The patient's response will be to attempt to grasp the object with his lips and suck it. The forced grasp reflex is obtained by placing two fingers on the patient's palm, the normal response being an involuntary grasping by the patient.

A pathologic jaw-jerk is an indication of corticobulbar disease and may be of value when the examiner is looking for evidence of disease above the foramen magnum in a patient with evidence of upper motor neuron signs in the arms and legs. A finger is placed against the patient's chin, slightly stretching the masseter muscles. The finger is tapped lightly with a reflex hammer; a positive response is a vigorous jaw-closure movement.

Abdominal reflexes are obtained by gently stroking the four abdominal quadrants and observing the movement of the umbilicus. They may be unilaterally reduced to absent on the side of an upper motor neuron lesion. The lower abdominal reflexes may be absent and the uppers present in a spinal cord lesion at the D-10 level. The abdominal reflexes are difficult to evaluate if the abdominal wall is flaccid.

AUTONOMIC AND SPHINCTER FUNCTION

The mechanism of urinary sphincter disturbances is probably better evaluated by history than by examination, but it is clearly of the greatest importance for localizing a lesion. The types of urinary incontinence caused by cerebral lesions are not specifically classifiable. Advanced dementia from any cause is associated with urinary incontinence, particularly at night when the patient is in bed. These patients usually do not show evidence of a neurogenic bladder when investigated but, rather, seem to void when and where they feel the urge instead of going to the toilet or asking for a urinal. Acute urinary retention or incontinence is common after cerebral infarctions or hemorrhage. Spinal cord lesions produce bladder "spasticity"; that is, the patient complains of urinary frequency and urgency and is incontinent if he cannot get to a toilet fast enough. Bladder capacity is decreased, which accounts for the frequency; and the heightened reflex responsivity of the detrusor muscle is responsible for the incontinent voiding. As the lesion progresses, there is associated urinary retention, particularly when the ascending sensory pathways in the spinal cord are destroyed. Lesions of the cauda equina or of the peripheral nerves affecting the bladder usually cause urinary retention, reduced bladder sensation, loss of desire to void, huge bladder capacity, and overflow incontinence.

The examination of any patient with a neurologic disorder includes careful palpation of the suprapubic area, looking for bladder distention. Rectal examination is done to evaluate anal sphincter tone, which is flaccid with cauda equina or peripheral nerve lesions, and may be with spinal cord lesions as well. With the finger in the anus and rectum, the examiner touches the penis with a pin to test the bulbocavernosus reflex. A normal response is a tightening of the perineal musculature, which can be felt by the palpating finger.

Absence of this reflex means that the S3–4 nerve roots or pudendal nerves are involved. A normal response is retained in spinal cord lesions. Integrity of the S3–4 reflex arc may also be tested by touching the perianal region with a pin. A normal response is a contracture or "wink" of the orifice.

In rare circumstances, a spinal cord level can be delineated by testing sweating function on the trunk.

SUGGESTED READINGS

Alpers BJ, and Grant FC: The clinical syndrome of the corpus collosum. *Arch Neurol Psychiatry* 25:67, 1931.

Bronisch FW: *The Clinically Important Reflexes.* Grune & Stratton, New York, 1952.

Bucy PC, and Kluver H: Anatomic changes secondary to temporal lobotomy. *Arch Neurol Psychiatry* 44:1142, 1940.

Calne DB, and Pallis CA: Vibratory sense: a critical review. *Brain* 89:723, 1966.

Carpenter MBJ: Athetosis and the basal ganglia. *Arch Neurol Psychiatry* 63:875, 1950.

Clinical Examination in Neurology. Mayo Clinic, Rochester, Minnesota. Saunders, Philadelphia, 1963.

Cogan DG: *Neurology of the Ocular Muscles,* 2nd edition, Charles C Thomas, Springfield, Illinois, 1956.

Cogan DG: *Neurology of the Visual System.* Charles C Thomas, Springfield, Illinois, 1966.

Critchley M: *The Parietal Lobes.* Arnold, London, 1953.

Dejong RN: *The Neurological Examination, Incorporating the Fundamentals of Neuroanatomy and Neurophysiology,* 3rd edition, Harper & Row, New York, 1967.

Denny-Brown D: The frontal lobes and their function. In: *Modern Trends in Neurology,* edited by D Williams. Butterworth, London, 1957.

Denny-Brown D: The nature of apraxia. *J Nerv Ment Dis* 120:9, 1958.

Fulton JF: *Functional Localization in the Frontal Lobes and Cerebellum.* Clarendon Press, Oxford, 1949.

Fulton JF: *Physiology of the Nervous System,* 3rd edition, Oxford University Press, New York, 1949.

Gerstmann J: Some notes on the Gerstmann syndrome. *Neurology (Minneap)* 7:866, 1957.

Glaser JS: *Neuroophthalmology.* Harper & Row, Hagerstown, Maryland, 1978.

Haymaker W: *Bing's Local Diagnosis in Neurological Diseases.* Mosby, St. Louis, Missouri, 1956.

Holmes G: The cerebellum of man (Hughlings Jackson Memorial Lecture). *Brain* 62:1, 1939.

Kremer M: Sitting, standing, walking. *Br Med J* 2:63, 121, 1958.

Lapides J, and Babbitt JM: Diagnostic value of bulbocavernosus reflex. *JAMA* 162:971, 1956.

Medical Research Council War Memorandum No. 7: *Aids to the Investigation of Peripheral Nerve Injuries.* Her Majesty's Stationery Office, London, reprinted 1965.

Papez JW: A proposed mechanism of emotion. *Arch Neurol Psychiatry* 38:725, 1937.

Penfield W, and Roberts L: *Speech and Brain Mechanisms.* Princeton University Press, Princeton, N.J., 1959.

Walshe F: The Babinski plantar response: its forms and its physiological and pathological significance. *Brain* 79:529, 1956.

Whitty CWM: The neurological basis for memory. In: *Modern Trends in Neurology,* edited by D Williams. Butterworth, London, 1962.

2

Cerebrovascular Diseases

Cerebrovascular diseases are the most important of all neurologic disorders for several reasons: (1) They are the most frequent, so every practitioner is faced with the problem regularly; even patients and families recognize the symptoms. (2) They rank third behind heart disease and cancer as a cause of death in the United States. (3) They are a major cause of disability in patients who survive. (4) Early recognition and management may be of great benefit to the patient. Great progress has been made during the past 25 years in understanding the clinical presentations and natural history of the various types of cerebral vascular disease, along with the development of increasingly sophisticated and accurate diagnostic tools, recognition of important risk factors, methods of prevention, improved understanding of the physiology of the cerebral circulation, recognition of the role of heart disease in cerebral embolization, and the great frequency and importance of extracranial vascular lesions in the production of stroke. Recent statistics reveal that the incidence of thrombotic and hemorrhagic stroke in the United States has decreased significantly during the past 5 years. The reason for this is not yet evident, but it may be related to greater public awareness of the importance of treating hypertension.

INCIDENCE AND RISK FACTORS

Evaluation of stroke incidence statistics indicates that we can expect about 500,000 new strokes of all kinds in the United States in 1980. Of this number, almost 40 to 50% of patients will die from the stroke or its complications during the first 30 days following the ictus. Of the survivors, 10% will require institutional care; 40% will require special care; 40% will have a mild residual disability; 10% will be unimpaired. These figures led to the inevitable conclusion that there are about 2.5 million persons living in the United States who have suffered a stroke, and of these about one-half require special services and care. These data apply only to actual cerebral infarction and intracerebral and subarachnoid hemorrhage; they do not include transient ischemic attacks, which have a much better prognosis.

There is no longer any doubt that hypertension is the major treatable risk factor in all types of stroke (ischemic or hemorrhagic), that the curve of stroke risk rises with increased blood pressure, and that effective treatment of hypertension reduces expected stroke incidence. The increased risk is measured at two to six times an age-controlled population, depending on the population group studied. Since hypertension is a treatable disease, it is evident that the capability of greatly reducing stroke incidence is already at hand and needs simply effective and universal application.

Other risk factors include aging, which exponentially increases stroke risk after age 60. Heart disease, particularly rheumatic heart disease and coronary artery disease, is a major risk; diabetes and certain types of serum lipid abnormalities are also important. Recent studies have convincingly demonstrated that birth control pills increase the risk of cerebrovascular disease. A good correlation with cigarette smoking has never been proved.

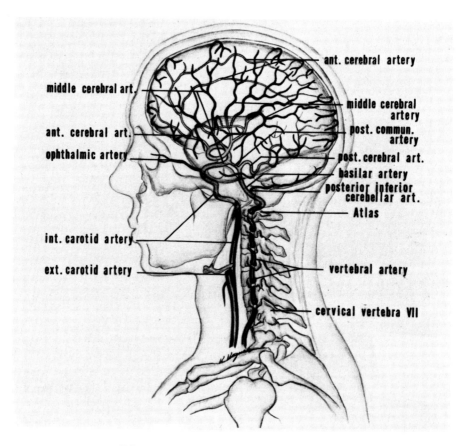

FIG. 2.1. Carotid and vertebrobasilar circulation.

VASCULAR ANATOMY

Figures 2.1 and 2.2 delineate the details of vascular anatomy required to understand the symptoms that result from occlusive cerebrovascular disease. The brain receives blood from two major circulations. Approximately two-thirds of the blood is delivered through the carotid arteries and one-third through the vertebral-basilar system. These two circulations are anatomically and dynamically joined at the base of the brain by the circle of Willis. The presence or absence of a complete circle may determine if a significant neurologic deficit develops in a patient following occlusion of a major extra-cranial vessel. It is well known, for example, that occlusion of one internal carotid artery may occur without any noticeable symptomatology or perma-nent neurologic sequelae. This is because blood is delivered to the involved cerebral hemisphere from the opposite carotid through the anterior commu-nicating artery or from the vertebrobasilar system via the posterior commu-nicating artery. *The existence of an anterior communicating artery or posterior communicating artery is thus of paramount importance in the outcome of extracranial occlusive vascular disease.*

One of the first branches of the internal carotid artery inside the skull is the ophthalmic artery, which supplies the retina and choroid. The carotid artery shortly thereafter bifurcates into the anterior and middle cerebral arteries, which supply the greater portion of the cerebral hemispheres. Terminal pial branches of the anterior and middle cerebral arteries anastomose with each other and with branches of the posterior cerebral artery on the surface of the cortex.

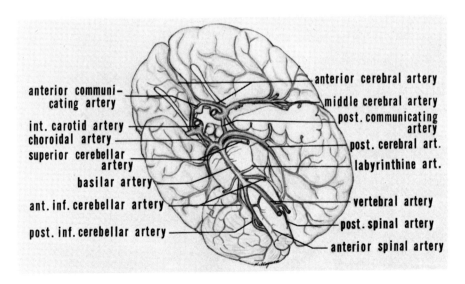

FIG. 2.2. Arterial supply of brain as seen from the inferior surface, showing the circle of Willis.

The vertebral arteries pass superiorly in special grooves of the transverse process of the cervical vertebrae, thereby making them potentially susceptible to injury or occlusion upon extreme rotation, flexion, or extension of the neck. They send important radicular branches to the cervical spinal cord and form the anterior spinal arteries. The two vertebral arteries unite on the ventral surface of the brainstem at the junction of the pons and the medulla to form the basilar artery (Fig. 2.2), which then proceeds along the ventral surface to the pons to divide, finally, into two posterior cerebral arteries. The branches of the vertebrobasilar system therefore supply the upper spinal cord, medulla, cerebellum, pons, portions of the midbrain and diencephalon, the posterior and medial portions of the temporal lobes, and the occipital lobes.

It is obvious, then, that the symptoms of cerebral ischemia can logically predict the vascular supply involved. Ischemic symptoms and signs from occlusive disease of an internal carotid artery or its branches are those of dysfunction of a cerebral hemisphere and include weakness or paralysis of the opposite side of the body, numbness or tingling of part or all of the opposite side of the body, dysphasia (disturbance of ability to speak or understand) if the dominant hemisphere is involved, visual field defects opposite the side of the lesion, and monocular blindness. The latter results from involvement of the ophthalmic artery or one of its major branches. Disease of the vertebrobasilar system results in vertigo, cranial nerve palsies, double vision, ataxia of gait or extremities, numbness and tingling around the mouth, and drop attacks (sudden transient weakness of both legs). There may also be visual field defects due to ischemia of the visual cortex in the occipital lobes.

CLASSIFICATION OF CEREBROVASCULAR DISEASES

Successful management of cerebrovascular diseases depends on an understanding of pathology and etiology as well as the clinical or functional state of the patient. It is useful to consider these separately for the sake of clarity.

Etiologic and Pathologic Classification

I. Infarction
    A. Thrombosis
        1. Arteriosclerosis
        2. Subintimal hyperplasia
        3. Inflammatory disease
    B. Embolism
        1. Extracranial vascular sources
        2. Cardiac sources

II. Hemorrhage (intracerebral or subarachnoid)
A. Hypertensive hemorrhage
B. Idiopathic hemorrhage
C. Berry (congenital) aneurysm
D. Arteriovenous anomaly
E. Mycotic aneurysm

Cerebral infarction is the end result of irreversible local ischemia. The term ischemia implies potential irreversibility of the insult. Infarctions of the brain are pale (ischemic) or hemorrhagic, the latter usually being secondary to embolism. Thrombosis implies the development of a clot in an artery secondary to local arterial disease, as opposed to embolism, which is a clot that has been carried by the blood from another source.

Arteriosclerosis of the extra- and intracranial cerebral arteries usually develops much later in life than arteriosclerosis in the coronary arteries and aorta. It occurs predominantly in the bifurcation of major arteries, one of the most common sites being the bifurcation of the common carotid artery, where arteriosclerotic plaques may not only cause vascular stenosis and occlusion but may be a major source of cerebral emboli (described in the section *Transient Ischemic Attacks*, below).

Another type of occlusive disease of small arteries or arterioles may develop in patients with prolonged hypertension, the pathologic process apparently being hyperplasia of the media and subintimal layers of the vessel, rather than atherosclerosis. The resulting infarction is usually small and the neurologic deficit less severe than in the atherosclerotic occlusive disease of large arteries (Fig. 2.3).

A third type of occlusive vascular disease is inflammatory. Although infrequent, it is important because arteritis requires a specific form of management. *Temporal arteritis* is an inflammatory granulomatous occlusion of the superficial temporal artery with occasional subsequent involvement of intracranial arteries, particularly the ophthalmic artery. It is the most frequent cause of ischemic optic neuritis. It occurs almost exclusively in middle-aged and elderly individuals, and there is usually a prodrome of malaise, generalized aching, weight loss, and anorexia, a syndrome termed *polymyalgia rheumatica*. This may last for several weeks and may be followed by recurrent headaches, usually of a vascular type, frequently in the temporal region. Neurologic signs develop in about 50% of these patients, particularly unilateral loss of vision. The diagnosis is clinical and depends on a high index of suspicion on the part of the physician. The superficial temporal artery is often tender and firm and the erythrocyte sedimentation rate (ESR) elevated, *but neither of these findings may be present*. If the diagnosis of polymyalgia rheumatica is suspected, the superficial temporal artery should be biopsied for verification. These patients often respond dramatically to oral steroids.

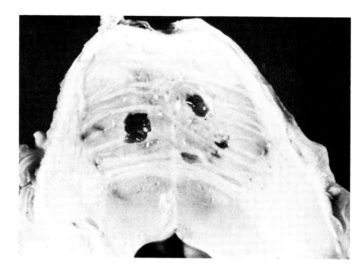

FIG. 2.3. Lacunar infarcts in pons. History of hypertensive cardiovascular disease and recurrent cerebrovascular accidents.

Early diagnosis and adequate treatment are essential if permanent neurologic sequelae are to be prevented (Fig. 2.4).

Cerebral embolism usually produces sudden onset of neurologic deficit. The precise character and severity of the deficit are related to the size and location of the vessel occluded by the embolism. Embolic occlusion of the entire internal carotid artery or the middle cerebral artery may, for example, result in infarction of a large part of the homolateral cerebral hemisphere,

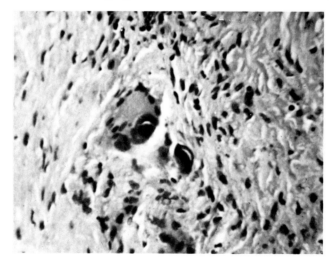

FIG. 2.4. Giant cell arteritis from biopsy of superficial temporal artery.

whereas small distal branch embolism may produce only minor and transient symptomatology. The embolism may originate from an arteriosclerotic plaque located in the carotid or vertebral circulation, or from a plaque located in the arch of the aorta or from the heart. Emboli are responsible for a significant percentage of cerebral infarctions. They are discussed in greater detail in the section *Management of the Acute Stroke*, below.

From the point of view of what the physician is called on to do by way of diagnosis and treatment, the most useful classification of strokes is based on the chronologic stage of the illness at the time the patient is seen.

Transient Cerebral Ischemic Attacks

By accepted definition, a transient cerebral ischemic attack (TIA) is a brief episode of neurologic deficit caused by ischemia; it lasts no more than 24 hr, and the patient recovers completely. In fact, the episode may last only a few seconds or as long as a day and still have the same pathologic significance. The important thing is that the physician usually sees the patient after the attack is over, so that no neurologic abnormalities may be observed, and all the information he can obtain about the problem must be obtained by history. The patient's symptoms depend on whether the TIA occurs in the carotid or the vertebrobasilar circulation, as previously described. If in the former, he may have transient weakness of one side of his body, numbness or tingling of an extremity, monocular blindness, or aphasia; and if in the latter, he may have transient diplopia, vertigo, dysarthria, weakness of one or more extremities, perioral numbness, or a drop attack (Table 2.1).

A patient who has recovered completely will have no neurologic deficit by the time he is examined. The examination should include auscultation over

TABLE 2.1. *Symptoms and signs in transient ischemic attacks*

Carotid origin
    Amaurosis fugax
    Hemiparesis or monoparesis
    Hemihypesthesia or dysesthesia
    Aphasia
Vertebrobasilar origin
    Vertigo
    Diplopia
    Dysarthria
    Dysphasia
    Ataxia
    Weakness of one or more extremities
    Cranial nerve palsies
    Perioral numbness
    Drop attacks
    Homonymous hemianopsia or cortical blindness
    Confusion
    Transient global amnesia

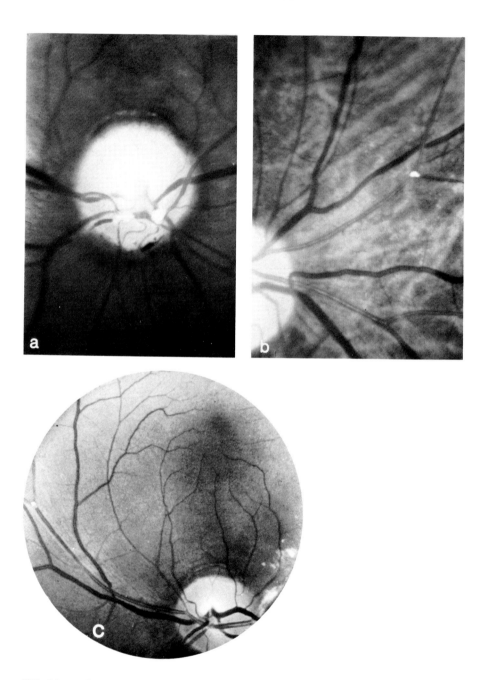

FIG. 2.5a–c: Bright plaques in retinal arterioles in patients with transient cerebral ischemic attacks. The presence of these plaques strongly implicates the role of embolization from carotid or vertebral atherosclerotic plaques of fibrin-platelet clots or cholesterol material from the interior of the plaques.

the anterior neck, with the examiner listening for a carotid bruit, which often denotes the presence of an arteriosclerotic plaque and the possible source of the transient ischemic episode. The examiner must also carefully inspect the fundi in a darkened room, looking for bright plaques in the retinal arterioles in patients with carotid TIAs, particularly if one of the complaints is transient monocular blindness (Fig. 2.5).

The pathogenesis of TIAs in most instances is embolization of a fibrin-platelet thrombus from an arteriosclerotic plaque on one of the major extra-cranial vessels or cholesterol emboli from an ulcerated arteriosclerotic plaque. Occasionally, the symptoms are hemodynamic in origin, related to reduced blood flow or perfusion pressure across the stenotic part of the artery. There is no evidence to suggest that these episodes are caused by spasm of cerebral arteries.

It is essential to distinguish between TIAs of the carotid and the ver-tebrobasilar circulation, because some of the former may be treated by carotid endarterectomy, whereas there is no surgical treatment for ver-tebrobasilar TIAs. For this reason, TIAs clinically diagnosed as originating in the carotid system usually require angiography, whereas vertebrobasilar TIAs do not.

The management of carotid TIAs is dependent on cause; in most instances angiography is required. There are other diagnostic techniques—in particu-lar, ophthalmodynamometry, oculoplethysmography, ultrasound, and Dop-pler scanning—but these noninvasive methods have not yet achieved the resolution which permits a definitive decision concerning carotid endarterec-tomy. Careful examination of the patient is important, particularly careful auscultation over the carotid bifurcation to listen for high-pitched bruits or to look for evidence of increased external carotid circulation. Emboli from the heart may also be a source of the TIA. In the end, however, angiography will be required to evaluate the extracranial and, if possible, the intracranial cerebral arteries before a final decision can be made in regard to endarterectomy.

The decision to proceed with angiography should be made only if carotid endarterectomy is a realistic goal. The importance of appropriate treatment of TIAs is emphasized by follow-up statistics which indicate that the cumulative probability of completed stroke after the first TIA compared to a comparable age-controlled population was three to four times as great during the first year. By the end of the fifth year, 40% of the TIA patients had cerebral infarctions compared to less than 10% of the controls.

Angiography carries a definite risk, particularly in elderly, hypertensive, and severely arteriosclerotic patients. The precise risk in figures is difficult to pin down, but approximately 1.5 to 2.0% morbidity can be expected in good hands. The angiogram should be as complete as is consistent with good medical principles. The risks of the procedure increase with the time required for the examination. Both carotids, as well as the intracranial arteries, must be

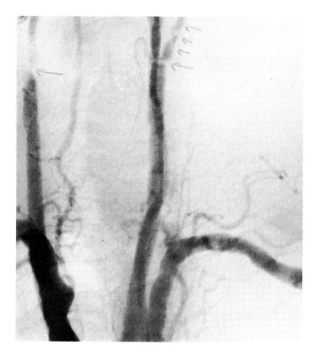

FIG. 2.6. Bilateral carotid stenosis. Aortic arch angiogram (subtraction technique). The stenotic lesions are flow-limiting.

visualized if possible. The transfemoral approach is probably the least traumatic and provides the most information in experienced hands. Contraindications for angiography include recent myocardial infarction, severe congestive heart failure, uncontrolled hypertension, and bleeding diathesis (Figs. 2.6 and 2.7).

Carotid endarterectomy should be performed for two types of lesion: (1) a severely stenosing (75%) nonulcerating plaque; and (2) a less-stenosing ulcerated plaque. It is not indicated for small stenosing plaques, lesions high in the internal carotid artery, or complete occlusion of the internal carotid artery.

It is important to keep in mind that at least 50% of individuals with carotid TIAs and all patients with vertebrobasilar TIAs do not have a surgically treatable lesion. The cause for the TIA in such patients may not be clearly established and may be due to intracranial arteriosclerosis or to emboli from cardiac sources. Treatment must therefore be directed at inhibiting the formation of intravascular clots. For this purpose two modalities are available: antithrombotic agents which inhibit platelet agglutination (e.g., aspirin or sulfinpyrazone) or anticoagulants.

A Canadian cooperative study demonstrated that aspirin, in doses of 0.6 g twice daily, reduced the risk of stroke or death by 48% in male patients with

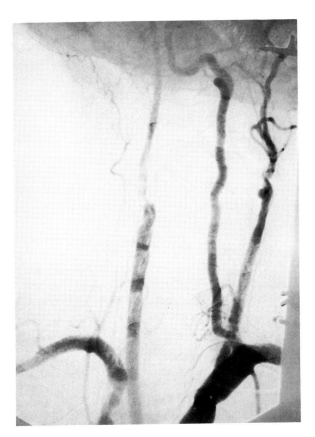

FIG. 2.7. Severe generalized extracranial vascular disease. Note the tortuosity and irregularity (plaques) of both subclavian arteries. The right internal carotid artery is completely occluded, and there is a 95% stenosing plaque at the origin of the right external carotid artery. The right vertebral artery is vestigial, whereas the left is much larger than usual. There is a plaque at the bifurcation of the left common carotid artery. The patient presented with TIAs of the right hemisphere.

TIAs but was of no benefit in women. Sulfinpyrazone, alone or in combination with aspirin, did not appear to be effective. Although there are some complications from aspirin, particularly abdominal pain and gastrointestinal bleeding, the benefit-risk ratio is quite high.

Anticoagulation as therapy for TIAs, either carotid or vertebrobasilar, remains an unsettled subject. The few controlled studies available have shown little evidence that anticoagulation of patients with TIAs statistically reduces the incidence of cerebral infarction, and there is no doubt that anticoagulants, even carefully monitored, greatly increase the risk of intracerebral bleeding. There are, no doubt, some patients who respond favorably to anticoagulants, but how to identify them remains a mystery.

Management of patients with asymptomatic carotid bruits has also been a controversial subject. Increasing numbers of conservative neurologists are recommending that these patients be considered for endarterectomy provided the bruit is high-pitched and well-localized over the carotid bifurcation and that the operating team has a morbidity record of less than 1%. The combined morbidity risk of angiography and surgery must be considered in these patients.

External-internal arterial anastomoses have received substantial attention in the literature of the past 10 years. The most frequently done procedure is superficial temporal-middle cerebral artery anastomosis. The major indications have been complete occlusion of an internal carotid artery with perfusion of the homolateral hemisphere from the opposite carotid and stenosis of the trunk of the middle cerebral artery. There is no longer any doubt that the operation can be successfully carried out, that it may improve perfusion of the hemisphere, and that the anastomoses usually remain patent. There are many reports of similar types of procedure on the vertebral circulation. What has not been proved is if these procedures prevent stroke. A major cooperative study is now under way to attempt to answer this question. Furthermore, recent studies of the natural history of patients with internal carotid artery occlusion and of patients with stenosis of the trunk of the middle cerebral artery have not confirmed that either of these conditions are compelling indications for shunt surgery. The incidence of infarction in the hemisphere homolateral to the lesion appears to be no greater than in the opposite hemisphere.

Differential diagnosis of TIAs includes any transient neurologic episode. In younger individuals the migraine prodrome with flashing scotomas and transient neurologic symptoms may closely simulate a TIA, but the diagnosis is usually obvious from the history of recurrent headaches. It should be remembered that brain tumors may produce temporary neurologic abnormalities and must therefore be considered in the differential diagnosis.

The recent development of computerized cerebral axial tomography has introduced a new dimension into neurologic diagnosis for it is atraumatic and allows a far better evaluation of the brain than does the isotope brain scan. Its value in the evaluation of a patient with TIAs lies in the identification or exclusion of nonischemic causes for the patient's symptoms, e.g., tumor, local atrophy, or any mass lesion. It does not allow identification of the offending vascular source of a true TIA.

PROGRESSING STROKE

The problem facing the attending physician is quite different when the patient has sudden onset of neurologic signs which continue to progress. This condition is called progressing stroke and demands immediate attention in order to minimize the extent of cerebral damage or prevent death. It may occur in either the carotid or vertebrobasilar systems. A typical situation is a middle-aged hypertensive man in whom mild weakness develops in the right upper extremity, followed after 1 hr by aphasia, progressive weakness of the entire right side, and finally increasing obtundation. This would represent a progressing stroke in the left carotid circulation. In the vertebrobasilar system, the clinical problem might be one of sudden onset of vertigo, nausea, and vomiting, followed by double vision and thereafter by progressive quadriparesis and difficulty swallowing. The pathogenesis of such critical problems is thought to be the progressive growth or extension of a thrombus in a major vessel, e.g., the middle cerebral or vertebral artery. As the thrombus extends, it occludes more branch vessels, thereby resulting in greater neurologic deficit. Another cause may be the development of edema in a cerebral hemisphere following infarction, with a resultant shift of midline structures toward the opposite side.

Unfortunately, the diagnosis in these patients may not be easy because a slowly expanding intracerebral hemorrhage may simulate a progressing thrombotic infarction. All such patients should undergo computerized axial tomography (CAT scan) of the brain; this procedure is atraumatic and provides by far the best means of excluding such surgically treatable lesions as intracerebral or subdural hematoma. If a CAT scan can be done promptly, lumbar puncture should be deferred, particularly if there has been rapid neurologic deterioration, as there may be some danger of transtentorial uncal herniation in the presence of an expanding hemisphere hematoma. If the cerebrospinal fluid (CSF) is to be examined, the tap should be done with a 20-gauge needle, the pressure measured, and the fluid immediately examined to look for bleeding. If the CSF is clear, hemorrhage can usually be excluded, but this is not invariably the case as some hemorrhages may not leak into the ventricles or subarachnoid space. Since the advent of the CAT scan, angiography is not required to determine if an intracerebral bleed is present.

Management of patients with progressing stroke is still a subject of dispute. Cerebral hemorrhage must be handled as discussed under *Intracerebral Hemorrhage*, below. The presence of massive edema, which can usually be determined by the CAT scan, requires treatment with hyperosmolar agents even though their value is not statistically proved. There can be no doubt that some of the patients treated with urea, mannitol, or glycerol improve, at least temporarily. Although there is tissue rehydration after urea and mannitol administration, it may be possible to keep the edema below the level at which herniation occurs.

If hemorrhage can be excluded and massive edema does not appear to be responsible for the patient's clinical deterioration, anticoagulation with constant drip intravenous heparin in doses of about 1,000 units per hour is indicated, in the opinion of this writer. The plasma recalcification time should be maintained at 2.5 times normal. The value of steroid administration in patients with progressing stroke has not been established.

THE COMPLETED STROKE

The patient with completed stroke, as the name implies, presents with a neurologic deficit which may have appeared abruptly or over a period of several hours, but which has stopped progressing and is not improving. The pathology is most likely an infarct, and the degree of recovery depends on the resolution of adjacent edema and recovery of function of injured but still viable neurons (Fig. 2.8). The etiology could be extra- or intracranial arterial thrombosis, embolism, or hypertensive arteriolar disease. Although the neurologic deficit at first appears to be fixed, many patients with completed stroke have a great deal of recovery. The earlier recovery begins, the better is the prognosis. In hemiplegia or severe hemiparesis, leg function usually recovers earlier and to a greater extent than that in the upper extremity. The principles of management of these patients is described below under *Management of Acute Stroke*. They present a different problem than that of the patient with a TIA or a progressing stroke, because evaluation for consideration of endarterectomy is not immediately necessary. The extent of the vascular work-up depends, to a great extent, on the degree of recovery. Patients who recover most of their neurologic function should be managed similarly to patients with

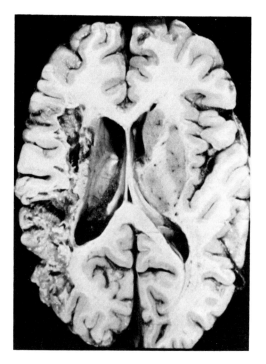

FIG. 2.8. Old (2-year) ischemic infarction, now atrophic and partially cystic, involving part of the left middle cerebral artery distribution. Note the huge dilatation of the left lateral ventricle (hydrocephalus *ex vacuo*).

TIAs because the objective is the same, i.e., to prevent further episodes of cerebral ischemia.

Cerebral Embolism

Although estimates vary, it is now accepted that embolism is responsible for about 30 to 40% of cerebral infarctions. Emboli usually produce or precipitate the onset of neurologic symptoms and signs. The size of the ischemic area or infarction depends on the artery which has been occluded. The infarctions are often hemorrhagic and may be accompanied by severe edema. The management of an infarct produced by an embolus is no different from any other completed stroke with the exception that it is important to seek the source of the embolus and to try to prevent additional embolization. The following cardiac causes of emboli should be considered:

1. *Rheumatic heart disease with atrial fibrillation and mitral stenosis.* The evidence of cerebral emboli is four to six times as great in the group of patients with this disease combination as in the normal population. Early treatment is by anticoagulation, usually beginning about 72 hr after the stroke. Subsequent therapy may be by valve replacement and cardioversion. Homograft valves usually do not cause emboli, but mechanical or plastic valves require long-term prophylactic anticoagulation.

2. *Atrial fibrillation due to arteriosclerotic heart disease.* Studies to establish the precise correlation to cerebral emboli are not available, but it is usually stated that such patients have a risk factor for emboli twice as great as normals. There is considerable dispute about effective therapy. Cardioversion is now infrequently used if the cardiac rate can be kept reasonably slow with digitalis, and many believe long-term anticoagulation is the best prophylaxis against emboli.

3. *Myocardial infarction and mural thrombosis.* This is a small but definite source for cerebral emboli. Diagnosis may be made by cardiac angiography or gated cardiac isotope flow studies, which may also be useful for demonstrating a ventricular aneurysm or asynergic section of ventricular wall. Long-term anticoagulants are used, although accurate figures for effectiveness are not available. Surgical repair of ventricular aneurysms is also a reasonable option in appropriate cases.

4. *Subacute bacterial endocarditis.* Cerebral embolization is not infrequent, and mycotic aneurysms may develop in cerebral arteries. Anticoagulation is contraindicated.

5. *Atrial or ventricular myxoma.* Diagnosis is made by echocardiography. Treatment is surgical removal.

6. *Prolapsed mitral valve.* This must be a rare cause of cerebral emboli, but it does cause ventricular arrhythmias and congestive heart failure. Myxomatous degeneration of the valve may be present. Diagnosis is by echocardiography.

7. *Sick sinus syndrome.* This probably is a rare cause of emboli but may well be responsible for syncope due to profound bradyarrhythmia.

MANAGEMENT OF ACUTE STROKE

There are four major steps to be considered immediately in the management of the patient with an acute stroke:

1. *Establish the diagnosis.* The differential diagnosis of acute thrombotic strokes must include the postictal state, metabolic encephalopathy, acute head injury, intracerebral hemorrhage, and subarachnoid hemorrhage. Each of the above conditions may simulate an acute thrombotic stroke, particularly if the patient is stuporous or poorly communicative and a good history is not available. The CAT scan is invaluable for distinguishing between infarction and intracerebral hemorrhage, a clinical distinction which is not always obvious (Figs. 2.9–2.11). In doubtful cases skull X-ray films should be obtained to look for skull fracture or other signs of trauma. Determinations of serum electrolytes, blood glucose, and arterial gases are important if there is any question of metabolic encephalopathy, and electroencephalography (EEG) if there is any question of the postictal state.

2. *Treat associated medical problems.* Patients with cerebrovascular disease often have advanced arteriosclerotic heart disease, and they should be screened for congestive heart failure and acute myocardial infarction, as well as for pulmonary insufficiency and gastrointestinal bleeding. The patients

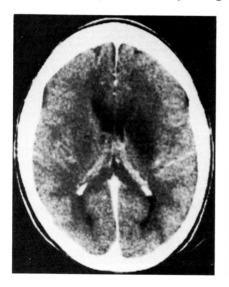 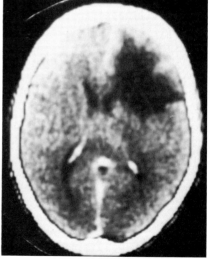

FIGS. 2.9, 2.10. Hemisphere infarction due to embolization from carotid plaque. No CAT abnormality was observed initially. This study, with contrast, was made 6 days postictus. The large area of decreased density adjacent to the lateral ventricle can readily be seen.

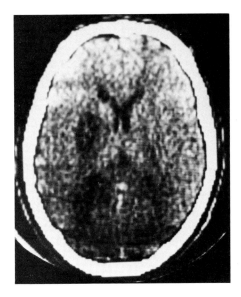

FIG. 2.11. Infarction of left basal ganglia. The area of decreased density in the left basal ganglia appeared 4 days after the infarction. Hemiplegic at first, the patient eventually recovered at least 80% of function of right extremities.

must be protected from the onset against aspiration and pulmonary embolism, which are major causes of death in patients with acute strokes.

3. *Look for cardiac sources of cerebral embolization.* This was already discussed (see Cerebral Embolism, above).

4. *Use anti-ischemic agents.* The various modalities and drugs utilized to treat cerebral ischemia have had the objectives of: (1) increasing collateral circulation, thereby improving blood flow within the area of ischemia; (2) reducing brain edema, thereby preventing compression of capillaries and small arterioles by swollen brain and inhibiting the shift of swollen brain from one intracranial compartment to another (herniation); and (3) reducing energy utilization by ischemic brain tissue, thereby diverting the diminished energy stores to the purpose of maintaining the viability of the cell structure.

Hyperosmolar agents: Many studies have shown that there is a rapid increase in brain water in experimental ischemia. This is thought to be due to power failure in the cells causing a loss of osmotic equilibrium. The increased cell water is clearly harmful to cell function and survival. Indeed brain edema is probably the most important neurologic cause of death in ischemic strokes.

Neither mannitol nor urea have been shown to improve survival rate or final morbidity in acute stroke, though there is no doubt that they may be temporarily useful in some patients when transtentorial herniation appears to be imminent. In order to reduce brain volume, therefore, hyperosmolar agents must produce an osmotic gradient between the blood and the brain. Such gradients are transient because the solutes eventually also enter the brain, and when the plasma level of the solute falls there may be a rebound of water back into the brain. Thus the improvement with most hyperosmolar agents tends to be transient.

Glycerol is a somewhat more complex drug in that it is metabolized by the brain, thereby causing little or no rebound swelling. The available evidence suggests that this drug may improve morbidity and mortality in stroke. It is best given orally or by naso-gastric tube in doses of 1.2 g/kg body weight. Because it elevates blood glucose significantly when given in large doses, glycerol may be dangerous if given to diabetics and can cause nonketotic hyperosmolar coma.

Low-molecular-weight dextran has been reported to reduce mortality in stroke patients. It probably acts by decreasing blood viscosity.

Steroids. There is no convincing evidence that adrenal cortical steroids are beneficial in reducing brain edema or improving tissue survival in either clinical or experimental stroke. The drugs most frequently used are dexamethasone in doses up to 36 mg daily and prednisone in doses up to 120 mg daily.

Barbiturates. There is substantial evidence that barbiturates improve functional recovery and diminish the size of the anticipated infarct in experimental stroke models. The dosages used (70 to 120 mg/kg) are much larger than are safe for humans, and there have been no properly controlled human studies. The theoretical mechanism for beneficial barbiturate action is that it acts as an antioxident, blocking the effect of free radicals (liberated within the cell by ischemia) on the cell membrane.

Increased perfusion pressure. Some evidence exists that increasing the mean arterial pressure (up to 130 mm Hg) by administration of levarterenol bitartrate (Levophed Bitartrate) or norepinephrine is beneficial in human stroke and experimental cerebral ischemia. The hypothesis is that ischemia impairs cerebrovascular autoregulation and that increased perfusion pressure increases flow in the ischemic zone. In any event, data suggest that hypertension associated with stroke should not be treated so vigorously that the blood pressure fall is precipitous.

Vasodilators. There are, in fact, few cerebral vasodilators. Drugs which dilate skin, muscle, or other organ blood vessels may have no effect on cerebral vessels. Nicotinic acid is one of these. Papaverine does cause modest cerebral vasodilatation but has no proved beneficial effect in acute stroke. Hypercapnia dilates cerebral vessels but has never been shown to alter the course of acute cerebral ischemia.

Other modalities which have been tried from time to time include hypercapnia, hypothermia, hyperbaric oxygenation, and aminophylline. No proved lasting benefits have been demonstrated.

Early rehabilitation is an essential feature of the management of the acute stroke. The patient should be moved out of bed into a chair as soon as possible, and passive and active exercises of the weak extremities initiated promptly.

It is important to keep in mind that patients may recover a great deal of neurologic function after a cerebrovascular accident; therefore every effort should be made to maintain vital functions even in those patients who appear to be neurologically devastated at the beginning of the illness. The earlier recovery begins, the better is the prognosis; but if there is no evidence of return of function at the end of 4 weeks, the prospect of good neurologic recovery is poor. Wisely used, rehabilitation in the form of physical and occupational therapy may be of great help in preventing contractures, increasing strength in weak extremities, and utilizing remaining function better. Speech therapy in the aphasic adult requires a great deal of dedication by the therapist and the patient. Nevertheless, many patients and their families subscribe to it.

There is no question, however, about the importance of exposing the patient to an enriched environment, with an opportunity to relate to family and friends, to be outdoors, and in general to have as much sensory input as possible.

The concerned physician must be sensitive to the impact of a stroke on a patient and the family. The loss of ability to function normally—to care for oneself, to work—result in profound alterations in self-image. Family roles are suddenly and unexpectedly altered. It is not surprising that anxiety and depression are common among the patients and their families. They need counseling, guidance, and occasionally assistance by appropriate pharmacologic management.

INTRACEREBRAL HEMORRHAGE

Primary cerebral hemorrhage is usually a major catastrophe, but it is important to remember that it is not invariably fatal, that spontaneous recoveries do occur, and that a small percentage of patients with intracerebral bleeding are salvageable by neurosurgical intervention. For these reasons, one has the obligation to consider every intracerebral bleed as a potentially treatable problem and to approach the problem in a constructive way.

The major cause of primary intracerebral hemorrhage is hypertension. Although blood dyscrasias or ruptured hamartomas (small congenital angiomas) may produce intracerebral hemorrhage, hypertensive vascular disease is probably the major culprit, so that the best treatment for brain hemorrhage is its prevention by the proper management of hypertension. Classically, the patient is middle-aged, with a history of poorly controlled hypertension. The onset of headache is followed by progression of neurologic

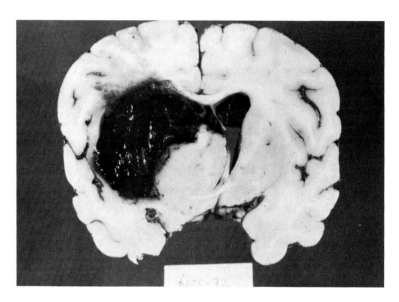

FIG. 2.12. Basal ganglionic hemorrhage with rupture into the lateral ventricle. Observe that the third ventricle has been compressed and pushed to the left.

signs, including confusion, hemiplegia, and unconsciousness over a period of minutes to hours. Sometimes the onset is dramatically sudden. Examination shows elevated blood pressure and very often also reveals signs of longstanding hypertension, e.g., cardiomegaly and hypertensive retinal vascular changes. There may be nuchal rigidity owing to the presence of blood in the subarachnoid space. The neurologic findings depend entirely on the location and extent of the hemorrhage. Massive basal ganglionic hemorrhage, with rupture into the ventricles, results in unconsciousness and hemiplegia (Fig. 2.12). Shortly thereafter, the patient may show signs of brainstem involvement either by extension of the hemorrhage into the brainstem through the cerebral peduncles or as a consequence of herniation of the temporal lobe beneath the tentorium. When the latter occurs, the pupil on the side of the lesion becomes dilated and fixed to light, and the patient shows decerebrate posturing upon stimulation. Decerebrate posturing is characterized by extension of the neck and back to a position of moderate opisthotonos, extension of the lower extremities, plantar flexion of the feet, and powerful inward rotation and extension of the upper extremities. Such posturing, an extremely grave prognostic sign, invariably means that the brainstem has been involved either primarily or secondarily. Under such circumstances, treatment is supportive: the arterial blood pressure is carefully reduced pharmacologically and adequate respiratory toilet is instituted and maintained.

Pontine hemorrhage is almost invariably fatal and may cause death within a few minutes of onset. The clinical presentation is usually an abrupt onset of unconsciousness, and examination reveals a comatose patient with spontaneous or easily induced decerebrate posturing and various eye signs, depending on the precise location and extent of the hemorrhage. The pupils are frequently pinpoint due to stimulation of the descending sympathetic fibers, but midposition unreactive pupils are also encountered. Skew deviation, internuclear ophthalmoplegia, or ocular bobbing are the commonest eye movement abnormalities observed. Treatment is supportive (Fig. 2.13).

The physician must be on the alert for a history which suggests that the hemorrhage is in the subcortical white matter of a hemisphere or in a cerebellar hemisphere for in both instances surgical excision of the hematoma is life-saving. In the former, the history is simply that of a rapidly developing intracerebral mass. The patient first experiences a headache; then, over the course of the next several hours, unilateral weakness or other cerebral hemisphere signs develop. Irritability, restlessness, unwillingness to follow instructions, and finally somnolence form the signature of a rapidly swelling cerebral hemisphere, which results in a shift of the 3rd ventricle and diencephalic structures and warns of impending transtentorial herniation. Surgical intervention by craniotomy, cortical excision, and aspiration of the blood clot may not only be lifesaving, the patient may also have remarkably little final neurologic disability.

Hemorrhage into a cerebellar hemisphere usually begins suddenly with vertigo and an inability to stand and walk properly often associated with occipital or cervical headache, nausea and vomiting, and double vision, followed by unconsciousness (Figs. 2.14 and 2.15). The time course is rapid—

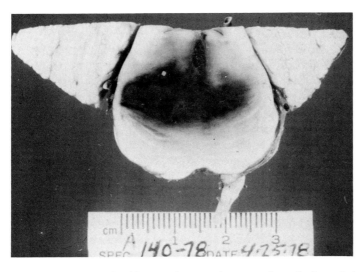

FIG. 2.13. Pontine hemorrhage. Rapid onset of unconsciousness, decerebrate posturing, loss of oculocephalic reflexes, and respiratory failure in a 50-year-old hypertensive man.

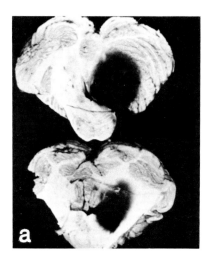
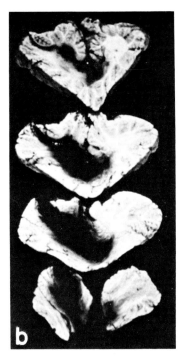

FIGS. 2.14, 2.15. Two fatal cerebellar hemorrhages. **2.14 (a):** The patient's history and physical findings merited immediate surgery, but it was delayed. **2.15 (b):** The hemorrhage was more extensive and bilateral, and the patient presented *in extremis.*

usually not more than 1 to 2 hr. The tip-off is the location of the headache, the cerebellar signs of ataxia and vertigo, and loss of conjugate eye movements. Under such circumstances, a posterior fossa hemorrhage must be considered. Operative intervention (posterior fossa craniotomy) cannot be delayed if the patient is to be salvaged. Time is of the essence.

The whole problem of evaluating a patient with an intracerebral or cerebellar hemorrhage has been altered by CAT scanning of the brain, which literally shows the entire dimensions of the blood clot as well as associated brain swelling, structural shifts, and ventricular blood from rupture of the hemorrhage into the ventricles. The clot has a greater density in the scan image, allowing ready identification. Any patient suspected of intracranial bleeding should have a prompt CAT scan if possible. The resultant image may well obviate the necessity for a lumbar puncture or angiography and will allow the physician to determine if surgical therapy is indicated (Figs. 2.16 and 2.17). *Indeed it has become increasingly evident that all patients with signs and symptoms of a stroke should have a CT scan as part of the evaluation because intracerebral hemorrhage may exactly simulate a thrombotic or embolic stroke.* The CAT scan provides so much information that follow-up angiogra-

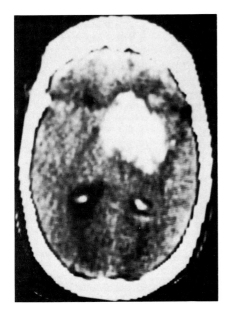 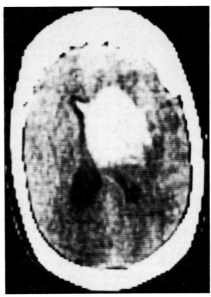

FIGS. 2.16, 2.17. Massive right basal ganglionic hemorrhage probably secondary to hypertension. The blood has remained almost entirely in the brain parenchyma and right lateral ventricle. There appears to be some early extension through the foramen of Monro on the left. This patient presented with abrupt onset of headache and progressive left hemiparesis. He became comatose within 2 hr and expired following cardiac arrest 24 hr after ictus.

phy is rarely required, except for instances where a ruptured aneurysm or arteriovenous anomaly is suspected.

HYPERTENSIVE ENCEPHALOPATHY

Hypertensive encephalopathy is an overused expression for a relatively rare disorder. True hypertensive encephalopathy is a medical emergency. It occurs in the malignant form of essential hypertension, acute glomerulonephritis, eclampsia, and pheochromocytoma. The signs are headaches, convulsive seizures, various types of neurologic deficit, and obtundation. Blood pressure is always dramatically elevated, blood urea nitrogen (BUN) is elevated, the fundi show at least grade 3 hypertensive retinopathy (arteriovenous nicking, arteriolar attenuation, exudates), and the CSF may be bloody. Identification of this process of necrotizing arteriolitis requires immediate therapy to reduce blood pressure: intravenous sodium nitroprusside, trimethaphan (Arfonad®), or other measures familiar to the attending physician. Sodium nitroprusside acts rapidly, but its effects disappear within 15 to 30 min after the infusion is completed. It is prepared by the hospital pharmacy by adding 60 mg sodium nitroprusside to 1,000 ml distilled water with 5% glucose. Because the solution is unstable, a fresh solution must be made every 12 hr if it is used continuously. Early treatment usually results in a good prognosis, and the patient recovers with minimal neurologic deficit. Failure to recognize the syndrome results in rapidly developing areas of brain necrosis and multiple small brain hemorrhages.

PRIMARY SUBARACHNOID HEMORRHAGE

The most common cause of primary subarachnoid hemorrhage (SAH) is ruptured "berry" aneurysm of one of the intracerebral arteries. These aneurysms occur at the bifurcations of major vessels, e.g., at the origin of the posterior communicating artery on the internal carotid artery, the anterior communicating artery, the trifurcation of the middle cerebral artery, and less frequently in arterial branching in the posterior circulation (Figs. 2.18–2.23). The aneurysm is a localized dilatation of the artery, probably resulting from a congenital defect in the internal elastic lamina or the media of the vessel, although it should be mentioned that the pathogenesis is not well understood. This defect permits gradual blistering of the vessel in a localized area, and

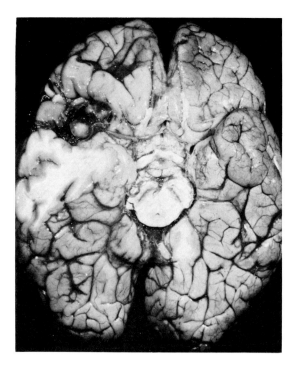

FIG. 2.18. Berry aneurysm at trifurcation of right middle cerebral artery. The temporal pole has been removed to expose the aneurysm and its bed, which is hemorrhagic. Note that the hemorrhage and swelling have compressed the right cerebral peduncle.

eventually rupture may occur. It is apparent from autopsy studies that unruptured aneurysms occur at increasing frequency with advancing age but are practically never seen during the first two decades of life. The mechanisms responsible for the actual rupture are not understood, although there is some evidence that hypertension may play an important role, as may temporary increases of arterial pressure. Aneurysmal rupture may occur when the patient is perfectly quiet, so a consistent relationship to activity has by no means been confirmed.

A typical onset is characterized by severe headache and stiff neck, followed by irritability and sleepiness. The neurologic deficits depend entirely on the location of the aneurysm and if it ruptures intracerebrally as well as into the subarachnoid space. Intracerebral rupture produces signs consistent with the location of the anatomic defect; the resulting intracerebral clot behaves as a mass lesion.

Because surgical treatment is predicated partially on the patient's clinical condition, it is convenient and important to grade the patient's neurologic status as follows:

Grade 1: alert, oriented, no motor or sensory deficit, with or without headache

Grade 2: moderate alteration in sensorium or focal deficit; severe headaches and meningeal signs

Grade 3: Obtunded and/or major focal deficit

Grade 4: Stuporous or comatose with or without major lateralizing findings

The neurologic signs occasionally suggest the site of the aneurysm. An aneurysm of the internal carotid artery at the origin of the posterior communicating artery may cause homolateral third nerve palsy (ptosis, dilated fixed pupil, laterally deviated eye). Abrupt onset of hemiparesis and/or aphasia points to an aneurysm at the trifurcation of the middle cerebral artery. Sudden onset of coma or decerebration are not of value for localizing the site of the bleed. Subhyaloid hemorrhages (blood located between the retina and the hyaloid membrane) are diagnostic of the presence of subarachnoid blood but do not denote etiology. These hemorrhages have a fluid level which distinguishes them from retinal hemorrhage.

In all instances the CSF is bloody, and when it is centrifuged the supernatant fluid is yellow (xanthochromic). Sometimes a traumatic tap may greatly confuse the issue and make it difficult to decide if subarachnoid hemorrhage has truly occurred. For that reason CSF examination should be done only on a sedated or cooperative patient; a total of three tubes should be examined to determine if there is a signficant difference in the red cell count between the first and third tubes; and the CSF should be centrifuged immediately to determine if xanthochromia is present. Delay in examination of the fluid results in a xanthochromic supernatant fluid even if the tap were traumatic.

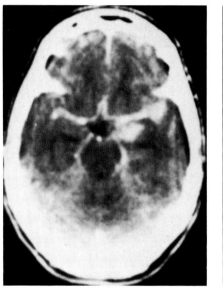 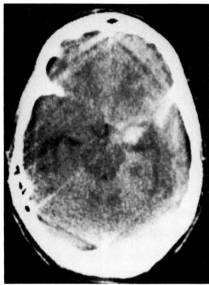

2.19, 2.20

FIGS. 2.19, 2.20, 2.21. CAT scan with contrast and carotid angiogram demonstrating a ruptured saccular aneurysm of the right internal carotid at the origin of the posterior cerebral artery. A clot is present in the middle fossa adjacent to the aneurysm. There is no evidence of arterial spasm in the angiogram. *(Cont.)*

Early management of patients with primary SAH is relief of pain, controlled lowering of blood pressure, and attention to tracheal toilet and other medical needs. Patients with grades 1 or 2 neurologic status can be considered surgical candidates, and complete angiography is performed on them within the first 7 to 10 days in preparation for surgery. There is still disagreement as to the value of ethylamino caproic acid (Amicar®) in preventing or deferring re-bleed of the aneurysm. Despite this lack of statistical certainty and the knowledge that the drug theoretically may promote phlebothrombosis, Amicar is nonetheless utilized in most major neurosurgical centers. It is given in doses of 24 to 48 g daily (1 to 2 g intravenously every hour). Approximately 20% of patients with SAH show multiple aneurysms by angiography. Locating the one that has bled is done by following various clues, including neurologic symptoms or signs, the presence of arterial spasm adjacent to one of the aneurysms, and clinical judgment.

The results of surgery of intracranial aneurysms have improved dramatically during the past 10 years as a result of:

1. Recognition of the importance of the patient's clinical state to the operative result. Patients with grades 3 or 4 neurologic status have poor surgical results.

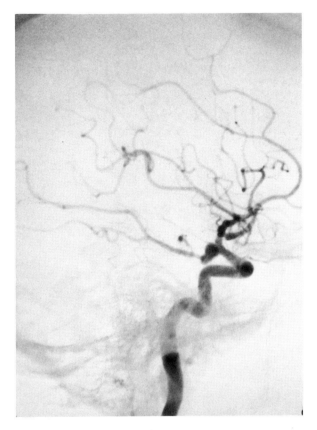

FIG. 2.21.

2. Improved neuroanesthesia with the ability to provide controlled hypotension.

3. Use of the operating microscope.

4. Use of an aneurysm clip which can be applied by a simple spring release.

5. Ability to control brain edema during surgery by dexamethasone and hyperosmolar agents if necessary.

Nevertheless, the experience and skill of the surgeon are extremely important. There is no doubt that operative results are better in the hands of a surgeon who performs these procedures frequently and regularly in contrast to one who operates on aneurysms only two or three times yearly.

There are a number of serious complications of SAH from ruptured aneurysm. Arterial spasm appears in a significant percentage of patients at the third day and again around the tenth day. This complication may cause cerebral infarction and/or massive cerebral edema. Although its cause is

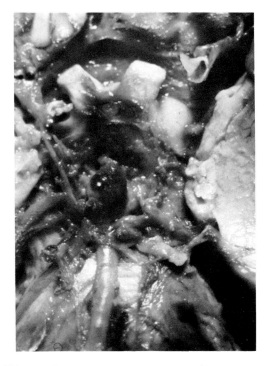

FIG. 2.22. Berry aneurysm at bifurcation of basilar artery.

unknown, it is thought to be somehow related to serotonin released from the subarachnoid blood and acting on receptor sites on the arterial surfaces. There is no known effective treatment. Some neurosurgeons advocate the combination of reserpine and kanamycin; others believe increased arterial pressure may be helpful.

About 40% of all patients with ruptured aneurysm die during the initial bleed. Re-bleeding occurs in a significant percentage at about the tenth to fourteenth day after the initial ictus. At least 50% of patients who re-bleed die and the morbidity for the remainder is increased. The optimal time for operation is a critical balance between allowing sufficient time for the patient's brain to recover from the initial bleed and the dangerous complication of waiting so long that re-bleeding occurs.

Hydrocephalus is another complication of SAH. It may occur relatively early (at 2 to 3 weeks) owing to fibrin obstruction of the foramina of Luschka and Magendie, or it may develop gradually as normal-pressure hydrocephalus several weeks to months after the bleed. In the latter instance, the cause is always impaired CSF reabsorption by the arachnoidal villi. Ventricular shunting may be necessary in both types of hydrocephalus.

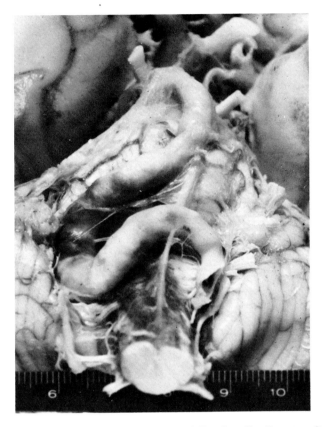

FIG. 2.23. Arteriosclerotic fusiform tortuous aneurysmal dilatation of basilar artery. Such a change is usually associated with longstanding hypertension. This type of aneurysm does not rupture but may cause symptoms by compressing cranial nerves.

An occasional patient may present with an SAH, but careful angiography reveals no aneurysm or other vascular abnormality. The angiogram should probably be repeated in these patients after a wait of 2 to 4 weeks because arterial spasm might prevent visualization of the aneurysm on a single occasion. Absence of a demonstrated aneurysm or vascular anomaly usually denotes a good prognosis.

CAT scans of the brain are useful in the evaluation of patients with SAH to exclude an intracerebral bleed or an arteriovenous anomaly. Rarely does the CAT scan reveal a berry aneurysm, but the presence of subarachnoid blood can be readily appreciated.

Surgery on asymptomatic aneurysms remains a controversial issue. Since the natural history of such aneurysms is not known, rational judgments are difficult.

Arteriovenous Malformations

Arteriovenous malformations and other types of intracranial angiomas may, like berry aneurysms, cause SAH. Many of these patients have had symptoms indicative of an intracranial lesion even prior to the occurrence of the bleed, so that the diagnosis is not infrequently made even though sub-

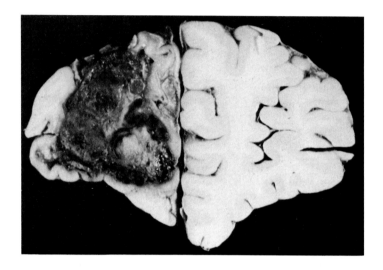

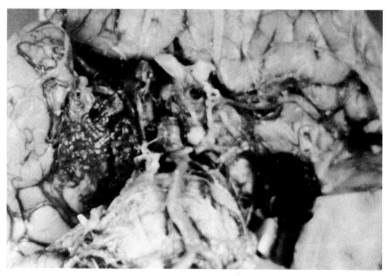

FIG. 2.24. Arteriovenous anomaly. This deep, extensive angioma caused seizures and persistent hemiparesis, and eventually ruptured.

arachnoid bleed has not occurred. Although there are several types of cerebrovascular anomalies, arteriovenous malformations comprise about 75% (Fig. 2.24). The other types include capillary and venous angiomas, cavernous angiomas, and capillary angiomas (Fig. 2.25).

These vascular anomalies, particularly the arteriovenous malformations (AVM), may cause focal or generalized epilepsy and in rare instances cause dementia. The epilepsy is due to the actual mass effect of the anomaly lying on the brain and the tissue destruction and gliosis which results from the lesion. The dementia said to be associated with large AVMs is presumed to be secondary to the vascular shunting which may draw substantial blood flow away from normal brain tissue with resultant neuronal loss and gliosis. Large arteriovenous shunts may result in congestive heart failure in children.

The severity of the bleeding which occurs from these vascular anomalies is usually much less than that from berry aneurysms, and the prognosis is much better. The necessity for surgical intervention is therefore less pressing. There is not universal agreement concerning the management of cerebrovascular anomalies. Many individuals are known to live essentially asymptomatically

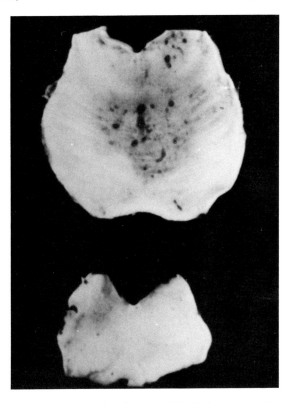

FIG. 2.25. Arteriovenous anomaly (angioma) of pons. This lesion produced a severe neurologic defect by causing local tissue infarction (rather than by rupture).

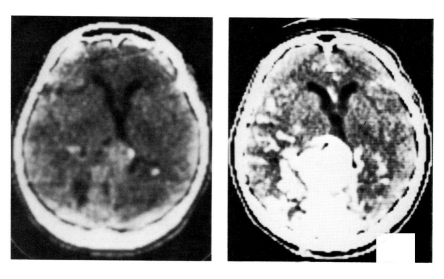

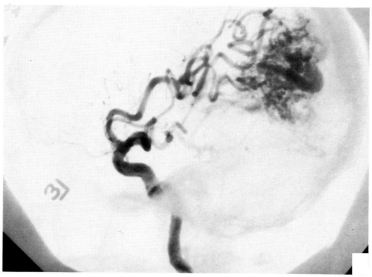

FIGS. 2.26, 2.27, 2.28. Huge occipital lobe arteriovenous anomaly. The contrast CAT scan shows the extent of the lesion and some of the dilated adjacent arteries and veins. The angiogram demonstrates that the major feeding vessel is from the middle cerebral artery. This patient presented with a history of progressively more frequent episodes of flashing lights in the right visual field, followed by abrupt onset of right homonymous hemianopsia. These episodes were not associated with headaches. There was no history of subarachnoid hemorrhage.

with large lesions, and there is usually little to gain from excision of an AVM which is causing epileptic seizures unless the seizures cannot be controlled medically. Documented histories of more than a single bleed certainly make the need to consider surgical intervention much more urgent. Other forms of therapy now include embolization of the feeding artery by glass or plastic beads introduced by intra-arterial catheter. The beads act as emboli which occlude feeding arteries and reduce the size of the AVM. In certain deeply located AVMs, there may be no other treatment available.

Diagnosis of cerebrovascular anomalies is by CAT scanning and angiography. The CAT scan may reveal an area of decreased density, parts of which may enhance after contrast injection (Figs. 2.26 and 2.27). Angiography reveals the details of the lesion. The angiographic study must be bilateral and complete, so that possible arterial feeders from anterior, middle, and posterior cerebral arteries can be identified (Fig. 2.28).

SUGGESTED READINGS

Physiology of Cerebral Circulation

Berne RM: Metabolic regulation of blood flow. *Circ Res* 14,15 (Suppl. 1):261, 1964.

D'Alecy LG, and Feigl EO: Sympathetic control of cerebral blood flow in dogs. *Circ Res* 31:267, 1972.

Fencl V, Vale JR, and Brock JA: Respiration and cerebral blood flow in metabolic acidosis and alkalosis in humans. *J Appl Physiol* 27:67, 1969.

Fieschi C: Regional cerebral blood flow in patients with brain infarcts. *Arch Neurol* 15:653, 1966.

Fieschi C, Agnoli A, Battistini N, et al: Derangement of regional cerebral blood flow and of its regulatory mechanisms in acute cerebrovascular lesions. *Neurology (Minneap)* 18:1166, 1968.

James IM, Millar RA, and Purves MJ: Observations on the extrinsic neural control of cerebral blood flow in the baboon. *Circ Res* 25:77, 1969.

Kogure K, Scheinberg P, Reinmuth OM, Fujishima M, and Busto R: Mechanisms of cerebral vasodilatation in hypoxia. *J Appl Physiol* 29:233, 1970.

Nelson E, and Rennels M: Innervation of intracranial arteries. *Brain* 93:475, 1970.

Paulson OB: Regional cerebral blood flow in apoplexy due to occlusion of the middle cerebral artery. *Neurology (Minneap)* 22:377, 1972.

Reivich M: Arterial PCO_2 and cerebral hemodynamics. *Am J Physiol* 206:25, 1964.

Roy CS, and Sherrington CS: On the regulation of the blood supply of the brain. *J Physiol (Lond)* 11:85, 1890.

Shinohara Y: Mechanism of chemical control of cerebral vasomotor activity. *Neurology (Minneap)* 23:186, 1973.

Sokoloff L: The action of drugs on the cerebral circulation. *Pharmacol Rev* 11:1, 1959.

Factors Influencing Stroke Including Risk Factors

Battacharji SK, Hutchinson EC, and McCall AJ: The circle of Willis: the incidence of developmental abnormalities in normal and infarcted brains. *Brain* 90:747, 1967.

Flora GC, Omae WT, and Nishimoru K: Clinical profile of the stroke patient. *Geriatrics* 24:95, 1969.

Garraway WM, Whisnant JP, Furlan AJ, Phillips LH, Kurland LT, and O'Fallon WM: The declining incidence of stroke. *N Engl J Med* 300:449, 1979.

Heyman A, Karp HR, Heyden S, et al: Cerebrovascular disease in the biracial population of Evans County, Georgia. *Stroke* 2:509, 1971.

Heyman A, Leviton A, Millikan CH, et al: Report of the Joint Committee for Stroke Facilities. XI. Transient focal cerebral ischemia: epidemiological and clinical aspects. *Stroke* 5:275, 1974.

Kurtzke JF: *Epidemiology of Cerebrovascular Disease.* Springer-Verlag, New York, 1969.

Clinical Syndromes of Occlusive Disease

Castaigne P, L'Hermitte F, Gautier JC, et al: Arterial occlusions in the vertebro-basilar system: a study of 44 patients with postmortem data. *Brain* 96:133, 1973.

Critchley M: The anterior cerebral artery and its syndromes. *Brain* 53:120, 1930.

Doniger DE: Bilateral complete carotid and basilar artery occlusion in a patient with minimal deficit: case report and discussion of diagnostic and therapeutic implications. *Neurology (Minneap)* 13:673, 1963.

Fisher CM: Lacunes: small, deep cerebral infarcts. *Lancet* 2:19, 1965.

Fisher CM: Pure sensory stroke involving face, arm, and leg. *Neurology (Minneap)* 15:76, 1965.

Fisher CM: A lacunar stroke: the dysarthria-clumsy hand syndrome. *Neurology (Minneap)* 17:614, 1967.

Fisher CM, and Adams RD: Transient global amnesia. *Acta Neurol Scand* 40 (Suppl 9):1, 1964.

Fisher CM, and Curry HB: Pure motor hemiplegia of vascular origin. *Arch Neurol* 13:30, 1965.

Gunning AJ, Pickering GW, Robb-Smith AHT, et al: Mural thrombosis of the internal carotid artery and subsequent embolism. *Q J Med* 33:155, 1964.

Kubick CS, and Adams RD: Occlusion of the basilar artery: a clinical and pathological study. *Brain* 69:73, 1946.

Landolt AM, and Millikan CH: Pathogenesis of cerebral infarction secondary to mechanical carotid artery occlusion. *Stroke* 1:52, 1970.

Lascelles RG, et al: Occlusion of middle cerebral artery. *Brain* 88:85, 1965.

Matthew NT, and Meyer JS: Pathogenesis and natural history of transient global amnesia. *Stroke* 5:303, 1974.

Newman M: The process of recovery after hemiplegia. *Stroke* 3:702, 1972.

Patel A, and Toole JF: Subclavian steal syndrome: reversal of cephalic blood flow. *Medicine (Baltimore)* 44:289, 1965.

Williams D: The diagnosis of the major and minor syndromes of basilar insufficiency. *Brain* 85:741, 1962.

TIAs: Mechanisms

Barnett HJM, Jones MW, Boughner DR, and Kostuk WJ: Cerebral ischemia events associated with prolapsing mitral valve. *Arch Neurol* 33:777, 1976.

Kendall RE, and Marshall J: Role of hypotension in the genesis of transient focal cerebral ischaemic attacks. *Br Med J* 10:344, 1963.

Marshall J: The natural history of transient ischemic cerebrovascular attack. *Q J Med* 33:309, 1964.

Siekert RG, and Jones HR Jr: Transient cerebral ischemic attacks associated with subacute bacterial endocarditis. *Stroke* 1:178, 1970.

Soloway HB, et al: Atheromatous emboli to central nervous system. *Circulation* 30:611, 1964.

Toole JF, Janeway R, Choi K, et al: Transient ischemic attacks due to atherosclerosis: a prospective study of 160 patients. *Arch Neurol* 32:5, 1975.

TIAs: Clinical Syndromes

David N, et al: Fatal atheromatous cerebral embolism associated with bright plaques in the retinal arterioles. *Neurology (Minneap)* 13:708, 1963.

Fisher CM: Observations of the fundus oculi in transient monocular blindness. *Neurology (Minneap)* 9:333, 1959.

Hollenhorst RW: Significance of bright plaques in the retinal arterioles. *JAMA* 178:23, 1961.

McDowell F, and Ejrup B: Arterial bruits in cerebrovascular disease: a follow-up study. *Neurology (Minneap)* 16:1127, 1966.

Whisnant JP, Matsumoto N, and Elveback LR: Transient cerebral ischemic attacks in a community: Rochester, Minnesota, 1955–1969. *Mayo Clin Proc* 48:194, 1973.

TIAs: Prognosis

Baker RN, Ramseyer JC, and Schwartz WS: Prognosis in patients with transient ischemic attacks. *Neurology (Minneap)* 18:1157, 1968.

Goldner JC, Whisnant JP, and Taylor WF: Long-term prognosis of transient cerebral ischemic attacks. *Stroke* 2:160, 1971.

TIAs and Strokes: Treatment

Anderson DC, and Cranford RE: Corticosteroids in ischemic stroke. *Stroke* 10:68, 1979.

Barnett HJM, McDonald JWD, and Sackett DL: Aspirin—effective in males threatened with stroke. *Stroke* 9:295, 1978.

Browne TR, and Poskanzer DC: Treatment of strokes. I. *N Engl J Med* 281:594, 1969.

Browne TR, and Poskanzer DC: Treatment of strokes. II. *N Engl J Med* 281:650, 1969.

Burrows EH, and Marshall J: Angiographic investigation of patients with transient ischemic attacks. *J Neurol Neurosurg Psychiatry* 28:533, 1965.

Canadian Cooperative Study Group. *N Engl J Med* 299:53, 1978.

Fields WS, Lemak NA, Frankowski RF, and Hardy RJ: Controlled trial of aspirin in cerebral ischemia. *Stroke* 8:301, 1977.

McHenry LC Jr: Cerebral vasodilator therapy in stroke. *Stroke* 3:686, 1972.

Millikan CH, and McDowell FH: Treatment of transient ischemic attacks. *Stroke* 9:299, 1978.

Patten BM, Mendell J, Bruun BF, et al: Double-blind study of the effects of dexamethasone on acute stroke. *Neurology (Minneap)* 22:377, 1972.

Peszcyzynski M, Benson DF, Collins JM, et al: Report of the Joint Committee for Stroke Facilities: II. Stroke rehabilitation. *Stroke* 3:373, 1972.

Report of the Joint Committee for Stroke Resources, January 1977.

Report of the Joint Committee for Stroke Facilities, March–April 1973.

Report of the Joint Committee for Stroke Resources, July–August 1977.

Rodvien R, and Mielke CH Jr: Platelet and antiplatelet agents in strokes. *Stroke* 9:403, 1978.

Samson DS, Hodosh RM, and Clark WK: Microsurgical treatment of transient cerebral ischemia. *JAMA* 241:376, 1979.

Smith AL, Hoff JT, Nielsen SL, and Larson CP: Barbiturate protection in acute focal cerebral ischemia. *Stroke* 5:1, 1974.

Whisnant JP, Anderson EM, Aronson SM, et al: Report of the Joint Committee for Stroke Facilities. V. Clinical prevention of stroke. *Stroke* 3:803, 1972.

Whisnant JP, Matsumoto N, and Elveback LR: The effect of anticoagulant therapy on the prognosis of patients with transient cerebral ischemic attacks in a community: Rochester, Minnesota, 1955 through 1969. *Mayo Clin Proc* 48:844, 1973.

Arteritis

Beevers DG, Harpur JE, and Turk KAD: Giant cell arteritis: the need for prolonged treatment. *J Chronic Dis* 26:571, 1973.

Erma M: The clinical manifestations of temporal arteritis. *Acta Med Scand* 179:691, 1966.

Hamilton CR Jr, Shelley WM, and Tumulty PA: Giant cell arteritis including temporal arteritis and polymyalgia rheumatica. *Medicine (Baltimore)* 50:1, 1971.

Harrison MJG, Bevan AT: Early symptoms of temporal arteritis. *Lancet* 2:638, 1967.

Strokes During Childhood

Banker BG: Cerebral vascular disease in infancy and childhood. *Arch Neurol* 17:313, 1967.

Schoenberg BS, Mellinger JF, and Schoenberg DG: Cerebrovascular disease in infants and children: a study of incidence, clinical features, and survival. *Neurology (Minneap)* 28:763, 1978.

Oral Contraceptives

Bickerstaff E, et al: Cerebral arterial insufficiency and oral contraceptives. *Br Med J* 1:726, 1967.

Cole M: Strokes in young women using oral contraceptives. *Arch Intern Med* 120:551, 1967.

Collaborative Group for the Study of Stroke in Young Women: Oral contraception and increased risk of cerebral ischemia or thrombosis. *N Engl J Med* 288:871, 1973.

Strokes: Diagnosis

Ginsberg MD, Greenwood SA, and Goldberg HI: Noninvasive diagnosis of extracranial cerebrovascular disease: oculoplethysmography-phonoangiography and directional Doppler ultrasonography. *Neurology (Minneap)* 29:623, 1979.

Glasgow JL, Currier RD, Goodrich JK, et al: Brain scans at varied intervals following C.V.A. *J Nucl Med* 6:902, 1965.

Emboli

Gilman S: Cerebral disorders after open-heart operations. *N Engl J Med* 272:489, 1965.

Steinmetz EF, Calanchini PR, and Aguilar MJ: Left atrial myxoma as a neurological problem: a case report and review. *Stroke* 4:451, 1973.

Angiography (Complications)

Faught E, Trader SD, and Hanna GR: Cerebral complications of angiography for transient ischemia and stroke: prediction of risk. *Neurology (Minneap)* 29:4, 1979.

Field JR, Robertson JT, and Desaussure RL Jr: Complications of cerebral angiography in 2,000 consecutive cases. *J Neurosurg* 19:775, 1962.

Hass WK, Fields WS, North RR, et al: Joint study of extracranial arterial occlusion. II. Arteriography, techniques, sites, and complications. *JAMA* 203:961, 1968.

Scheinberg P, and Zunker E: Complications in direct percutaneous carotid arteriography. *Arch Neurol* 8:676, 1963.

Endarterectomy

Bauer RB, Meyer JS, Fields WS, et al: Joint study of extracranial arterial occlusion. III. Progress report of controlled study of long-term survival in patients with and without operation. *JAMA* 208:509, 1969.

Blaisdell W: Extracranial arterial surgery in the treatment of stroke. In: *Cerebral Vascular Diseases*, edited by FH McDowell and RW Brennan, pp. 3–26. Grune & Stratton, New York, 1973.

Easton JD, and Sherman DG: Stroke and mortality rate in carotid endarterectomy: 228 consecutive operations. *Stroke* 8:565, 1977.

Fields WS, Maslenikov V, Meyer JS, et al: Joint study of extracranial arterial occlusion. V. Progress report of prognosis following surgery or nonsurgical treatment for transient cerebral ischemic attacks and cervical carotid artery lesions. *JAMA* 211:1993, 1970.

Heyman A, et al: Long term results of carotid endarterectomy for treatment of cerebral ischemia and infarction. *Circulation* 36:212, 1967.

Hypertensive Encephalopathy

Ziegler DK, et al: Hypertensive encephalopathy. *Arch Neurol* 12:472, 1965.

Cerebral Hemorrhage

Aurell M, and Hood B: Cerebral hemorrhage in a population after a decade of active antihypertensive treatment. *Acta Med Scand* 176:377, 1964.

Cuatico W, Adib S, and Gaston P: Spontaneous intracerebral hematomas: a surgical appraisal. *J Neurosurg* 22:569, 1965.

Fisher CM: Clinical syndromes in cerebral hemorrhage. In: *Pathogenesis and Treatment of Cerebrovascular Disease*, edited by WS Fields, pp. 318–342. Charles C Thomas, Springfield, Illinois, 1961.

Fisher CM: The pathology and pathogenesis of intracerebral hemorrhage. In: *Pathogenesis and Treatment of Cerebrovascular Disease*, edited by WS Fields, p. 562. Charles C Thomas, Springfield, Illinois, 1961.

Fisher CM: Acute hypertensive cerebellar hemorrhage. *J Nerv Ment Dis* 140:38, 1965.

Freytag E: Fatal hypertensive intracerebral hematomas: a survey of the pathological anatomy of 393 cases. *J Neurol Neurosurg Psychiatry* 31:616, 1968.

Hyland HH: Non-aneurysmal intracranial hemorrhage. *Neurology (Minneap)* 11:165, 1961.

Ivamoto HS, Numoto M, and Donaghy RMP: Surgical decompression for cerebral and cerebellar infarcts. *Stroke* 5:365, 1974.

McKissock W, Richardson A, and Taylor J: Primary intracerebral hemorrhage: a controlled trial of surgical and conservative treatment in 180 unselected cases. *Lancet* 2:221, 1961.

McKissock W, Richardson A, and Walsh L: Spontaneous cerebellar hemorrhage: a study of 34 consecutive cases treated surgically. *Brain* 83:1, 1960.

Richardson EP Jr, and Dodge PR: Epilepsy in cerebral vascular disease: a study of the incidence and nature of seizures in 104 consecutive hemorrhages. *Epilepsia* 3:49, 1954.

Subarachnoid Hemorrhage

Lee MLK, and Cheung EMT: Moyamoya disease as a cause of subarachnoid haemorrhage in Chinese. *Brain* 96:623, 1973.

Locksley HB: Natural history of subarachnoid hemorrhage, intracranial aneurysms and arteriovenous malformations. In: *Intracranial Aneurysms and Subarachnoid Hemorrhage*, edited by AL Sahs, G Perret, HB Locksley, and H Nishioka, Chap 5. Lippincott, Philadelphia, 1969.

Locksley HB, Sahs AL, and Knowles L: Report on the cooperative study of intracranial aneurysms and subarachnoid hemorrhage. Sect. V, Parts I and II. Natural history of subarachnoid hemorrhage, intracranial aneurysms, and arteriovenous malformations. *J Neurosurg* 25:219, 321, 1966.

Locksley HB, Sahs AL, and Sandler R: Subarachnoid hemorrhage unrelated to intracranial aneurysm and A-V malformation. In: *Intracranial Aneurysms and Subarachnoid Hemorrhage*, edited by AL Sahs, G Perret, HB Locksley, and H Nishioka. Chap 13. Lippincott, Philadelphia, 1969.

McKissock W, and Paine KWE: Subarachnoid hemorrhage. *Brain* 82:356, 1959.

McKissock W, et al: An analysis of the results of treatment of ruptured intracranial aneurysms. *Acta Neurol Scand* 40:200, 1964.

Aneurysms

Crompton MR: The pathogenesis of cerebral aneurysms. *Brain* 89:797, 1966.

Hassler O: On the etiology of intracranial aneurysms. In: *Intracranial Aneurysms and Subarachnoid Hemorrhage*, edited by WS Fields and AL Sahs, pp. 25–39. Charles C Thomas, Springfield, Illinois, 1965.

Krayenbuhl HA, Yasargil MG, Flamm ES, and Tew JM: Microsurgical treatment of intracranial saccular aneurysms. *J Neurosurg* 37:678, 1972.

Locksley HB: Natural history of subarachnoid hemorrhage, intracranial aneurysms and arteriovenous malformations. In: *Intracranial Aneurysms and Subarachnoid Hemorrhage*, edited by AL Sahs, G Perret, HB Locksley, and H Nishioka, Chap 5. Lippincott, Philadelphia, 1969.

Locksley HB, Sahs AL, and Knowles L: Report on the cooperative study of intracranial aneurysms and subarachnoid hemorrhage. Sect. V, Parts I and II. Natural history of subarachnoid hemorrhage, intracranial aneurysms, and arteriovenous malformations. *J Neurosurg* 25:219, 321, 1966.

McKissock W: Multiple intracranial aneurysms. *Lancet* 1:623, 1967.

McKissock W, Paine KW, and Walsh LS: An analysis of the results of treatment of ruptured intracranial aneurysms: report of 772 consecutive cases. *J Neurosurg* 17:762, 1960.

Sahs AL: Observations on the pathology of saccular aneurysms. In: *Intracranial Aneurysms and Subarachnoid Hemorrhage*, edited by AL Sahs, G Perret, HB Locksley, and H Nishioka, Chap 4. Lippincott, Philadelphia, 1969.

Skultety FM, and Nishioka H: The results of intracranial surgery in the treatment of aneurysms. In: *Intracranial Aneurysms and Subarachnoid Hemorrhage*, edited by AL Sahs, G Perret, HB Locksley, and H Nishioka, Chap 10. Lippincott, Philadelphia, 1969.

Richardson AE, Jane JA, and Payne PM: Assessment of the natural history of anterior communicating aneurysms.

Sundt TM, and Whisnant JP: Subarachnoid hemorrhage from intracranial aneurysms: surgical management and natural history of disease. *N Engl J Med* 299:116, 1978.

Winn HR, Richardson AE, O'Brien W, and Jane JA: The long-term prognosis in untreated cerebral aneurysms. II. Late morbidity and mortality. *Ann Neurol* 4:418, 1978.

Angiomas

Crawford JV, and Russell DS: Cryptic arteriovenous and venous hematomas of brain. *J Neurol Neurosurg Psychiatry* 19:1, 1956.

Locksley HB, Sahs AL, and Sandler R: Subarachnoid hemorrhage unrelated to intracranial aneurysm and A-V malformation. In: *Intracranial Aneurysms and Subarachnoid Hemorrhage*, edited by AL Sahs, G Perret, HB Locksley, and H Nishioka, Chap 13. Lippincott, Philadelphia, 1969.

McCormick WF, and Nofzinger JD: "Cryptic" vascular malformations of the central nervous system. *J Neurosurg* 24:865, 1966.

Perret G, et al: Arteriovenous malformations. *J Neurosurg* 25:467, 1966.

Svien HJ, and McRae JA: Arteriovenous anomalies of the brain: fate of patients not having definitive surgery. *J Neurosurg* 23:23, 1965.

Books: General

Toole JF, and Patel AN: *Cerebrovascular Disorders*. McGraw-Hill, New York, 1967.

Walton JN: *Subarachnoid Hemorrhage*. Livingstone, London, 1956.

Wylie EJ, and Ehrenfeld WK: *Extracranial Occlusive Cerebrovascular Disease*. Saunders, Philadelphia, 1971.

3

Dementia

Dementia is not easily definable because it encompasses an exceptionally broad spectrum of symptoms and signs and is caused by many diseases primary to the central nervous system (CNS) as well as systemic diseases and drugs or toxins which secondarily affect the nervous system. Primary to the definition is the concept that dementia is a disorder of mental functioning of organic cause, the nature of that disorder varying from the mildest disturbance of judgment or memory to an inchoate state of mental functioning in which the patient has lost all cognitive functions. The difficulties inherent in any such definition, rendering it temporal, are apparent, because the term dementia traditionally excludes "functional" or "nonorganic" disorders such as depression, the schizophrenias, manic-depressive insanity, severe neuroses, and personality disorders. In fact, there is considerable evidence that some or all of these psychiatric disorders which profoundly affect mental functioning have an organic basis which, at least in some instances, may be a disorder of one or more of the brain's putative neurotransmitters. Indeed there are clearly organic causes of emotional disorders. Nevertheless, for the purposes of this presentation, dementia is arbitrarily defined in its orthodox and neurologic context and the so-called "functional" disorders are not discussed.

Dementia is of great interest to physicians who are interested in brain function. It is particularly fascinating to realize that such enormous devastation of mental function can occur without there being evidence, with some exceptions, of the localization of the responsible lesion. It is possible to localize with reasonable accuracy lesions of the nervous system causing a variety of motor disorders, visual abnormalities, sensory changes, and aphasias, but dementia is said by some authors to be a disturbance of the integrative function of the whole brain, rather than a loss of one of its parts. The fact is that the pathology of dementia may be diffuse and varied, but it may be too early and too romantic to view it as a defect of the brain as an entity. Our tendency is to regard dementia as a uniquely human disease, but perhaps that also is a defect in our own perception of function of the "lesser" primates and

[handwritten margin note: ↓ memory ↓ judgement ↓ mental functioning]

other animals; their dementia may be framed in the context of the demands of their society. Who is to say that other animals do not think creatively; they can certainly learn to handle complicated problems, and they clearly manifest affection and loyalty.

Perhaps we should accept the empiricism of our definition and state simply that demented patients have disturbances of what we choose to call "higher cortical functions," e.g., memory, orientation in time and space, calculation, reading comprehension, judgment, ability to reason, and affect. So long as we are honest and recognize that some of these terms have vague meanings and must also be defined arbitrarily, we can at least deal with the practicalities of the clinical problem without assigning physiologic meanings for which evidence does not exist. We thereby avoid somewhat the pretentiousness of ignorance.

The view that the brain lesions causing dementia are nonlocalizable can also be partially disputed. Memory disturbances have been shown to have an anatomic localization, generally in the limbic system and specifically in the mammillary bodies and medial dorsal nuclei of the thalami. The classical clinicoanatomic studies demonstrating this were made in a unique clinical model, i.e., the Wernicke-Korsakoff syndrome. Dyscalculia can occur without other stigmata of dementia as a result of a tumor, infarct, or contusion of the dominant supramarginal and angular gyri, and acquired dyslexia may occur from similar pathology in the splenium of the corpus callosum on the dominant side. Finally, disturbance of communication, particularly comprehension, is often described as a part of a dementing syndrome, yet it is known that impaired comprehension (fluent aphasia) may occur as a consequence of a highly localized lesion in the dominant superior temporal gyrus.

Thus we are beset with inconsistencies, but they are not insurmountable if we are rigidly empiric in our approach to the clinical problem. We must, for example, recognize that a demented patient may develop significant disturbances of language function (aphasia), but by the same token we must avoid confusing an aphasic patient with one who is demented and we must be aware that evaluation of mental status, and thereby the determination of dementia, is difficult to impossible on the severely aphasic patient.

CLINICAL PICTURE OF DEMENTIA

It must be kept in mind that dementia is a symptom complex; it is not a disease per se but, rather, is caused by a large number of disorders affecting the brain. Just as important is the concept that the spectrum of symptoms and signs in dementia is extremely broad, ranging from what appears to be a mild disorder of affect to the most profound loss of all higher cortical functions. Understanding this, the perceptive physician may be suspicious of dementia in an individual who shows the following:

1. Decreased effectiveness in work
2. Impaired ability to deal with social pressures and less control of emotional behavior
3. A tendency to be withdrawn
4. Changes in personal habits and deterioration of dress
5. Superficiality
6. Increased intensity of emotionality
7. Irritability
8. Paranoia
9. Inappropriate sexuality

The similarity of these symptoms to those seen in depressive states or a thought disorder is obvious. It points out the great importance of not labeling a patient as having a "psychiatric" disorder without reasonable confirmation by prior history, clinical course, or psychological testing. As important, it emphasizes the importance of always considering the diagnosis of depressive state, a treatable condition, in a patient whose withdrawn condition seems to label him as demented. The borderline between neurologic and psychiatric disease is tenuous and shifting, and the physician must always be on the lookout for a treatable illness on either side of this line.

There is a group of organic diseases which almost invariably produce disturbances of function that are considered to be emotional. These include:

1. Familial hepatolenticular degeneration (Wilson's disease)
2. Huntington's disease
3. Temporal lobe epilepsy
4. Frontal lobe lesions
5. Drug ingestion—particularly amphetamine overdose
6. CNS lues
7. Nondominant hemisphere lesions

Although the symptoms in each of these disorders are different—ranging among apathy, aggressivity, paranoid delusions, denial of illness, altered sexuality, heightened emotionality, and a sense of destiny—the disorders are frequently misdiagnosed as emotional or psychiatric disorders and proper management is delayed, sometimes to the point of irreversibility of pathology.

The second important feature of the symptom complex of dementia, aside from its variability and capacity to be confused with psychiatric disease, is that there is a longitudinal progression of symptoms. From the subtle alterations in personality described above, most dementing diseases progress with varying rapidity to the more obvious stigmata:

1. Disturbances of orientation in space and time. The patients confuse directions and may not be able to find their way to a simple destination. Missed appointments because of confusion of time are frequent.

2. Progressive loss of memory, particularly recent memory. This defect is in reality an impairment in the patient's ability to acquire new information. The effect is to greatly impair the patient's effectiveness at work or in social activities. It reflects itself in loss of reading skills, the patient being unable to recall what he has read.

3. Dyscalculia. Many patients are unable to make change with money or keep any records involving numbers.

4. Judgmental alterations. The patient's thinking becomes even more concrete. He may be unable to appreciate the allusions in a joke, makes obvious judgmental errors at work and home, and has difficulty reasoning out a problem; his mental status testing reveals an inability to interpret or understand the meaning of simple proverbs or to identify similarities.

5. Eventually the patient may become apathetic, show greatly distorted situational responses and blunting of feelings, and become indifferent to his surroundings, family, and friends.

6. In the latter stages of dementia due to any cause, neurologic dysfunction other than alterations of mental status are observed. These include aphasias, apraxias, cortical release phenomena, sphincter incontinence, and eventually decline in the state of consciousness.

INCIDENCE

Studies in northern Europe have shown that about 4% of all individuals above the age of 65 are sufficiently demented to require institutional care, and an additional 11% have sufficient disorder of mental functioning that they cannot function normally and need assistance with some of the activities of daily living. It is further estimated that about two-thirds of elderly individuals currently institutionalized in all public and private hospitals in the United States are there because of dementia. The number of demented elderly in nursing homes and old age homes is staggering. A case can be readily made that dementia is the greatest public health problem in most industrialized nations in which the median age of survival has increased progressively during the last generation. Faced with increasing numbers of elderly, the magnitude of the problem is frightening, not only in human cost but in the enormous economic burdens which the demented elderly impose on the remainder of the population. In a less complex agrarian society, families could absorb their elderly demented without significant upheaval or displacement. Three generations living under one roof was a common occurrence. In a mobile urban environment, the problem posed by the demented parent or spouse rends families, embitters the last years of a spouse, and produces practical problems of management which often require that the patient be placed in some type of institution for care, draining the financial reserves of the family.

It is not generally recognized that dementia is probably the fourth commonest cause of death in the United States. Patients with Alzheimer's disease have a median life span of about 7 years from diagnosis as compared to about 23 years in a nonaffected age-controlled population. Life expectancy in patients with dementia of every cause is about one-third that of nondemented controls of similar age.

One must not infer from this that dementia invariably accompanies old age because it does not. It is true that most elderly persons have diminished intellectual capacity, a part of the aging process that does not interfere significantly with their lives. It is accepted that psychomotor skills, particularly those which involve rapid movements and perceptual integrative abilities, decline at an accelerated rate compared to verbal abilities in the elderly.

CAUSES OF DEMENTIA

It is beyond the scope of this book to discuss all the causes of dementia in detail. Our major objective is to establish for the reader a perspective of this symptom complex which will be useful in differential diagnosis, to point out that the great majority of patients with dementia are suffering from a disorder of unknown cause (i.e., presenile dementia, or Alzheimer's disease, and senile dementia of the Alzheimer type), and finally and most importantly to call attention to the treatable causes of dementia. In the management of the demented patient, the physician's most important objective is to look for a treatable cause.

Dementing Diseases in Which There is Clinical and Pathological Evidence of Diffuse CNS Disease

Dementing diseases with evidence of diffuse CNS disease are presently untreatable. They may be classified as follows:

I. Genetic and probably genetic basis
   A. Huntington's disease
   B. Spinocerebellar degeneration
   C. Progressive myoclonic epilepsy
II. Due to slow virus infections
   A. Progressive transmissible subacute spongiform encephalopathy, sometimes referred to as Jakob-Creutzfeldt disease
   B. Progressive multifocal leukoencephalopathy, presumably caused by an opportunistic papovavirus
   C. Subacute sclerosing panencephalitis (rubeola virus is considered the etiologic agent)

III. Probable enzymatic defects
  A. Metachromatic leukodystrophy (caused by a defect in aryl-sulfatase A)
  B. Lipid storage diseases
IV. Unknown cause
  A. Progressive supranuclear palsy
  B. Striatonigral degeneration
  C. Schilder's disease

Dementing Diseases in Which Dementia is the Only or the Most Prominent Neurologic and Medical Abnormality

Alzheimer's disease (presenile dementia) and *senile dementia of the Alzheimer type* fall into this category. The terminology is used to avoid a specific inference that the cause of the two conditions is the same, although the pathology is identical. The clinical distinction is that presenile dementia begins during early midlife, whereas the senile form usually has its onset at age 65 or later. About 75 to 80% of all demented patients fall into these diagnostic categories. The etiology is unknown.

The characteristic pathology of Alzheimer's disease and senile dementia includes shrunken brain, senile plaques, neurofibrillary tangles, and gran-ulovacuolar degeneration (Fig. 3.1). The senile plaques occur almost ex-clusively in the cortex and consist of bulbous, rounded, grossly enlarged neuronal processes. Alzheimer's neurofibrillary degeneration consists of al-teration of the normal, delicate intraneuronal fibrils into thickened, densely staining fibers which are twisted and distorted within the neuronal perikaryon, frequently tangling around the nucleus. The origin of the gran-ulovacuolar degeneration seen in Alzheimer's disease has not been clarified by electron microscopic studies.

What is Alzheimer's disease? Is it a true disease process or simply an acceleration of the normal aging process? All extant data suggest that the correlation between the clinical picture of dementia and the classical pathol-ogy of Alzheimer's is quantitative only. The studies of Tomlinson, Blessed, and Roth on the brains of nondemented and demented old people showed that:

1. Brain weights in the two groups were not significantly different, all being within the range for normal adults. Brains of patients with presenile dementia and Huntington's disease frequently weighed less than 1,000 g.

2. Marked generalized atrophy and severe atrophy of the temporal con-volutions and hippocampus occurred only in the dements, but considerable diffuse atrophy can occur in normal old people.

3. Moderate ventricular enlargement was more common in the dements.

4. There were much larger numbers of senile plaques and Alzheimer's neurofibrillary changes in the dements. The authors concluded that there was

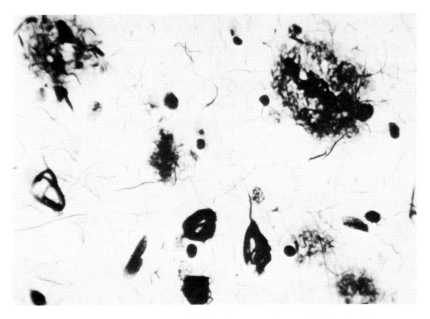

FIG. 3.1. Alzheimer's disease. Senile plaques and neurofibrillary tangles.

a quantitative correlation between the degree of dementia and the number of neurofibrillary tangles.

Neuronal counts are not significantly different in patients with Alzheimer's disease and normal old people. Neurofibrillary tangles occur not only in normal old people and patients with Alzheimer's disease but also in punchdrunk fighters and patients with parkinsonism and progressive supranuclear palsy, as well as those with Down's syndrome who survive to the third or fourth decades.

During the past several years experimental studies by Crapper and others have shown that there is increased aluminum content in the brains of patients with Alzheimer's disease, and that experimental aluminum encephalopathy is associated with neurofibrillary degeneration. This interesting relationship has yet to be further validated. Recent interesting studies by Davies and others demonstrated that there is a selective reduction of choline acetylase and acetylcholinesterase in the amygdala, hippocampus, and cortex of brains of patients with Alzheimer's disease. There appears to be a selective reduction of those enzymes involved in the metabolism of acetylcholine mainly in the regions of greatest density of neurofibrillary tangles. The concept that the symptoms of Alzheimer's disease may be a manifestation of cholinergic deficit in certain parts of the brain emerges.

Dementias Caused by Definable Toxic, Metabolic, or Deficiency States or by Some Associated Illness or Injury

Dementias caused by toxic, metabolic, or deficiency states or by an illness or injury comprise the treatable causes for dementia, although not all are treatable. See Table 3.1 for a list of the treatable causes of dementia. Those causes not specifically treatable include:

1. Multi-infarct dementia. This is not a frequent cause of dementia but certainly does occur in patients who have had repeated small brain infarctions, either embolic or thrombotic. Other neurologic signs and a history of repeated strokes are almost invariably present.
2. Chronic posttraumatic encephalopathy.
3. Postmeningoencephalitis encephalopathy.

TREATABLE DEMENTIAS

It is difficult to know which of the treatable dementias to discuss first because none are common. In general the physician must be on the lookout for any clue—from the history, physical examination, or laboratory work—which might point to a treatable lesion.

Frontal Lobe Tumors

Meningiomas of the frontal lobe (Fig. 3.2), particularly those originating in the orbital surface, are curable if detected early enough. The patients manifest a personality change characterized by deterioration in dress and personal habits, inability to control emotional behavior, inappropriate sexuality, poor judgment, irritability, and finally apathy. Examination may reveal anosmia and disturbance of gait characterized by staggering. Diagnosis is often sus-

TABLE 3.1. *Treatable dementias*

Frontal lobe tumors
Myxedema
CNS syphilis *(lues)*
Bilateral subdural hematomas
Wilson's disease
Normal-pressure hydrocephalus
Hepatocerebral degeneration
Nutritional disorders
Vitamin B_{12} deficiency
Hypercalcemia
Addison's disease
Lead encephalopathy
Bromidism
Fungal meningitis

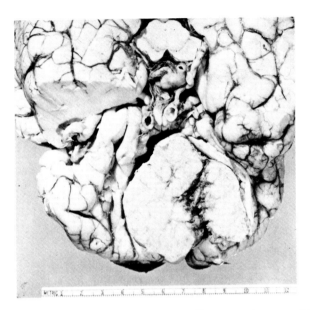

FIG. 3.2. Meningioma of frontal lobe. Elderly woman with progressive nonagitative dementia characterized by personality change, withdrawal, depression, and ultimately stupor. Subfrontal and frontal menigiomas can achieve great size without producing obvious motor abnormalities and must always be considered in the differential diagnosis of dementia.

pected by the history and physical examination, and confirmed by computerized axial tomography (CAT) scan, skull x-rays, and appropriate contrast studies.

Myxedema

Classical myxedema is easy to recognize. The patient's skin is puffy and pasty; the voice is hoarse and deep-pitched; the lateral portions of the eyebrows are absent; prolonged relaxation phase of the deep tendon reflexes and pseudomyotonia are common. The patients are often withdrawn or apathetic. The dementia may be mild or profound and has no special characteristics. Thyroid function studies should be part of every dementia work-up. The cerebrospinal fluid (CSF) in patients with hypothyroid disease often has an elevated protein level. The CAT scan is usually normal.

Nutritional Diseases

Wernicke-Korsakoff syndrome (Fig. 3.3). This is usually associated with severe alcoholism. The patients are often alert and communicative, although they have a severe disturbance of recent memory and frequently confabulate. Other signs are invariably present, including ophthalmoplegias, ataxia,

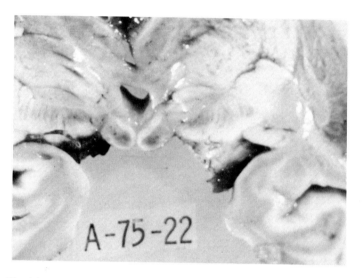

FIG. 3.3. Wernicke-Korsakoff syndrome. The mammillary bodies show extensive necrosis. Lesions were also seen in the thalamus and periaqueductal region.

nystagmus, and peripheral neuropathy. The patients have a variable and unpredictable response to treatment with thiamine HC1.

Pellagra, due to niacin deficiency. Pellagra is now rare in the United States except in cases of obstructive gastrointestinal disorders, dietary faddism, or widespread carcinoma. The dementia is often accompanied by dermatitis and diarrhea.

B_{12} *deficiency.* Dementia is rare in the absence of spinal cord involvement. The major CNS affliction is in the dorsal and lateral columns of the spinal cord, but very rarely a patient presents with predominantly a disturbance of intellectual function. Vitamin B_{12} blood levels should be a part of every dementia work-up.

Other Metabolic Causes of Dementia

1. Addison's disease
2. Hypercalcemia of any cause
3. Acquired hepatocerebral degeneration
4. Uremia
5. Cushing's syndrome

Wilson's Disease (Copper Encephalopathy, Familial Hepatocerebral Degeneration)

Awareness of Wilson's disease, a rare entity, is important because it frequently begins as a behavior disturbance which can easily be misinterpreted as being psychiatric. If the patients are mistreated with psychotropic drugs, the involuntary movements they develop may be thought to be drug-related and their true significance not appreciated. The typical presentation is disturbed mentation, poor judgment, bizarre behavior, involuntary choreiform movements, and ataxia. Diagnosis is made by finding a Kayser-Fleischer ring around the periphery of the cornea by direct or slit-lamp examination and by a decrease in serum ceruloplasmin and serum copper and an increase in urinary copper excretion. The disease can be successfully treated if therapy is begun before permanent brain damage has occurred. Penicillamine, a chelating agent which binds copper, is given in doses of 1 to 2 g daily for life. Asymptomatic affected siblings should be identified and treated prophylactically.

Cerebral Intoxicants

Although many materials are toxic to the nervous system, only a few produce the syndrome of dementia. Chronic intoxication by arsenic or lead may result in dementia, but other findings are always present to suggest the diagnosis.

Chronic arsenic encephalopathy, rarely seen today except in attempted homicides, is characterized by lethargy, headache, vertigo, and weakness, along with dementia; and examination almost invariably shows evidence of peripheral neuropathy. The poisoning may produce renal and hepatic involvement as well as anemia. Transverse white striae (Mee's lines) on the nails appear about 1 month after the initial poisoning. The diagnosis is suspected because of the accompanying neuropathy, and the diagnosis is confirmed by finding an elevated urinary arsenic level (>0.1 mg arsenic in 24 hr) or an increased arsenic content in hair (>0.1 mg in 100 g). Treatment is by British anti-Lewisite (BAL).

The symptoms and signs of lead intoxication differ in children and adults. In children the syndrome is encephalitic with projectile vomiting, papilledema, lethargy, irritability, and convulsions. In adults, chronic lead poisoning results in weakness, pallor, tremulousness, headaches, vomiting, and convulsions. Dementia is usually late and is accompanied by a variety of motor abnormalities, but particularly bilateral wrist drop from radial nerve palsies. Sensory neuropathy is rarely seen. Chronic lead poisoning in adults is no longer common; sources are the burning of lead-containing storage batteries for fuel, ingestion of moonshine or exterior paint, and absorption from the lead pellets in old gunshot wounds. The main cause in children in slum areas has been chewing sticks of glazed putty that have fallen from old windows or ingestion of leaded paint from old furniture, particularly cribs. Diagnosis is suspected from the stippling of red blood cells and increased urinary coproporphyrins, and is established when δ-aminolevulinic acid is increased in the blood and lead is increased in stools, urine, and CSF. Treatment is tricky, and assistance from a toxicologist should be obtained if possible. It is accomplished by chelation by a combination of BAL with additional calcium disodium verse-nate (Ca EDTA).

Bromidism remains an important cause of dementia. It results in irritability, drowsiness, insomnia, disorientation, memory disturbances, and occasion-ally delusions and hallucinations. In addition, the patients show slurred speech and ataxia. Bromide levels above 150 mg% in the blood are considered to be toxic. Treatment involves removing the source of the bromide and giving the patient 4 to 5 liters of fluid daily, along with large doses of sodium chloride (up to 100 g daily).

CNS Infections

Lues

One must not forget that parenchymatous and vascular syphilis of the brain still exist, and that true paresis may present as a progressive dementia. When it occurs in the absence of other stigmata of lues, the dementia is usually of a special type, wherein the individual becomes garrulous and often quite expan-sive and agreeable, manifesting delusions of grandeur. The expansive nature of the delusions may result in all sorts of wild financial promises made by the patient, all beyond his ability to keep. Other signs of syphilis may be absent. Patients with paresis do not necessarily have Argyll-Robertson pupils or other signs of tabes. If the diagnosis is suspected, the serum fluorescent treponema antibody test (FTA) should be done. This is far more reliable than the Venereal Disease Research Laboratories test (VDRL) and establishes the diagnosis of syphilis unequivocally. The CSF may be normal or show the classic changes of lymphocytic pleocytosis, elevated protein, normal sugar, and increased gamma globulin. These patients should respond well to therapy, which con-sists of a total of 8 to 10 million units of penicillin given over a 2- to 4-week interval (either benzanthine penicillin G, 2.4 million units weekly for 4 weeks, or procaine penicillin G, 600,000 units daily for 15 days).

Fungal Meningitis

Rarely a patient with fungal meningitis (cryptococcosis, aspergillosis) or *Toxoplasma* meningitis may present because of progressive dementia, other signs either being absent or unobtrusive. It is for this reason that careful CSF examination is necessary for patients with unexplained dementia. The pres-ence of an abnormal number of cells in the CSF requires an India ink prepara-tion, fungal cultures, and appropriate skin, serum, and CSF complement-fixation tests.

Normal-Pressure Hydrocephalus

The original description of normal-pressure hydrocephalus, a form of communicating hydrocephalus, by Adams and co-workers in 1965 was accompanied by great optimism that this apparently treatable disorder was a common cause of dementia. Experience has not substantiated the original spate of enthusiasm for ventriculoatrial shunting, particularly as criteria for the diagnosis of the disorder have crystallized.

Patients with this syndrome are thought to have a disturbance in CSF absorption caused by dysfunction of the Pacchionian villi or a defect in the normal movement of CSF in the cisterns of the subarachnoid space. The causative lesions include subarachnoid hemorrhage or meningoencephalitis, or it may be idiopathic. The prognosis of recovery after shunting is much better if there is a history of a precipitating cause.

The classic symptoms are psychomotor retardation, disturbance of gait, dementia, and urinary incontinence. The gait disturbance is caused by an apraxia of walking. The patient's legs are not weak, but they "stick to the floor" and he often falls backward, being unable to initiate proper walking movements.

The diagnosis is difficult to establish, and it is even more difficult to be certain that the patient will respond to a shunting procedure. CAT scans show dilated ventricles and relatively little sulcal widening (cortical atrophy) (Figs. 3.4 and 3.5). Cisternography following injection of labeled indium into the lumbar subarachnoid space classically reveals sequestration of the label in the ventricles with no migration over the cerebral cortex. Pneumoencephalography shows dilated ventricles and no air over the cortex. The patients almost invariably demonstrate worsening of their symptoms immediately after the pneumoencephalogram.

If all diagnostic criteria are present, the likelihood of improvement after ventriculoatrial or lumbar-peritoneal shunt is enhanced, *but there are no absolute diagnostic signs, either clinical or laboratory*. Unfortunately, shunting is not an innocuous operation. Complications include kinking and obstruction of the shunt tubing, infection, hemorrhage, and the complications of any operative procedure that requires general anesthesia.

SUBDURAL HEMATOMA

Although subdural hematomas usually produce a motor abnormality, they may on occasion cause a confusing, dementing syndrome characterized by drowsiness, gait disturbance, urinary incontinence, and dementia. The CAT scan may be difficult to interpret properly, particularly if the subdurals are bilateral, thereby causing no mass effect, and isodense, which means that

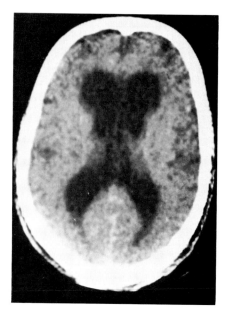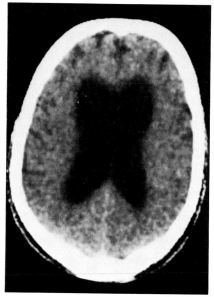

FIGS. 3.4, 3.5. Normal-pressure hydrocephalus. A 58-year-old woman presented with moderate dementia, difficulty in walking, urinary incontinence, and a history of subarachnoid hemorrhage 1 year previously. Ventricles, including the fourth and temporal horns, are symmetrically enlarged. There is little sulcal widening. Cisternogram showed sequestration of label in the ventricles with none appearing over the cortex even after 72 hr.

there is no obvious difference in density between the brain parenchyma and the hematoma. Cerebral angiography is occasionally required for diagnosis. Treatment is by surgical drainage.

The diagnostic work-up of a patient with dementia should include studies to exclude those diseases listed in Table 3.1. CAT scanning has been particularly helpful because it shows not only mass lesions but also widening of the cortical sulci, and ventricular dilatation can be appreciated. The presence of widened sulci and interhemispheric spaces, frontal and temporal atrophy, and ventricular dilatation is powerful evidence for a degenerative parenchymatous process, not surgically or medically treatable (Figs. 3.6 and 3.7).

ACUTE DEMENTIAS

This is the proper context in which to discuss briefly the problem of acute dementia or delirium. The clinical picture is that of rapid onset—often while the patient is in the hospital—of confusion, restlessness, rambling and incoherent speech, tremulousness, and even psychotic behavior such as delusions or hallucinations. In special circumstances there may be accompanying lethargy or extreme drowsiness and, depending on the etiology, motor abnor-

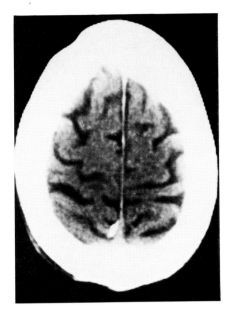 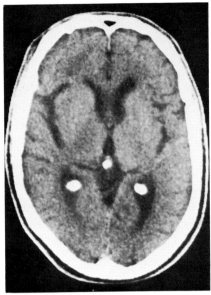

FIGS. 3.6, 3.7. Cerebral CAT scan without contrast from a 52-year-old woman with progressive global dementia. The clinical diagnosis was presenile dementia of the Alzheimer type, a clinical diagnosis of exclusion. The ventricles are generous and the Sylvian fissures enlarged, as is the suprapineal cistern. There is widening of the cortical sulci. This CAT picture cannot be used to make a clinical diagnosis without clinical evidence of the disease because occasional patients with cortical atrophy by CAT scan have no apparent dementia.

malities. The first considerations in such patients are acute intoxication by drugs or alcohol, an acute infectious process (including encephalitis), high fever from any source, withdrawal state (as in delirium tremens), hypoxia, hypoglycemia, hypercapnia, seriously altered blood electrolytes (particularly hyponatremia), Wernicke-Korsakoff syndrome, acute hyperthyroidism, impending hepatic coma, hypercalcemia, and the acute hyperosmolar state associated with high blood sugar. Even a distended bladder may cause an otherwise ill but nondemented patient to become restless, confused, and delirious. In many instances the clinical pictures resulting from various causes are similar and indistinguishable, making diagnosis dependent on a few specific observations and laboratory data. For example, the presence of chronic lung disease and rapid respiration requires immediate arterial blood gas determinations to exclude hypoxia, even though the patient is not clinically cyanotic. If hypoxia is complicated by hypercapnia, the physician recognizes at once that respiratory assistance is required.

Acute dementia associated with motor abnormalities is common. Asterixis (arm flap) is most commonly seen in hepatic encephalopathy. Akathisia (restless movements, inability to sit still) is seen in phenothiazine toxicity, although a similar type of restlessness is observed in Wernicke-Korsakoff syndrome, early delirium tremens, or acute hyperthyroidism. Seizures may occur in the hyperosmolar state, which may also cause obtundation and signs of corticospinal tract disease. Similar abnormalities may accompany hyponatremia or water intoxication, and profound motor weakness and absent reflexes occur in hypercalcemia.

The onset of acute dementia should prompt the treating physician to look for acute infection, check the medications the patient is receiving, look carefully for telltale motor or respiratory abnormalities, and obtain blood samples for determination of blood gases, electrolytes, and sugar.

SUGGESTED READINGS

Mechanisms

Agranoff BW, Davis RE, and Brink JJ: Chemical studies on memory fixation in goldfish. *Brain Res* 1:303, 1966.

Alfrey AC, et al: The dialysis encephalopathy syndrome—possible aluminum intoxication. *N Engl J Med* 294:184, 1976.

Brain WR: Disorders of memory. In: *Recent Advances in Neurology and Neuropsychiatry*, edited by WR Brain and M Wilkinson, 8th edition, pp 1–12. Churchill, London, 1969.

Brody H: Organization of the cerebral cortex: a study of aging in the human cerebral cortex. *J Comp neurol* 102:511, 1955.

Bruyn GW, Mink CJK, and Calje JF: Biochemical studies in Huntington's chorea. *Neurology (Minneap)* 15:455, 1965.

Corsellis JAN: The pathology of dementia. *Br J Hosp Med* 2:695, 1969.

Drachmann DA, and Arbit J: Memory and the hippocampal complex. II. *Arch Neurol* 15:52, 1966.

Geschwind N: Disconnexion syndromes in animals and man. Part I. *Brain* 88:237, 1965.

Geschwind N: Disconnexion syndromes in animals and man. Part II. *Brain* 88:585, 1965.

Hachinski VC, et al: Multi-infarct dementia—a cause of mental deterioration in the elderly. *Lancet* 2:207, 1974.

Obrist WD, Chivian E, Cronqvist S, and Ingvar DH: Regional cerebral blood flow in senile and presenile dementia. *Neurology (Minneap)* 20:315, 1970.

Selkoe DJ, and Shelanski ML: *The Neurochemistry of Aging. Xth Princeton Conference on Cerebral Vascular Disease*, edited by P. Scheinberg, Raven Press, New York, 1976.

Victor M, Adams RD, and Collins G: *The Wernicke-Korsakoff Syndrome (Contemporary Neurology Series)*. Davis, Philadelphia, 1971.

Diagnosis

Folstein MF, Folstein SE, and McHugh PR: "Mini-mental state": a practical method for grading the cognitive state of patients for the clinician. *J Psychiatr Res* 12:189, 1975.

Fox JH, et al: Use of computerized tomography in senile dementia. *J Neurol Neurosurg Psychiatry* 38:948, 1975.

Menzer L, et al: Computerized axial tomography: use in the diagnosis of dementia. *JAMA* 234:754, 1975.

Robinson DS, et al: Aging, monoamines and monoamine-oxidase levels. *Lancet* 1:290, 1972.

Weiner H, and Schuster DB: The electroencephalogram in dementia—some preliminary observations and correlations. *Electroencephalogr Clin Neurophysiol* 8:479, 1956.

Wells CE (ed): *Dementia (Contemporary Neurology Series)*. Davis, Philadelphia, 1971.

Signs and Symptoms

Bieber I: Grasping and sucking. *J Nerv Ment Dis* 91:31, 1940.

Brain WR: Disorders of memory. In: *Recent Advances in Neurology and Neuropsychiatry*, edited by WR Brain and M Wilkinson, 8th ed, pp 1–12. Churchill, London, 1969.

Fisher CM, and Adams RD: Transient global amnesia. *Acta Neurol Scand [Suppl 9]* 40:1, 1964.
Harrison TR, Adams RD, et al: *Principles of Internal Medicine*, 4th ed. McGraw-Hill, New York, 1962.
Wells CE (ed): *Dementia (Contemporary Neurology Series)*. Davis, Philadelphia, 1971.

Alzheimer's Disease

Blessed G, Tomlinson BE, and Roth M: The association between quantitative measurements of dementia and of senile changes in the cerebral grey matter of elderly subjects. *Br J Psychiatry* 114:797, 1968.
Bowen DM, Smith CB, and Davison AN: Molecular changes in senile dementia. *Brain* 96:849, 1973.
Bowen DM, Smith CB, White P, Goodhardt MJ, Spillane JA, Flack RHA, and Davison AN: Chemical pathology of the organic dementias. I. Validity of biochemical measurements on human post-mortem brain specimens. *Brain* 100:397, 1977.
Crapper DR, Krishnan SS, and Quittkat S: Aluminum, neurofibrillary degeneration and Alzheimer's disease. *Brain* 99:67, 1976.
Gonatas NK, Anderson W, and Evangelista I: The contribution of altered synapses in the senile plaque: an electron microscopic study in Alzheimer's dementia. *J Neuropathol Exp Neurol* 26:25, 1967.
Gordon EG, and Sim M: The EEG in pre-senile dementia. *J Neurol Neurosurg Psychiatry* 30:285, 1967.
Grundke-Iqbal I, Johnson AB, Terry RD, Wisniewski HM, and Iqbal K: Evidence that Alzheimer neurofibrillary tangles originate from neurotubules. *Lancet* March 17:578, 1979.
Heston LL, Lowther DLW, and Leventhal CM: Alzheimer's disease. *Arch Neurol* 15:225, 1966.
Katzman R: The prevalence and malignancy of Alzheimer's disease. *Arch Neurol* 33:217, 1976.
McDermott JR, Smith AI, Iqbal K, and Wisniewski HM: Brain aluminum in aging and Alzheimer's disease. *Neurology (Minneap)* 29:809, 1979.
Roth M: The natural history of mental disorders arising in the senium. *Br J Psychiatry* 101:281, 1955.
Roth M, Tomlinson BE, and Blessed G: Correlation between scores for dementia and counts of "senile plaques in cerebral grey matter of elderly subjects." *Nature* 209:109, 1966.
Smith CM, and Swash M: Possible biochemical basis of memory disorder in Alzheimer's disease. *Ann Neurol* 3:471, 1978.
Suzuki K, Katzman R, and Korey SR: Chemical studies on Alzheimer's disease. *J Neuropathol Exp Neurol* 24:211, 1963.
Terry RD: Dementia: a brief and selective review. *Arch Neurol* 33:1, 1976.
Tomlinson BE, Blessed G, and Roth M: Observations on the brains of demented old people. *J Neurol Sci* 11:205, 1970.

Miscellaneous Causes

Astrom KE, Mancall EL, and Richardson EP, Jr: Progressive multifocal leukoencephalopathy: a hitherto unrecognized complication of chronic lymphocytic leukemia and Hodgkin's disease. *Brain* 81:93, 1958.
Bannister R, Gilford E, and Koren R: Isotope encephalography in the diagnosis of dementia due to communicating hydrocephalus. *Lancet* 2:1014, 1967.
Beam AG: Wilson's disease. In: *The Metabolic Basis of Inherited Disease*, edited by JB Stanbury, JB Wyngaarden, and DS Fredrickson, 2nd edition. McGraw-Hill, New York, 1966.
Brownell B, and Oppenheimer DR: An ataxic form of subacute presenile polioencephalopathy (Creutzfeld-Jacob disease). *J Neurol Neurosurg Psychiatry* 28:350, 1965.
Burger PC, and Vogel FS: The development of pathologic changes of Alzheimer's disease and senile dementia in patients with Down's syndrome. *Am J Pathol* 73:457, 1973.
Corsellis JAN, Bruton CJ, and Freeman-Browne D: The aftermath of boxing. *Psychol Med* 3:270, 1973.
Critchley M: Neurologic changes in the aged. *J Chronic Dis* 3:459, 1956.
Davies FL: Mental abnormalities following subdural hematoma. *Lancet* 1:1369, 1960.

Fisch M, Goldfarb AJ, Shahinian SP, and Turner H: Chronic brain syndrome in the community aged. *Arch Gen Psychiatry* 18:759, 1968.

Fraser TN: Cerebral manifestations of Addisonian pernicious anemia. *Lancet* 2:458, 1960.

Gibbs CJ, Jr, and Gajdusek DC: Infection as the etiology of spongiform encephalopathy (Creutzfeld-Jacob disease). *Science* 165:1023, 1969.

Hirano A, Kurland LT, Krooth RS, and Lessell S: Parkinson-dementia complex, an endemic disease on the island of Guam. I. Clinical features. *Brain* 84:642, 1961.

Ironside R, Bosanquet FD, and McMenemey WH: Central demyelinization of the corpus callosum (Marchiafava-Bignami disease). *Brain* 84:212, 1961.

Jellinek EH: Fits, faints, coma, and dementia in myxedema. *Lancet* 2:1000, 1962.

Karpati G, and Frame B: Neuropsychiatric disorders in primary hyperparathyroidism. *Arch Neurol* 10:387, 1964.

Locke S, Merrill JP, and Tyler HR: Neurological complications of uremia. *Arch Intern Med* 108:519, 1961.

Mawdsley C, and Ferguson FR: Neurological disease in boxers. *Lancet* 2:795, 1963.

Plum F, Posner JB, and Hain RF: Delayed neurologic deterioration after anoxia. *Arch Intern Med* 110:18, 1962.

Robinson KC, Kallberg MH, and Crowley MF: Idiopathic hypoparathyroidism presenting as dementia. *Br Med J* 2:1203, 1954.

Sanders V: Neurologic manifestations of myxedema. *N Engl J Med* 266:547, 599, 1962.

Steele JC, Richardson JC, and Olszewski J: Progressive supranuclear palsy. *Arch Neurol* 10:333, 1964.

Strachan RW, and Henderson DG: Dementia and folate deficiency. *Q J Med* 60:189, 1967.

Victor M, Adams RD, and Cole M: The acquired (non-Wilsonian) type of chronic hepatocerebral degeneration. *Medicine (Baltimore)* 44:345, 1965.

Victor M, Adams RD, and Collins G: *The Wernicke-Korsakoff Syndrome (Contemporary Neurology Series)*. Davis, Philadelphia, 1971.

Wadia N, and Williams E: Behçet's syndrome with neurological complications. *Brain* 80:59, 1957.

Wells CE (ed): *Dementia (Contemporary Neurology Series)*. Davis, Philadelphia, 1971.

Normal-Pressure Hydrocephalus

Adams RD, Fisher CM, Hakim S, Ojemann RG, and Sweet WH: Symptomatic occult hydrocephalus with "normal" cerebrospinal fluid pressure. *N Engl J Med* 273:117, 1965.

Bannister R, Gilford E, and Koren R: Isotope encephalography in the diagnosis of dementia due to communicating hydrocephalus. *Lancet* 2:1014, 1967.

Hakim S, and Adams RD: The special clinical problem of symptomatic hydrocephalus with normal cerebrospinal fluid pressure: observations on cerebrospinal fluid hemodynamics. *J Neurol Sci* 2:307, 1965.

Books: General

Critchley M: *The Parietal Lobes*. Arnold, London, 1953.

Karp H: Dementias in adults: In: *Clinical Neurology*, edited by AB Baker and LH Baker, Vol 2, pp 1-22. Harper & Row, Hagerstown, Maryland, 1975

Pearce J, and Miller E: *Clinical Aspects of Dementia*. Bailliere Tindall, London, 1973.

Wells CE (ed): *Dementia (Contemporary Neurology Series)*. Davis, Philadelphia, Pennsylvania, 1971.

4

Disorders of Movement, Tone, and Coordination

It is difficult to devise a logical heading under which to discuss in an organized fashion all disturbances of motor activity and the various diseases which cause them. Obviously disorders of motor activity occur in a large percentage of patients with whom clinical neurology is concerned. Decrease in motor strength may occur as a consequence of disease of primary motor neurons (pyramidal system) and their axons in the cerebral hemisphere's brainstem, or spinal cord. Such weakness is usually characterized by increased tone of the extremities (spasticity), hyperactive deep tendon reflexes, and pathologic reflexes (Babinski). Weakness caused by lesions of the lower motor neurons (cranial nerve nuclei, anterior horn cells) or their axons usually cause weakness associated with decreased muscle tone and diminished deep tendon reflexes. Lesions of the myoneural junction (myasthenia gravis or myasthenic syndrome) cause weakness or fatigability with no special alteration in tone and, in the instance of the myasthenic syndrome, decreased deep tendon reflexes. Muscle disease (polymyositis) usually causes weakness of the midline muscles (neck and trunk) and proximal muscle groups in the extremities. The diseases responsible for these various forms of diminished muscle strength are dealt with in other chapters. The major thrust of this chapter is to discuss the motor abnormalities caused by central nervous system (CNS) lesions which do not involve the pyramidal pathways.

The diseases themselves have various etiologies. The term "degenerative" is often used to describe them, but that term has little meaning except to express our ignorance of the true pathophysiology. It simply implies that certain CNS tissues have "degenerated" without obvious cause. Many of the disorders are also traditionally classified as "extrapyramidal disease" or "cerebellar system disease," implying a distinction of action and function which probably do not exist, but which is rather based upon localization of the most significant pathology in each instance. It is not unreasonable to think of the pyramidal, extrapyramidal, and cerebellar motor systems as being comprised of separately identifiable anatomic structures, but their functional integration in the brain as well as in the spinal cord through local feedback systems in which the α-motor neuron is markedly influenced by the γ-loop, as well as from sensory structures in muscle and skin, clearly denote that the traditionally used classifications are arbitrary at best and can be misleading at worst.

It should be stated that we actually know little about the mechanisms responsible for the performance of motor acts. Traditionally, the motor cortex and pyramidal system have been ascribed the role of initiating a purposeful motor act and being responsible for the conscious or volitional aspects of that performance, whereas the extrapyramidal and cerebellar systems are said to modulate, integrate, control, stabilize, and adjust these movements as well as the unconscious postural adjustment necessary to their performance. yet even after complete surgical ablation of one entire motor cortex, monkeys are capable of relearning all normal purposeful activity using the once-paralyzed extremities, with the possible exception of the finest finger activity. Indeed, sensory cortex ablation appears to produce a more devastating disturbance of movement. Motor performance should be thought of as a composite of input and output from all the sensory and motor systems, and the traditional practice of thinking in terms of pyramidal and extrapyramidal movement abnormalities is patently incomplete and naive.

In this context, we think of involuntary movements as any that are not willed by the performer. They usually not only interfere with accurate intended motor performance but also with the patient's resting state. Clinical-pathological correlations have provided most of our insight into the presumed origin or anatomic substrate of involuntary movements, but, in fact, the pathology of most such disturbances is rarely precisely localized and usually involves many groups of neural structures. The correlation of pathologic localization with clinical phenomenology does not even allow an understanding of the role played by the diseased structure in movement, although the evidence now suggests that in health the diseased nuclei are concerned with inhibition of movement. We have gradually learned to assign specific types of movement abnormalities to certain neural structures; and although incomplete and imprecise, it can yet be a useful device in the evaluation of the clinical problem.

CLINICAL CLASSIFICATION OF MOVEMENT DISORDERS

Fasciculations, Myokymia, and Clonic Facial Hemispasm

Disorders manifested by fasciculations, myokymia, and clonic facial hemispasm share a common responsible pathology in the *lower motor neuron*. *Fasciculations* are fine muscle twitches, usually not felt by the patient as a movement but readily observable. Small areas of the muscle move; rarely is there any actual movement of an extremity. Fasciculations are the hallmark of disease of the bulbar nuclei or anterior horn cells, although they may occur in nerve root or peripheral nerve lesions.   *Lou Gehrig's disease*

Primary motor neuron disease (amyotrophic lateral sclerosis; ALS) is the most frequent etiology of widespread fasciculations. This is a disease of unknown etiology, usually occurring in middle life, but its homologue may occur during infancy (Werdnig-Hoffmann disease) or during adolescence or young adult life (Kugelberg-Welander syndrome). ALS is characterized by progressive, fairly rapid, asymmetrical extremity and bulbar weakness and atrophy with fasciculations and severe muscle wasting. Upper motor neuron signs may also be present, particularly early in the disease. These consist of spasticity, increased deep tendon reflexes in the lower extremities, and positive Babinski signs. Sphincter dysfunction and loss of sensation practically never occur. The differential diagnosis should include cervical spondylosis, spinal cord tumor, syringomyelia, and benign fasciculations. The diagnosis can be established by electromyography, which reveals widespread fasciculation potentials and evidence of denervation. X-rays of the cervical spine and myelography may be necessary to exclude cervical spondylosis, although the clinical distinction is usually apparent. There is no effective treatment. Guanidine HC1 has not been shown to be effective therapy.

Myokymia is a restricted discrete muscle undulation which often has no pathologic significance. Fatigue or emotional stress may induce myokymia of the orbicularis oris. Persistent myokymia of facial muscles is indicative of serious pathology in the pons, usually either *multiple sclerosis* or *brainstem glioma*.

Clonic facial hemispasm is a rapid twitch of all muscles on one side of the face, followed by persistent muscle spasm. It may be precipitated by chewing or talking. There are probably multiple etiologies for this syndrome. It may be caused by an aberrant artery or vein compressing the roots of the facial nerve as it leaves the brainstem, or rarely a tumor is responsible. Surgical exposure and nerve decompression has been reported to be helpful in some of these patients, although there is not universal acceptance of this approach. Carbamazepine (400 to 800 mg daily) has also been reported to be successful in some instances.

Flexor and Extensor Spasms

Flexor and extensor spasms of the lower extremities are almost invariably accompanied by other evidence of spinal cord disease or injury. The patients usually demonstrate spasticity of the involved extremities, a sign of an upper motor neuron lesion. Spasticity may occur in upper motor neuron lesions anywhere in the CNS, of course, not only in the spinal cord. It is usually described as progressively increasing resistance of an extremity to continuous passive stretch, followed by a sudden cessation of resistance. This has been termed the clasp-knife phenomenon. The physiologic explanation of this phenomenon is complex and still debated. In simplest terms, it appears to be due to a decreased threshold for synaptic excitation at the anterior horn cell, most likely as a consequence of isolation from descending inhibitory motor input by the lesion.

Flexor and extensor spasms may be painful. Treatment should be attempted with diazepam (10 mg q.i.d.), phenytoin (300 to 400 mg daily), or amitriptyline (100 mg q.h.s.). Treatment of spasticity may make it more difficult for the patient to walk, because it helps brace the extremities. If the patient is in a wheelchair, therapy for spasticity may be useful. Two drugs presently available are dantrolene sodium and baclofen. The latter is a γ-aminobutyric acid derivative. Surgery or phenol injection intrathecally should be considered only as a last resort.

Tremor

The most ubiquitous of the involuntary movements, tremor occurs in a wide variety of diseases as well as in normal individuals under circumstances of emotional or physical stress. It is easier to describe tremor than to define it. It is produced by fairly regular contractions of paired agonistic and antagonist muscle groups and results in a back-and-forth oscillation of the involved part, usually at a rate of about four cycles per second; it may involve a single finger, a part of or an entire extremity, the head, the jaw, or all these structures at once. The most frequent movement is flexion-extension of the digits and hands or feet, but pronation-supination movements of the forearms and lateral or vertical movements of the head or jaw are not uncommon.

There is considerable consistency between the type of tremor observed and the physiologic or pathologic stress which produces it. One approach to classification of tremors is their association with the state of voluntary activity of the extremities.

The most frequent cause of *resting tremor* is parkinsonism, but *benign familial tremor* may also affect the resting extremities and the head. The tremor of parkinsonism usually involves the distal portions of the extremities, most often the fingers and hands. The thumb and finger move in apposition ("pill-rolling tremor"), and pronation-supination of the forearm is common. The foot tremor is usually a simple flexion-extension or slight lateral movement. The tremor is inhibited by voluntary movement. Parkinsonism tremor is almost invariably associated with other stigmata of the disease, so diagnosis is usually not difficult.

Benign familial tremor may appear at rest. It is much finer and usually less rhythmic than the tremor of parkinsonism; the pill-rolling characteristic is not present, nor are other signs of parkinsonism, e.g., akinesia or rigidity. Usually familial tremor is accentuated by action or by voluntary movement of the extremities, and titubation of the head is a common accompaniment. Despite the name, there may be no family history, and there appears to be no consistent pathology. Usually these patients are concerned that they have parkinsonism, and a definitive negative diagnosis is a great relief to them. The tremor occasionally becomes rather pronounced and interferes substantially with motor function. Propranolol in doses of 50 to 200 mg daily is helpful in some instances, whereas other patients find that mild sedation or an alcoholic beverage suppresses the tremor.

Postural tremor is one that appears predominantly in sustained posture of an extremity. The commonest cause is stress or anxiety, in which instance it is probably caused by the action of released norepinephrine on central and peripheral synaptic receptor sites. The physiologic tremor of stress is rapid and irregular. A similar tremor appears in the hyperthyroid state. Postural tremor is also observed in metabolic and toxic encephalopathies (withdrawal from drugs or alcohol, hyponatremia, liver or renal failure). In some of the above instances postural tremor may be associated with the distinctive up-and-down flapping movements called asterixis.

As the name implies, *intention tremor* occurs primarily during voluntary purposeful activity of the extremity. Although intention tremors are characteristic of cerebellar system disease, it is important to recognize that the resting or action tremors of parkinsonism or benign familial tremor may also be associated with a component of intention tremor. The intention tremor of cerebellar disease is a loss of the normal coordinative activities of agonistic and antagonistic muscles during voluntary movement. This might better be termed ataxia of the extremities or incoordination of movement. The ataxia is usually most marked when several joints are involved in the movement, as in finger-to-nose, finger-to-finger, or heel-to-shin testing. Such ataxia of movement may also occur in the presence of severe peripheral sensory loss; in such instances it is due to loss of appropriate proprioceptive clues from the joints.

Intention tremor of cerebellar disease is accompanied by other signs of disease of the cerebellar hemisphere, including hypotonia, impairment of check movements of the extremities, and an inability to perform rapid alternating movements of the extremities (dysdiadochokinesis). In addition, dysarthria (in which speech is slurred or has a scanning quality), nystagmus, ocular dysmetria, and disequilibrium of gait are common. In lesions of the midline cerebellar structures (flocculonodular lobule) or the anterior lobe of the cerebellum, severe truncal ataxia and disequilibrium of gait, in which the patient staggers and walks with legs spread wide apart, may be quite prominent in the absence of extremity ataxia or intention tremor.

The various disorders causing cerebellar lesions include the following:

1. Spinocerebellar degeneration (Figs. 4.1 and 4.2)
2. Cerebellar tumors (see Chapter 15)

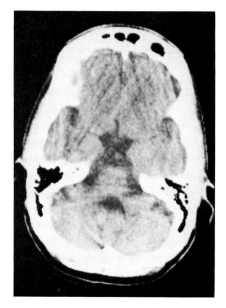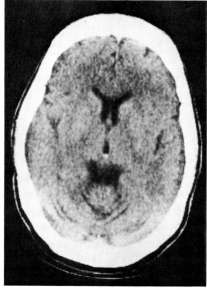

FIGS. 4.1, 4.2. CAT scan of patient with spinocerebellar degeneration. Note widening of cerebellar folia, shrunken brainstem, and enlarged basilar and ambient cisterns.

3. Alcoholic degeneration of the anterior lobe of the cerebellum
4. Cerebellar infarction or hemorrhage
5. Multiple sclerosis
6. Cerebellar abscess

In some disorders the tremor is difficult to classify. *Hepatolenticular degeneration* (Wilson's disease) causes resting, postural, and intention tremors of the extremities, as well as tremors of the lips and tongue. These are associated with ataxia, spasticity, chorea, and progressive dementia. Mixed tremors also occur in Huntington's disease, CNS lues, acquired hepatocerebral degeneration, and mercury poisoning.

Rigidity

Rigidity is a disturbance of motor activity which can markedly impair function without causing weakness. The clinical distinction between rigidity and spasticity (previously described in this chapter) is by no means always simple, nor is there yet universal agreement as to the precise differences in the physiologic mechanisms responsible for each. Rigidity is characterized by resistance to passive motion at a joint (usually the wrist, elbow, or knee) during flexion and extension. Diffuse frontal cortical or white matter lesions may produce a type of rigidity called *gegenhalten*, or *paratonia*, characterized by a waxy rigidity which increases in intensity as the examiner attempts to extend or flex the extremity. These patients invariably manifest other signs of diffuse brain disease, e.g., altered awareness, dementia, and cortical release signs.

True rigidity is believed to be caused by disease in the substantia nigra and other extrapyramidal structures, and is due to an imbalance between the alpha and gamma motor systems, but there is no universal acceptance of any extant physiologic explanation. Electromyography reveals that there is no recruitment during muscle contraction in patients with parkinsonian rigidity. It is also evident that surgical lesions in the ventral lateral nucleus of the thalamus or the medial portion of the globus pallidus reduce or abolish rigidity (and tremor) in the opposite extremities of some patients with Parkinson's disease. Biochemically, rigidity is associated with depletion of brain dopamine, particularly in the corpus striatum.

Parkinson's Syndrome (Parkinsonism)

There is some justification for using the term syndrome to describe parkinsonism. The diagnosis is made on the basis of a group of symptoms and signs—in particular diminution of spontaneous and associated movements, rigidity, tremor, hypokinesia, and a characteristic gait abnormality—but the fact is that some of these may not be present in any given patient early in the disease, and in some patients a significant extraocular movement disorder may be present. By far the most characteristic and consistent findings are rigidity and decreased spontaneous and associated movements. Tremor may be absent or be the prominent sign of the disease. It is also true that there are several etiologies for the clinical complex described above, but these (described below) usually have special characteristics which distinguish them from the idiopathic or degenerative type; the latter is sometimes called paralysis agitans and comprises more than 95% of the patients with the syndrome.

Parkinsonism is a frequent disorder of middle and old age, usually beginning during the middle to late fifties. There are more than 200,000 patients with parkinsonism in the United States, and about 40,000 new cases appear each year.

Etiology of parkinsonism

The etiology is unknown. Some believe that the syndrome results in some way from a prior viral encephalitic process, particularly von Economo's encephalitis lethargica. Although it is true that almost all individuals in the United States and western Europe with parkinsonism were alive during the great influenza pandemic between 1917 and 1930, it is rare to find a patient who recalls having influenza or encephalitis. Parkinsonism occasionally follows other forms of viral encephalitis. If it is somehow related to an encephalitic process which occurred more than 50 years prior, the mechanism of that relationship is obscure; slow virus seems a very unlikely explanation.

Other conditions which may be confused with idiopathic parkinsonism include:

1. _Drug-induced_ parkinsonism. The most important drugs are the phenothiazine derivatives, including chlorpromazine (Thorazine), prochlorperazine (Compazine), trifluoperazine (Stelazine), and perphenazine (Trilafon). Parkinsonian symptoms are dose-related and can usually be controlled readily by anticholinergic drugs. In addition to rigidity, tremor, and hypokinesia, akathisia (a feeling of restlessness) and dystonic movements are common.

2. _Postencephalitic_ parkinsonism. There is some question that this is truly a separate entity. It occurs at an earlier age than the idiopathic variety and is associated with oculogyric crises, markedly seborrheic skin, and sialorrhea. Oculogyric crises are uncommon. The patient's eyes suddenly turn upward (rarely downward) and may remain fixed for minutes to hours. These are usually well controlled by anticholinergic drugs.

3. _Arteriosclerotic parkinsonism_. There is no evidence that cerebral infarctions produce typical parkinsonism, but repeated lacunar infarctions may cause gait disorders and rigidity.

4. _Manganese poisoning_. This may occur in manganese miners. The patients are usually demented, show loss of motivation, and exhibit rigidity.

5. _Parkinsonism-dementia complex_. There is a question that this syndrome is anything more than parkinsonism in conjunction with senile dementia of the Alzheimer's type.

6. _Shy-Drager syndrome (primary dysautonomia)_. These patients usually present with orthostatic hypotension and sphincter disorders secondary to disease of the sympathetic nervous system; they later develop difficulty walking and rigidity. The etiology is unknown. There is marked degeneration of CNS sympathetic neurons and pathways, and the disease usually runs its course within 2 to 4 years.

7. _Progressive supranuclear palsy_. This is a disease of unknown etiology. It is characterized by progressive restriction of eye movements, often beginning with impaired down gaze, and resulting in gait abnormality. Oculocephalic reflexes remain intact. The patients become increasingly rigid and hypokinetic, and usually become demented late in the disease. Some patients seem to show temporary improvement on L-DOPA.

Symptoms and signs of parkinsonism

Patients with parkinsonism may present with a variety of complaints; these are most frequently because of tremor or difficulty in walking, in particular with a feeling of insecurity and poor balance. Changes in handwriting, difficulty in getting up from a chair or turning over in bed, inability to perform fine hand movements, sialorrhea, and slowness in all types of motor activity are also common early complaints. Many patients complain that their feet occasionally seem to freeze to the floor, particularly when they encounter an obstacle or threshold. Families note a change in facial expression, particularly that the patient appears sad, and they remark that he appears to be bent forward when standing or walking.

The extent of abnormality in the physical examination depends on the stage of the disease. In early parkinsonism the diagnosis may be difficult, depending on subtle findings, e.g., early rigidity of one extremity or a decrease in arm swing on one side when walking. As the disease progresses, the neurologic abnormalities become more florid. Mental status examination is often normal, but a significant number of patients show evidence of depression. Dementia is usually not considered a part of the Parkinson syndrome, but careful mental status evaluation not infrequently reveals signs of organic mental disorders.

The patients move infrequently while sitting, and the face is expressionless or mask-like, with reduced frequency of eye blinking. Voice volume is reduced, and speech is monotonous and poorly enunciated. Repetition of syllables and phrases is frequent (palilalia). Sialorrhea is commonly observed. Tremor is usually evident while the patient sits with his hands in his lap. It is typically rhythmic and pill-rolling in character, and decreases when the patient uses his extremities. The same rate tremor may involve the feet, head, jaw, or tongue. The handwriting is characteristic, not appearing in any other motor disorder. The patient writes with small letters, crowding them on each other, the result called micrographia. When asked to walk, he may have difficulty getting up from a sitting position, particularly if the chair is deep. On standing the patient characteristically assumes a simian posture, with head bent forward, knees slightly flexed, and arms flexed at the elbows; he may be unable to initiate a gait because his feet feel frozen to the floor. When walking, the arm swing is diminished to absent, and his steps are small and shuffling and may increase in rate (festination) so that the patient is almost running forward. He moves and turns like a robot and appears to have a precarious balance. The feet often stick to the floor when the patient encounters an obstacle, and gait can be initiated again only after many false starts. A slight shove may cause the patient to move backward in an exaggerated fashion (retropulsion).

Examination of the face and cranial nerves usually reveals abnormally oily skin. Seborrheic dermatitis is common. Hypomimia has been noted. Extraocular movements may be normal, but defects in convergence and restriction of upward gaze are common. Less commonly, slowness and limitation of lateral gaze movements (pseudo-ophthalmoplegia) are observed. Blepharospasm is infrequent but may be produced by tapping the patient's forehead with a reflex hammer.

Passive movements of the extremities are met by a ratchety cogwheel type of rigidity, most prominent at the wrist, elbow, and ankle. The tremor is as previously described. Adequate motivation calls forth normal strength, but fine or repetitive movements are slowly and incompetently performed. Deep tendon reflexes are normal. Plantar responses are flexor. Sensory examination is normal.

There is no specific laboratory test to aid the diagnosis. The electroencephalogram (EEG) may be normal or show mild nonspecific diffuse changes. There is no characteristic computerized axial tomography (CAT) scan, although mild cortical atrophy is not uncommonly observed. The differential diagnosis of parkinsonism includes essential tremor, depression, myxedema, progressive supranuclear palsy, phenothiazine or reserpine toxicity, hepatocerebral degeneration, low-pressure hydrocephalus, Shy-Drager syndrome, and multiple cerebral lacunar infarcts.

Pathology of parkinsonism

Depigmentation of the substantia nigra, readily observable grossly (Fig. 4.3), is the only consistent pathology of idiopathic parkinsonism, although cell loss in basal ganglionic nuclei is also usually present. Other structures containing pigmented nuclei (locus ceruleus and dorsal motor nuclei of the vagus) show cell loss. Hyaline cytoplasmic changes in the substantia nigra (Lewy bodies) are characteristically observed in idiopathic parkinsonism and no other condition. Their origin and exact composition are unknown. Cortical

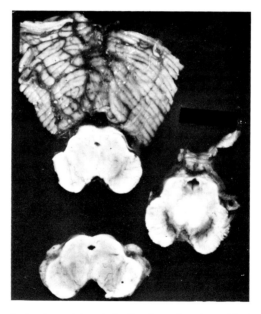

FIG. 4.3. Loss of melanin pigment in substantia nigra of patient with Parkinson's syndrome. Compare to normal control on right.

atrophy is more prevalent in patients with parkinsonism than in a normal age-controlled population.

The biochemical pathology of parkinsonism is pertinent to therapy of the disorder; the dopamine content of the basal ganglia is greatly reduced from normal. Metabolites of dopamine, particularly homovanillic acid, are also reduced in the brains and cerebrospinal fluid (CSF) of patients with Parkinson's disease. Other putative neurotransmitters, norepinephrine, γ-aminobutyric acid, and serotonin, as well as the enzymes responsible for the metabolism of their precursors, are also reduced in the basal ganglia of parkinsonian patients. Aromatic DOPA decarboxylase, which metabolizes DOPA to dopamine in the brain, is deficient to absent in the caudate, putamen, and substantia nigra of patients with parkinsonism.

Therapy of parkinsonism

Treatment of parkinsonism cannot cure the disorder but can greatly alleviate the patient's symptoms and signs. Unfortunately, there is evidence that the disease progresses despite the most effective therapy, which becomes progressively less effective after an average of 6 years. Pharmacologic management is directed at replacing the dopamine by the administration of L-DOPA, which is converted into dopamine by DOPA decarboxylase in the brain. Dopamine itself does not cross the blood-brain barrier and is therefore of no therapeutic value as a drug. The reason for the eventual loss of effectiveness of L-DOPA is not known, but it may be due to a deficiency of brain DOPA decarboxylase.

There is some evidence that there is a dopamine-acetylcholine imbalance in the basal ganglia of parkinsonian patients, the relative excess of acetylcholine seeming to be responsible for some of the symptoms of the disorder. Anticholinergic drugs are often helpful, particularly as a supplement to L-DOPA, and formed the basis for therapy of parkinsonism prior to the discovery of the effectiveness of L-DOPA.

Amantadine hydrochloride (Symmetrel) is variably effective. It is believed to increase dopamine release from certain striatal neurons. It is administered in doses of 100 mg twice daily and may be given alone or together with L-DOPA; however, its effectiveness seems to diminish after 2 to 3 months. Side effects are uncommon, but complaints of insomnia, restlessness, and hallucinations have been reported.

Drugs which act directly on the postsynaptic dopaminergic receptor sites are called dopamine agonists. Apomorphine is such an agent. It relieves parkinsonian rigidity and tremor, but the side effects of emesis, hypotension, and uremia are intolerable. Bromocriptine, an ergot compound recently approved by the Food and Drug Administration (FDA) in the United States for use in the short-term management of amenorrhea/galactorrhea associated with hyperprolactinema due to varied etiologies excluding demonstrable pituitary tumors, is manufactured by Sandoz Pharmaceuticals under the name Parlodel. Although the drug has not received FDA approval for treatment of parkinsonism, extensive studies have been carried out. The consensus is that this dopamine agonist is probably not as effective as L-DOPA in the management of the average patient with parkinsonism but that it may be effective when L-DOPA effectiveness is decreasing, that it is marginally useful in handling the on–off syndrome, and that its most valuable use might be at the initiation of therapy in a patient previously untreated, with the objective of delaying the use of L-DOPA and thereby prolonging its therapeutic effectiveness. Unfortunately, side effects, particularly vomiting, anxiety, and hallucinations, are frequent at therapeutic levels, and the drug is extremely costly.

Although no pharmacologic therapy may be indicated in some patients whose symptoms are mild, L-DOPA is the drug of choice in most patients with parkinsonism. Use of DOPA decarboxylase inhibitors with levodopa has replaced the use of L-DOPA alone as the preferred treatment because the patient takes only one-fourth the amount of L-DOPA with this regimen, thereby reducing the side effects of nausea, vomiting, and orthostatic hypotension. In addition, the combination of DOPA decarboxylase inhibitors and L-DOPA is often more effective in controlling the patient's symptoms.

L-DOPA itself is manufactured by several pharmaceutical concerns and is available in 125-, 250-, and 500-mg tablets or capsules. It must be begun with a low dosage, gradually building up to a therapeutic level. The effective dosage varies from 2 to 12 g daily. The medication should be taken at meals or after a snack to reduce the likelihood of gastric irritation. Side effects include anorexia, nausea, vomiting, dyskinesias (grimacing, tongue movements, tonic posturing of the extremities or head, and motor restlessness), orthostatic hypotension, cardiac arrhythmias, and episodes of confusion, agitation, and hallucinations. Most of these complications, with the probable exception of orthostatic hypotension, are dose-related and can be relieved by decreasing the drug. Patients who have taken L-DOPA in any form for several years may develop sudden changes in their clinical status, varying from akinesia to good mobility within a few moments. This is called the "on–off" phenomenon. It is a feared complication because it is difficult to treat. It is usually managed by varying the dosage of the drug, particularly using smaller, more frequent doses. Sometimes a drug holiday (removal of all medications for 10 days) is helpful.

The DOPA decarboxylase inhibitor approved by the FDA is carbidopa (γ-methyldopa hydrazine); it is marketed with levodopa in a combination tablet (Sinemet), available in two tablet sizes: 10 mg carbidopa/100 mg L-DOPA and 25 mg carbidopa/250 mg L-DOPA. As previously mentioned, this combination tablet is the preferred drug therapy for most parkinsonian patients. The carbidopa does not pass the blood-brain barrier but acts to inhibit peripheral DOPA decarboxylase, making a larger amount of L-DOPA available to the brain and reducing the amount of L-DOPA which must be ingested.

Treatment should be initiated with small doses, one 10/100 tablet three or four times daily, gradually increased to the point of maximal improvement or the development of side effects. Dyskinesias are common and represent an endpoint in therapy at which the dosage can be reduced. It is rare for a patient to require more than five or six 25/250 tablets daily, and half this amount suffices for the average patient.

The anticholinergic drugs available include the following with their recommended daily dosages:

Trihexyphenidyl (Artane)	1.5 to 15 mg
Benztropine mesylate (Cogentin)	0.5 to 6 mg
Biperiden (Akineton)	2 to 8 mg
Procyclidine (Kemadrin)	5 to 50 mg

The potential effectiveness of any of these drugs cannot be predicted in advance. In many instances anticholinergic drugs do not augment the effectiveness of L-DOPA and should not be used. They produce some unpleasant side effects, including dryness of the mouth, visual blurring to pupillary dilatation, confusion, hallucinations, and urinary retention. They are contraindicated in patients with glaucoma.

Patients with parkinsonism are frequently depressed, and appropriate pharmacologic therapy, particularly tricyclic antidepressants, should be utilized if indicated. Pyridoxine should be avoided in patients receiving L-DOPA because it somehow interferes with its effectiveness. Monoamine oxidase inhibitors should not be used in conjunction with L-DOPA because severe hypertension may result.

Surgical treatment of parkinsonism, specifically cryothalamotomy, is rarely necessary, although it may yet be useful in the management of severe unilateral tremor.

The question of physical therapy for patients with parkinsonism is one that requires individualization. The patients should be encouraged to be active and to participate as fully as possible in all activities of daily living. It is a mistake, however, to create a sense of compulsion about physical activity, for this often turns the patient's spouse and family into nags, with resulting mutual irritation and frustration. The patients need gentle persuasion, reasons for motivation, and an understanding of their accompanying mental as well as physical problems, rather than a drill sergeant approach.

Hemiballism

Hemiballism is an uncommon disorder in which an entire upper extremity or both extremities on one side move abruptly and purposelessly in a flailing or flinging fashion. It resembles severe choreoathetosis, but the primary component of the movement originates in the proximal muscles of the extremities. Occasionally the trunk is also observed to twist and jerk. The causative lesion is usually either infarction or hemorrhage in the region of the subthalamic nucleus of Luys opposite the involved extremities. The appearance is frightening and may be exhausting to the patient, but drastic or surgical therapeutic measures are rarely required. Most cases subside spontaneously within a few days to several months. Therapy consists of simple sedation or the use of chlorpromazine in doses up to 500 mg daily or haloperidol (2 to 8 mg daily).

Myoclonus

Myoclonus is a movement disorder which is seen in a wide variety of disease states and for which no consistent anatomic pathology can be identified. It is best described as an abrupt involuntary contraction of a muscle or group of muscles. It is unpredictable, brief in duration, and asymmetrical in distribution. It is frequently precipitated by sensory stimulation, e.g., a loud noise, a touch, or a sudden flash of light. It is a symptom common to many syndromes and appears in a variety of forms. The classification is usually clinical.

Myoclonus of Metabolic Encephalopathy

This type of myoclonus accompanies any severe metabolic encephalopathy, viz., hepatic encephalopathy, uremia, hyponatremia, hypercalcemia, hypoglycemia, and cerebral anoxia. Action myoclonus, which occurs on attempted directed motor activity, occurs particularly in the posthypoxic state and can be alleviated by clonazepam, which is also used in the treatment of myoclonic epilepsy.

"Viral" Myoclonus

This term has been applied to the myoclonus observed in patients with known CNS virus infections, viz., subacute spongiform encephalopathy (Jakob-Creutzfeldt disease), subacute sclerosing panencephalitis, and epidemic encephalitis. The clinical picture in each is different. Subacute transmissible spongiform encephalopathy, so named because of the vacuolar appearance of the parenchymatous lesions observed pathologically and because it has been transmitted to chimpanzees by intracerebral inoculation of brains of involved patients, is better known as Jakob-Creutzfeldt disease. It is characterized by progressive rigidity, spasticity, resting tremors, myoclonic jerks, and profound dementia, progressing relentlessly to death within 1.5 to 24 months. The method of transmission from patient to patient is not known, but it is known that it may be contracted by direct inoculation of a subject with infected tissue and that the responsible "virus" is practically indestructible by heat and may lie dormant for an indefinite period of time. There is no useful treatment.

Subacute sclerosing panencephalitis usually occurs in children but has been reported in adults. It is thought to be due to invasion of the brain by a rubeola or measles-like virus. It is usually progressive but may be remitting, and is characterized by progression from ataxia to paralysis, myoclonic jerks, blindness, spasticity, and dementia. The EEG shows characteristic recurring diffuse bursts of spike and slow wave complexes.

In epidemic encephalitis the course is quick, and the patient is acutely ill and often unconscious. Diagnosis depends on careful viral studies of the blood and CSF.

Myoclonus of Idiopathic Epilepsy

Myoclonic jerks of individual extremities may be present on the day or two preceding a generalized seizure or may be associated with petit mal or akinetic seizures.

Infantile Myoclonic Epilepsy (Salaam Attacks)

These attacks occur between the third and eighth months of life, and are characterized by jack-knife movements of the trunk and temporary unresponsivity. They are associated with a characteristic EEG abnormality of spike or polyspike discharges on a background of irregular high-voltage activity called hypsarrhythmia. Although the attacks may cease or be replaced by other seizure activity, these children are almost invariably retarded. Early treatment with ACTH is recommended.

Progressive Myoclonic Epilepsy

1. Lafora body disease (Unverricht disease) is a familial dementing myoclonic epilepsy associated with rigidity and, in the late stages, paralysis of all limbs. The myoclonus is stimulus-sensitive, and the pathology is characterized by neuronal inclusions, which have the appearance of corpora amylacea. These Lafora bodies are located in the cerebral and cerebellar cortex.

2. Systemic degenerative diseases, particularly the heredofamilial ataxias.

3. Myoclonus associated with leukodystrophies or lipidoses. This usually appears during adolescence and is rapidly progressive. The patients have seizures, spasticity, paralysis, and myoclonus.

Palatal Myoclonus

This represents a precise clinical picture, quite different from other forms of myoclonus. The myoclonic contraction of the orobronchiorespiratory muscles is regular and rhythmic, and persists during sleep. No specific anatomic lesion can be ascribed to all the various forms of myoclonus. Lesions have been described in the spinal cord, cerebral hemisphcres, and brainstem. In palatal myoclonus the lesions, which may be caused by infection, neoplasm, oi encephalitis, are located in the olivary nuclei, dentate nuclei, and central tegmental pathways.

Tics

It is difficult to define or categorize tics because they have no specific pathologic substrate and may develop without any known organic cause. They are hyperkinesias of various sorts, usually brief, e.g., nose-sniffing, eye-blinking, shoulder-shrugging, head-turning, facial grimacing, hand posturing, tongue protrusion, grunting, barking, coughing. There has been a great deal of interest in these movements as they occur quite commonly, particularly during childhood, and in many instances are thought to be psychogenic in origin. Indeed, many tics are transitory, improving with lessening of tension or simply the passage of time, whereas others persist into adult life. Some investigators believe that EEG patterns and family histories of epilepsy suggest that there is an organic basis for the so-called functional tics of childhood, but no pathologic changes have been incriminated.

Even the remarkable disorder called Gilles de la Tourette generalized tic disease, characterized by generalized tics, compulsive ejaculation of inarticulate sounds, and coprolalia, has no known pathologic basis. This extraordinary malady begins during childhood and progresses intermittently. These children retain a pronounced degree of infantilism throughout their lives. When the disease has its onset in adult life, the patients often show psychopathic stigmata, including strong streaks of paranoia. In addition to coprolalia, echolalia (repetition of words heard), palilalia (repetition of one's own words), and echopraxia (imitation of acts) accompany the tics. A similar type of generalized tic syndrome has been described in cases of encephalitis lethargica. This observation plus the frequent finding of EEG abnormalities in Gilles de la Tourette syndrome suggest that there is an organic basis for the disorder. Many of these patients show a good response to haloperidol, a known dopamine-receptor-blocking agent. This drug has little effect on most other types of tic.

Torticollis

Torticollis is an abnormal involuntary contraction of neck muscles, result-ing in more or less sustained movements or abnormal postures of the head (Fig. 4.4). It may occur in a variety of specific disease states, e.g., athetosis, dystonia, Huntington's disease, parkinsonism, and dystonia musculorum deformans. Most clinicians label it as a form of dystonia. The etiology of

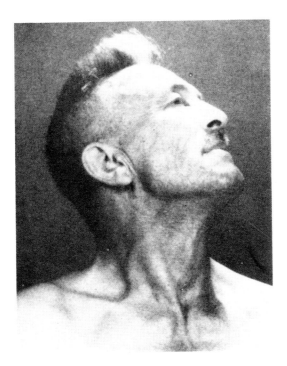

FIG. 4.4. Spasmodic torticollis. (Reproduced with permission from "Torticollis," by F. Podivinský. In: *Handbook of Clinical Neurology,* Vol. 6. North-Holland, Amsterdam, 1968.)

torticollis unassociated with other CNS abnormalities has been debated for many years, many considering it to be of psychogenic origin. It is now thought to be an organic disease because nerve cell changes and degeneration, gliosis, and occasional perivascular round cell infiltrations have been described in the striatum and globus pallidus, but actual pathophysiologic correlation is still lacking. Treatment is with anticholinergic drugs used in parkinsonism, phenothiazines, or simple sedatives. Although a variety of surgical treatments have been suggested, their efficacy is unproved.

Chorea

There is a group of involuntary movement disorders, reasonably familiar, which have as their commonality pathologic changes in the corpus striatum (caudate and putamen). *Chorea* (from the Greek word for dance) describes brief involuntary movements involving mainly the distal portions of the extremities as well as the face. Facial involvement causes characteristic grimaces which are unsustained, and mild chorea resembles simple restlessness, somewhat like tics; however, unlike tics, they do not occur repeatedly in the same place. The movements are sometimes so smooth and graceful, although inappropriate, that they appear to be well coordinated and willful. The uncoordinated contractions of the intercostal muscles, tongue, and palatal muscles frequently cause an explosive type of speech. As the disease progresses the patient shows a typical syncopated dance-like gait from which the name of the movement disorder is derived. Each movement, smooth and direct in itself, appears to be interrupted by another unrelated one, so that voluntary motor activity may be significantly impaired. The involuntary movements interject into the willed ones, causing them to be delayed and awkward. Fingers clench and unclench, arms and legs flex and extend abruptly and inappropriately, the tongue protrudes suddenly, and the eyes deviate into an unwanted position; all may be precipitated or worsened by emotional or sensory stimuli. Evaluation of motor strength is difficult because of the offending movements. If the patient is asked to grasp the examiner's hand or fingers tightly, the involuntary movements show themselves as intermittency of the force of the grasp.

The causes of chorea include the following.

Iatrogenic Chorea—Induced by L-DOPA or Phenothiazines

The hyperkinesia produced by L-DOPA or phenothiazines is usually more complex than simple chorea; there is often an admixture of dystonic posturing and athetosis. The movements are ordinarily dose-related and, particularly in the case of L-DOPA, can be titrated by small variations in the amount of drug ingested. *Tardive dyskinesia* is a type of choreiform and dystonic hyperkinesia which develops in some patients who are receiving long-term phenothiazine treatment for psychiatric diseases and which persists after the offending drug has been discontinued. It is theorized that tardive dyskinesia is caused by the development of hypersensitivity in some of the dopaminergic receptor sites, which accordingly respond excessively to circulating dopaminergic chemicals, producing almost incessant choreic and dystonic movements of the patient's extremities, trunk, face, and tongue. Management of these patients can be challenging. Prolonged abstinence from the offending drug may help, but often it is necessary to use phenothiazine to control the movements.

Huntington's Disease

Huntington's disease is doubly tragic, not only because of the chorea-athetosis and dementia which characterize the clinical picture, but because of the agonizing suspense in which the offspring of an affected parent must live, not knowing if he has inherited the dread gene. Because it is a mendelian dominant disorder, each child of an affected parent has a 50% chance of having the disease. Even though rare cases have been reported without known family history, the grandchild of an affected person will not get the disease if his own parents were unaffected. Unfortunately, there may be no manifestations of the illness until middle life, far past the child-producing age, so unless genetic counseling is rigidly followed the strain persists and proliferates.

The abnormal movements are choreiform, athetoid, and dystonic. The dementia is not unique in character, although hostility, suspicion, and irritability are frequent components. There may be great variability in the severity of the disease within the same family.

The pathology is characterized by astrocytic replacement of the striatal small neurons. There is striking atrophy of the heads of the caudate nuclei and the putamina (Fig. 4.5). The shrinkage of the caudate can often be confirmed by pneumoencephalography. Cortical atrophy is also present as a result of neuronal degeneration. The most consistently observed biochemical change is a striking reduction in the putative transmitter gamma-aminobutyric acid (GABA) in the basal ganglia, particularly the putamen, but how this produces the symptoms remains unclear.

The only effective therapy is by the administration of one of the butyrophenones (haloperidol), beginning with doses of 1 mg four times daily and increasing to tolerance. Many patients show a significant reduction in the involuntary movements, although the dementia is unaffected.

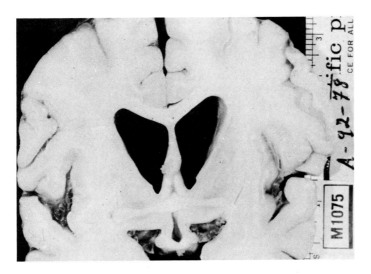

FIG. 4.5. Huntington's disease. Note atrophy of caudate nuclei with dilated ventricles.

Sydenham's Chorea

Sydenham's chorea has become an uncommon disorder. It occurs mainly in conjunction with rheumatic fever (although the association may be difficult to establish) and during pregnancy (chorea gravidarum). There is no consistent pathology in the brain. Treatment is usually symptomatic with mild sedation or haloperidol. Fortunately the illness is self-limited.

Dystonia

Dystonic movements are inappropriate, frequently deforming, powerful prolonged muscle contractions which in severe instances result in distortion of the proximal parts of the limbs and the trunk (Fig. 4.6). The origin of the disorder cannot be ascribed to any one CNS structure, although degenerative changes in the striatum are consistently present. A variety of diseases can *drugs* cause dystonic movements, and as mentioned above they may be produced by certain drugs, e.g., phenothiazines. Indeed, mild dystonia and athetosis are commonplace complications of L-DOPA therapy, suggesting that the neuropharmacologic basis for the movements is an imbalance between dopaminergic and other neural transmitter receptor sites or among the various neurons that produce the neurotransmitters.

Dystonia musculorum deformans is the name applied to a relatively rare progressive disorder, usually beginning during childhood, with its highest concentration in Ashkenazi Jews whose family origins were in southern Lithuania and northern Poland. The gene distribution must be worldwide, however, because the disease (or its counterpart) has been observed in Japanese, Chinese, Negroes, Arabs, and South American Indians.

Dystonic postures are at first labile and then gradually become more fixed (Fig. 4.6). The first sign of the disease may be a sensation of muscular pulling or stiffness. A foot may become rotated inward and produce an equinovarus posture or show sustained plantar flexion, forcing the patient to walk on tiptoe. In the upper extremities, forced flexion or extension of the fingers or forearm muscles may produce the syndrome of true writer's cramp, in which the quality of the writing deteriorates as a function of time. Progression of the disorder results in the severe truncal and extremity distortions and deformities which are characteristic of the advanced disease. Although facial muscle involvement is usually not extreme, it may appear early as blepharospasm or grimacing. Dysarthria does occur, but the patient is able to chew and swallow normally; not infrequently there is a remarkable disparity between the distorted appearance of the patient and his retained ability to execute skilled movements.

The disorder is usually associated with normal intelligence; children with milder forms of the disease not infrequently complete their education in a

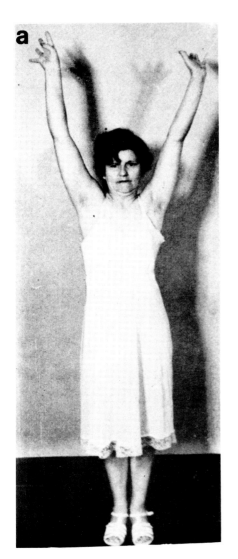 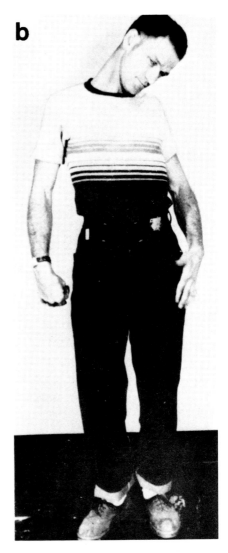

FIG. 4.6. Dystonia. **a:** Early dystonia with minimal discrete posturing of the hands. **b:** More advanced state with persistent neck and trunk deformity. (Reproduced with permission from "Dystonia Musculorum Deformans," by W. Zeman and P. Dyken. In: *Handbook of Clinical Neurology,* Vol. 6. North-Holland, Amsterdam, 1968.)

creditable manner. Haloperidol is helpful in some patients, and stereotactic cold lesions of portions of the thalamus have also been reported to produce improvement in a substantial number of patients.

Athetosis

Athetosis refers to writhing, unwanted movements of the distal extremities. The hand or foot is in a position of forced flexion with hyperextension and spreading of the fingers and toes (Fig. 4.7). Facial grimacing and tongue and truncal movements are frequent, and speech may be distorted to the point of being incomprehensible. Athetosis usually is the result of perinatal brain injury, particularly by hypoxia–ischemia from prolonged difficult labor, and kernicterus. It is rarely seen *de novo* during adult life, although some posthypoxic encephalopathic states resemble it. The pathology is confined primarily to the striatum, producing a marbled appearance of the diseased nuclei ("status marmoratus"). In kernicterus the globus pallidus is particularly involved.

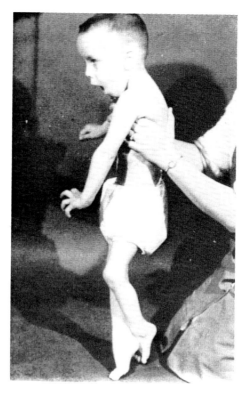

FIG. 4.7. Athetosis. Note the posturing of the distal portions of the extremities and the face. (Reproduced with permission from "Athetotic Syndromes," by E. A. Spiegel and H. W. Baird. In: *Handbook of Clinical Neurology,* Vol. 6. North-Holland, Amsterdam, 1968.)

SUGGESTED READINGS

Parkinsonism: Pathology

Andén NE, Carlssen A, et al: Demonstration and mapping out of nigroneostriatal dopamine neurons. *Life Sci* 3:523, 1964.

Duvoisin RC, and Yahr MD: Encephalitis and parkinsonism. *Arch Neurol* 12:227, 1965.

Eadie MJ, and Sutherland JM: Arteriosclerosis in parkinsonism. *J Neurol Neurosurg Psychiatry* 27:237, 1964.

Parkinsonism: Biochemical or Pharmacological

Barbeau A: Some biological disorders in Parkinson's disease—a review. *J Neurosurg* 24:162, 1966.

Jasper HH: Discussion on anatomical and physiological aspects of Parkinson's disease. *J Neurosurg* 24:235, 1966.

Marttila RJ, and Rinne UK: Changing epidemiology of Parkinson's disease: predicted effects of levodopa treatment. *Acta Neurol Scand* 59:80, 1979.

Poirier LJ, and Sourkes TL: Influence of the substantia nigra on the catecholamine content of the striatum. *Brain* 88:181, 1965.

Parkinsonism: Symptoms and Signs

Barbeau A: long-term assessment of levodopa therapy in Parkinson's disease. *Can Med Assoc J* 112:1379, 1975.

Hoehn MM, and Yahr MD: Parkinsonism: onset, progression, and mortality. *Neurology (Minneap)* 17:427, 1967.

Kaada BR: The pathophysiology of Parkinsonian tremor, rigidity, and hypokinesia. *Acta Neurol Scand [Suppl 4]* 39:39, 1963.

Lance JW, Schwab RS, and Peterson ER: Action tremor and the cogwheel phenomenon in Parkinson's disease. *Brain* 86:95, 1963.

Pollock M, and Hornabrook RW: The prevalence, natural history and dementia of Parkinson's disease. *Brain* 89:429, 1966.

Parkinsonism: Treatment

Barbeau A: L-DOPA therapy in Parkinson's disease. *Can Med Assoc J* 101:791, 1969.

Calne DB: Developments in the pharmacology and therapeutics of parkinsonism. *Ann Neurol* 50:119, 1977.

Calne DB, Reid JL, Vakil SD, Rao S, Petrie A, Pallis CA, Gawler J, Thomas PK, and Hilson A: Idiopathic parkinsonism treated with an extracerebral decarboxylase inhibitor in combination with levodopa. *Br Med J* 3:729, 1971.

Cooper IS: *Parkinsonism. Its Medical and Surgical Therapy.* Charles C Thomas, Springfield, Ill., 1961.

Cooper IS: Surgical treatment of parkinsonism. *Annu Rev Med* 16:309, 1965.

Cooper IS: *Involuntary Movement Disorders.* Harper & Row (Hoeber), New York, 1969.

Cotzias GC, Van Woert MH, and Schiffer LM: Aromatic amino acids and modification of parkinsonism. *N Engl J Med* 276:374, 1967.

Cotzias GC, Papavasiliou PS, and Gellene R: Modification of parkinsonism—chronic treatment with L-DOPA. *N Engl J Med* 280:337, 1969.

Duvoisin RC: Cholinergic-anticholinergic antagonism in parkinsonism. *Arch Neurol* 17:124, 1967.

Fahn S, and Calne DB: Considerations in the management of parkinsonism. *Neurology (Minneap)* 28:5, 1978.

Gron U: Bromocriptine versus placebo in levodopa treated patients with Parkinson's disease. *Acta Neurol Scand* 56:269, 1977.

Lees, et al: Bromocriptine in parkinsonism. *Arch Neurol* 35:503, 1978.

Lesser RP, Fahn S, Snider SR, Cote LJ, Isgreen WP, and Barrett RE: Analysis of the clinical problems in parkinsonism and the complications of long-term levodopa therapy. *Neurology (Minneap)* 29:1253, 1979.
Lieberman A, Kupersmith M, Estey E, and Goldstein M: Treatment of Parkinson's disease with bromocriptine. *N Engl J Med* 295:1400, 1976.
Marsden CD, and Parkes JD: "On-off" effects in patients with Parkinson's disease on chronic levodopa therapy. *Lancet* 2:292, 1976.
Parkes JD, Baxter RCH, Curzon G, Knill-Jones RP, Knott PJ, Marsden CD, Tattersall R, and Vollum D: Treatment of Parkinson's disease with amantadine and levodopa: a one-year study. *Lancet* 1:1083, 1971.
Rivera-Calimlim L, Tandon D, Anderson F, and Joynt R: The clinical picture and plasma levodopa metabolite profile of parkinsonian nonresponders. *Arch Neurol* 34:228, 1977.
Schwab RS, England AC Jr, Poskanzer DC, and Young RR: Amantadine in the treatment of Parkinson's disease. *JAMA* 208:1168, 1969.

Tremor

Aronson NI: Neurophysiology of tremor. *J Neurosurg* 24:207, 1966.
Critchley M: Observations on essential (heredofamilial) tremor. *Brain* 72:113, 1949.
Dupont E, Hansen HJ, and Dalby MA: Treatment of benign essential tremor with propranolol. *Acta Neurol Scand* 49:75, 1973.
Marshall J: Observations on essential tremor. *J Neurol Neurosurg Psychiatry* 25:122, 1962.

Hepatolenticular Degeneration

Barnes S, and Hurst EW: Hepato-lenticular degeneration. *Brain* 48:279, 1925.
Cumings JN: The copper and iron content of brain and liver in the normal and hepato-lenticular degeneration. *Brain* 71:410, 1948.
Denny-Brown D: Hepato-lenticular degeneration (Wilson's disease). *N Engl J Med* 270:1149, 1964.
Scheinberg IH, and Sternlieb I: Wilson's disease and the concentration of caeruloplasmin in serum. *Lancet* 1:1420, 1963.

Sydenham's Chorea

Aron AM: Treatment of Sydenham's chorea. *Mod Treatm* 5:351, 1968.
Aron AM, Freeman JM, and Carter S: The natural history of Sydenham's chorea: review of the literature and long-term evaluation with emphasis on cardiac sequelae. *Am J Med* 38:83, 1965.

Torsion Dystonia and Torticollis

Barrett RE, Yahr MD, and Duvoisin RC: Torsion dystonia and spasmodic torticollis: results of treatment with L-DOPA. *Neurology (Minneap)* 20:107, 1970.
Eldridge R: The torsion dystonias (dystonia musculorum deformans). *Neurology (Minneap)* 20:1, 1970.
Gilbert GJ: The medical treatment of spasmodic torticollis. *Arch Neurol* 27:503, 1972.
Johnson W, Schwartz G, and Barbeau A: Studies on dystonia musculorum deformans. *Arch Neurol* 7:301, 1962.
Larsson T, and Sjögren T: Dystonia musculorum deformans: a genetic and clinical population study of 121 cases. *Acta Neurol Scand [Suppl 17]* 42:1, 1966.
Sorensen BF, and Hanby WB: Spasmodic torticollis. *Neurology (Minneap)* 16:867, 1966.

Huntington's Disease

Barbeau A, Chase TN, and Paulson GW (eds): Huntington's chorea, 1872–1972. In: *Advances in Neurology,* Vol. 1, Raven Press, New York, 1973.

Bird ED, Mackay AVP, Rayner CN, and Iversen LL: Reduced glutamic-acid-decarboxylase activity of post-mortem brain in Huntington's chorea. *Lancet* 1:1090, 1973.
Bird MT, and Paulson GW: The rigid form of Huntington's chorea. *Neurology (Minneap)* 21:271, 1971.
Blinderman EE, Weidner W, and Markham CH: The pneumoencephalogram in Huntington's chorea. *Neurology (Minneap)* 14:601, 1964.
Byers RK, and Dodge JA: Huntington's chorea in children; report of four cases. *Neurology (Minneap)* 17:587, 1967.
James WE, Mefferd RB Jr, and Kimbell I Jr: Early signs of Huntington's chorea. *Dis Nerv Syst* 30:556, 1969.
Klawans HL Jr: A pharmacologic analysis of Huntington's chorea. *Eur Neurol* 4:148, 1970.
Lyon RS: Drug treatment in Huntington's chorea. *Br Med J* 1:1308, 1962.
Perry TL, Hansen S, and Lkoster M: Huntington's chorea: deficiency of gamma-aminobutyric acid in brain. *N Engl J Med* 288:337, 1973.

Jakob-Creutzfeldt Disease

Bratan J: Jakob-Creutzfeldt disease: treatment by amantadine. *Br J Med* 4:212, 1971.
Gajdusek DC, and Gibbs CJ Jr: Transmission of two subacute spongiform encephalopathies in man (kuru and Creutzfeldt-Jakob disease) to New World monkeys. *Nature* 230:588, 1971.
Gibbs CJ Jr, and Gajdusek DC: Infection as the etiology of spongioform encephalopathy (Creutzfeld-Jakob disease). *Science* 165:1023, 1969.

Ballism

Carpenter MBJ: Ballism associated with partial destruction of the subthalamic nucleus of Luys. *Neurology (Minneap)* 5:479, 1955.

Tardive Dyskinesia

Carruthers SG: Persistent tardive dyskinesia. *Br Med J* 3:572, 1971.
Kivalo E, and Weckman N: The effect of haloperidol on some dyskinetic syndromes. *Scand J Clin Lab Invest 23 (Suppl 108):*64, 1969.
Schmidt WR, and Jarcho LW: Persistent dyskinesias following phenothiazine therapy. *Arch Neurol Psychiatry* 14:369, 1966.

Progressive Supranuclear Palsy

Steele JC, Richardson JC, and Olszewski J: Progressive supranuclear palsy; heterogenous degeneration involving the brain stem, basal ganglia and cerebellum with vertical gaze and pseudobulbar palsy, nuchal dystonia and dementia. *Arch Neurol* 10:333, 1964.

Chronic Hepatic Encephalopathy

Victor M, Adams RD, and Cole M: The acquired (non-Wilsonian) type of chronic hepato-cerebral degeneration. *Medicine (Baltimore)* 44:345, 1965.

Books: General

Denny-Brown D: *The Basal Ganglia and Their Relation to Disorders of Movement.* Oxford Univ. Press, Oxford, 1962.
Cooper IS: *Involuntary Movement Disorders.* Harper & Row (Hoeber), New York, New York, 1969.
Liversedge LA: Involuntary movements—a clinical review. In: *Modern Trends in Neurology,* Vol. 3, edited by D Williams, Chap 4. Butterworth, London, 1962.

5

Brain and Spinal Cord Injuries

Trauma to the nervous system, particularly the brain, is lamentably common. The frequency, enormous cost in lives, disability, and economic loss certainly indicate that injuries to the nervous system be considered a public health problem of major proportions. Indeed, accidents are the major cause of death and disability between the ages of 1 and 37 years. Approximately 25% of the population of the United States is accidentally injured each year. Of these 50 million injuries, 3 million involve the head; and well over a half million of these are caused by automobile accidents. Although there are no good statistics to indicate the outcome of the 3 million annual head injuries, it is generally agreed that injuries to the head are the major cause of death and serious disability from accidents of all types.

The statistical importance of head trauma can hardly be overrated, as anyone who has ever worked in a big city hospital emergency room can testify. What is not generally appreciated is that less than 20% of head-injured patients require neurosurgical intervention, and it is estimated that over 85% of patients with head injuries are first seen and evaluated by nonneurologic physicians. Every physician should therefore be alert to the signs that demand immediate consultation:

1. Prolonged unconsciousness
2. Any lateralizing neurologic deficit, e.g., hemiparesis
3. Progressive or intermittent drowsiness after a period of alertness
4. Convulsive seizure
5. Anisocoria
6. Missile wounds of head
7. Evidence of depressed skull fracture

It is estimated that more than 10,000 people in the United States annually incur spinal cord injuries sufficiently severe to cause about 50% of the victims to be paraplegic and the other 50% quadriplegic. Automobile accidents are by far the most frequent cause of spinal cord injuries, but diving and motorcycle accidents also rank high. Like head injuries, spinal cord injuries are largely preventable; yet serious legislative efforts to reduce the likelihood of trauma have not been forthcoming, in most instances blocked by special interest lobbies.

CLASSIFICATION OF CLOSED HEAD INJURY

There is no entirely satisfactory or consistent nomenclature for classifying closed head injuries, and practical management of the patient depends on the important variables mentioned above. *Cerebral concussion,* traditionally defined as a clinical syndrome produced by a blunt head injury (blow or fall), is characterized by immediate and transient impairment of neural function, specifically loss of consciousness, which may be associated with alarming cardiorespiratory changes (bradycardia, hypotension, transient arrest of respiration), temporary loss of muscle tone, areflexia, and a positive Babinski reflex. Usually there is a significant lapse of time between the moment the patient opens his eyes and appears awake and when he is fully alert and responsive. Most patients have a gap in memory which extends from a variable period prior to the trauma to the time when full responsivity has occurred.

It is evident, however, that closed head trauma may result in a state in which the patient is "stunned"; he does not completely lose consciousness but may have a transient disturbance of vision, loss of equilibrium, and inability to think clearly. Such patients have obviously suffered temporary neuronal derangement secondary to the trauma and their injury should probably also be classified as concussion.

The important distinguishing feature of *concussion* is the duration of the syndrome. If the unconsciousness lasts more than 30 min and the period of confusion more than several hours, the likelihood is great that pathologically visible brain tissue injury has occurred.

The mechanism of concussion is still debatable, but there is evidence that it is the consequence of rapid acceleration or deceleration of the head, a deformity of the skull, or both, which jostles the brain about within the skull and stretches and distorts the brainstem. The instantaneous loss of consciousness reflects injury to the reticular activating substance of the brainstem. This is known to be accompanied by temporary electrical silence in the electro-encephalogram (EEG), loss of autoregulatory capacity of cerebral arteries, and evidence of temporary failure of the blood-brain barrier. These physiologic disturbances are transient; otherwise they would encourage the development of brain edema, which is the major cause of death early in the course of closed head trauma.

Contusion and *laceration* of the brain are pathologic terms often used to describe a clinical state. They are said to occur when closed head injury results in prolonged unconsciousness or is associated with localizing neurologic deficit other than loss of consciousness, viz., convulsive seizure, hemiparesis, aphasia, cranial nerve abnormalities, or subarachnoid bleeding. Such brain injuries are severe and require prompt neurosurgical evaluation, even though no surgical treatment may be needed. There may be no way to distinguish clinically between contusion (bruising) of the brain and actual laceration, but the distinction is not important in practical management.

Although the prognosis of uncomplicated head trauma (i.e., those not requiring surgical removal of blood clots) is often proportional to the duration of unconsciousness, it must be emphasized that patients comatose for weeks may make remarkable recoveries, so that care must not be abandoned prematurely. This is particularly true in children, who have a marvelously flexible brain and often regain normal function after severe closed head injury and protracted unconsciousness. Retrograde amnesia of varying severity is common after cerebral contusion or laceration and not infrequent after simple concussion.

The presence of cranial nerve abnormalities (e.g., extraocular palsies, facial palsy, and deafness) almost invariably denotes basilar skull fracture. This does not necessarily worsen the prognosis for recovery from cerebral trauma, although the cranial nerve deficit may be permanent. Patients who demonstrate disturbances of eye movements have an injury to one or more of the 3rd, 4th, and 6th cranial nerves, and the movement defect is due to a "blow-out" fracture of the orbit. Unless these fractures are repaired, the ocular gaze defect may be permanent.

PRINCIPLES OF MANAGEMENT OF CLOSED HEAD INJURY

1. *Establish an adequate airway.* This takes precedence over all else. It can be accomplished by turning the patient on his side and making the head somewhat dependent to allow drainage of blood, vomitus, and mucus from the mouth and nasopharynx. This measure can be assisted by aspiration if necessary. If there is evidence of airway obstruction, an endotracheal tube should be passed immediately; if not, tracheostomy must be performed. Whatever must be done to establish an airway is performed and must take top priority, for hypoxia will not only rapidly injure the brain further but may result in cardiac arrest.

2. *Evaluate the extent of the injury.* If the patient is in shock, therapy must be instituted at once; this may include initiating an intravenous infusion and the administration of vasopressors and oxygen, as well as starting a search for a source of bleeding. The presence of cyanosis denotes hypoxia and may be secondary to a crushing or penetrating chest wound, which may require release of air from a tension pneumothorax or other emergency management.

3. *Evaluate the extent of the head injury once the immediate threats to the patient's life are dealt with.* The search for head trauma includes inspection for depressed skull fracture and looking for cerebrospinal fluid (CSF) rhinorrhea and blood behind the tympanic membranes, both of which denote basilar

skull fracture. X-ray films of the skull should be obtained early if the additional time or movement of the patient does not constitute a hazard, but it should be remembered that the only really compelling reasons for x-ray films of the skull are suspicion of depressed fracture or epidural hematoma. Otherwise, the presence of a skull fracture does not determine therapy. Cervical spine x-rays should be taken early to look for fracture and unnecessary movement limited until the neck has been immobilized.

The extent of intracranial trauma should be evaluated as promptly as is consistent with good medical management by a CAT scan. This enables the treating physician to distinguish, in many instances, between epidural hemorrhage, acute subdural hematoma, intracerebral hemorrhage, and localized brain swelling with mass effect. The CAT scan has largely replaced angiography as the most important diagnostic tool in the critical evaluation of the patient with severe head injury. Rarely angiography is necessary to make the distinctions described above.

An epidural hematoma (Fig. 5.1) occurs only in the presence of a fracture in the squamous portion of the temporal lobe, the fracture lacerating the middle meningeal artery, one of the distal branches of the external carotid artery. The result is arterial bleeding into the epidural space, a circumstance which is almost invariably fatal unless the clot is surgically removed and the bleeding

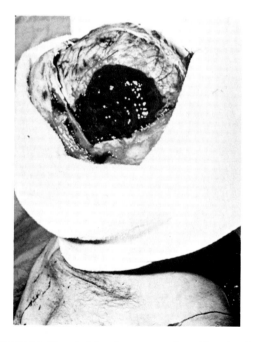

FIG. 5.1. Epidural hematoma. The skull has been opened, and the clot (from laceration of the middle meningeal artery) can be seen lying on the surface of the dura in the midtemporal region.

stopped. The "classic" history of epidural hematoma is closed head injury, usually associated with brief unconsciousness, followed by a lucid interval, and, after a period of hours, by drowsiness, headache, opposite hemiparesis, obtundation, and coma. The epidural clot causes massive shift of the midline structures to the opposite side, followed usually by transtentorial herniation and fatal brainstem compression.

A high index of suspicion is an important ingredient in the diagnosis of epidural hematoma. Persistent drowsiness or any focal neurologic deficit requires immediate investigation by CAT scan and, if necessary, angiography. The only useful treatment is to evacuate the clot and stop the arterial bleeding.

Any of the signs of acute epidural hemorrhage may be simulated by cerebral contusion accompanied by brain swelling. This is not infrequently accompanied by an *acute subdural hematoma* (Fig. 5.2). The distinction is of great importance because the treatment for epidural hemorrhage is always surgical removal of the clot as promptly as it is discovered, whereas many acute subdural hematomas are small and do not require surgical excision. Small amounts of subdural bleeding occur with head trauma severe enough to cause brain contusion and swelling; the rule is that the acute subdural hematoma should be drained only if it is thought to produce a mass effect. In many

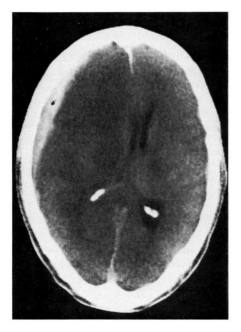

FIG. 5.2. Acute subdural hematoma. This CAT scan was made without contrast 24 hr after head trauma. The crescent-shaped area of increased density is a collection of fresh blood which extended from the middle fossa almost to the vertex. The ventricles are pushed sharply to the opposite side. Death from transtentorial herniation is a major cause of death in injuries of this sort.

instances the patient's symptoms and signs are the result of the contusion, and associated swelling and the subdural blood is incidental.

Treatment of the swollen contused brain is by hyperosmolar agents and dexamethasone (Decadron). Mannitol is the preferred agent, in doses of 250 ml of 20% solution given intravenously over 30 to 60 min and repeated in 4 to 6 hr if necessary. Dexamethasone is given intravenously in doses up to 100 mg daily. The usual dose is 16 mg at once followed by 8 mg every 4 to 6 hr. Patients receiving these drugs require careful observation of blood electrolytes and fluid volume.

The nonsurgical management of the patient with severe closed head injury, persistent unconsciousness, and signs of hemisphere swelling varies in different centers. The important underlying principles are the same, i.e., use of an intensive care unit or special nursing with adequate monitoring for blood gases, electrocardiography, arterial pressure, and changes in clinical neurologic status. Because of the possibility of convulsions, intravenous dilantinization (15 mg/kg i.v. over a period of 20 min) is appropriate. The daily maintenance dosage averages 300 mg. Induced hypothermia (body temperature kept at 95° to 96°F) is felt by some to inhibit brain swelling and to reduce energy requirements of the injured brain. Use of this modality requires a team skilled in recognizing its complications, which include cardiac arrhythmias and metabolic acidosis. At least one group in the United States has studied the effects of large doses of phenobarbital given intravenously, the rationale being that barbiturates inhibit the development of infarction in experimental cerebral ischemia. The evidence suggests that barbiturates, in doses large enough to produce an isoelectric EEG, sustained over a 24- to 36-hr period, improves the prognosis in terms of mortality and quality of survival in patients who are comatose following severe closed head injury. It goes without saying that such treatment requires skilled and experienced intensive care.

The question of acute subdural hematoma was alluded to above. Surgical removal should be reserved for those large enough to cause a mass effect, always keeping in mind that the underlying brain contusion may be responsible for the patient's clinical state.

The problem of chronic subdural hematoma should properly be considered apart from the acute complications of head injury, for it usually heralds its presence days to weeks after the injury. A subdural hematoma is a collection of blood in the subdural space following tearing or rupture of bridging veins. Its effect is caused by compression of the brain, shift of the midline structures, and finally herniation of the uncus of the temporal lobe beneath the tentorium and compression of the brainstem. The latter is usually the final stage in an unrecognized subdural hematoma and frequently heralds a fatal outcome.

The symptoms and signs of a subdural clot are similar to those of any slowly expanding intracranial mass and depend originally on its location. There may be no history of trauma, or the trauma that caused the lesion may have been so

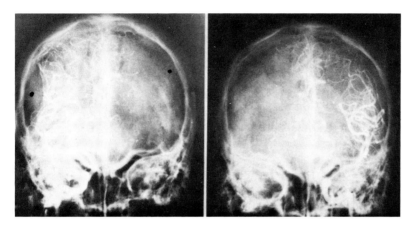

FIG. 5.3. Bilateral subdural hematoma. The arteriogram shows a chronic subdural collection on the right (medial surface convex) and an acute subdural collection on the left (concave medially). The result is no shift of midline structures.

minor as to have been ignored. The most frequent symptoms and signs are headache, drowsiness, psychomotor retardation, and hemiparesis.

The presence of a chronic subdural hematoma (Fig. 5.3) may not be suspected clinically, particularly in an elderly patient. Fortunately, the CAT scan allows the diagnosis to be made simply and atraumatically. Some chronic subdural hematomas are small and produce no symptoms or signs. Such patients should be followed carefully in the hope that the clot will resolve spontaneously. Treatment of symptomatic chronic subdural hematoma is surgical removal. Although there is some controversy over the most effective surgical technique, most data indicate that aspiration through burr holes is at least as effective as more radical procedures.

Epileptic convulsions following head injury merit special comment. The occurrence of an epileptic seizure, either focal or generalized, after closed head trauma does not necessarily signify a poor prognosis, particularly if the seizure is brief and the patient has no other neurologic signs. Seizures may occur after simple concussion or may result from cerebral contusion or laceration. Recurrent seizures early after trauma denote serious brain injury and must be brought under control.

Posttraumatic epilepsy occurs much more frequently following penetrating head injuries than after closed head injuries; the incidence in the latter is about 5%. The first attack usually occurs within 6 months posttrauma. (It is difficult to ascribe a seizure disorder which begins more than 2 years following a head injury to the trauma.) The type of seizure may be focal or generalized, and temporal lobe seizures may also occur. The characteristic EEG change is a focus of spike waves in an area of slow wave activity. Trauma does not produce petit mal seizures. Treatment is the same as for any patient with epilepsy.

The causes of death in head injury include severe brain injury, usually contusion or laceration, involving vital areas; cerebral edema; subdural hematoma; epidural hematoma; severe metabolic disturbances, particularly the hypo-osmolal state; multiple injuries to other parts of the body, overlooked because the patient is comatose; coincidental cerebral and coronary vascular lesions in elderly or hypertensive subjects; pulmonary complications, particularly aspiration. There is undoubtedly a small group of patients with head injury who die because of uncontrolled cerebral edema without morphologic evidence of an otherwise fatal brain lesion. The management of this problem is described above. All patients with significant head injury should be hospitalized and carefully observed for any evidence of brain compression, either by edema or clot formation.

Although there may be no lateralizing defects, many patients have significant and unpredictable sequelae from closed head injury. If the patient has been unconscious for more than a few minutes, there is often a period of amnesia for the accident itself and for events immediately preceding and following it. There is some correlation between the severity of brain damage and the length of the retrograde amnesia, which usually becomes shorter as the patient recovers. Permanent alteration of intellectual function is rare in simple concussion but not infrequent following brain contusion and prolonged unconsciousness. Certainly impaired mental function may be present for several months following apparent recovery from moderately severe head injury, and may result in frustration and personality change if the patient attempts to return to preinjury activities (e.g., work or school) too quickly.

The large incidence of liability suits that are now filed following accidents of all sorts adds another dimension to the difficulty of evaluating symptoms of patients who have suffered cerebral concussion. Headache, a feeling of giddiness, and easy fatigability are not uncommon postconcussion symptoms. These usually occur if there has been significant trauma and the period of unconsciousness has lasted more than a few seconds. In most instances the patient improves progressively and becomes symptom-free within a few weeks. Unfortunately, it is not uncommon to hear similar complaints from patients many months after minor head trauma. The possible influence, unconscious or otherwise, of a lawsuit on such patient's symptomatology must be considered.

Treatment of the postconcussion syndrome is symptomatic, using simple analgesics and encouraging the patient to gradually increase physical activity. In rare instances orthostatic hypotension is present, requiring the use of elastic stockings, mild vasopressors, and encouragement to be active.

SPINAL CORD INJURY

Although injury to the spinal cord clearly requires neurologic attention as promptly as possible, every physician should be aware of some general principles of diagnosis and management, particularly because he may be called on to handle such a patient immediately after trauma. There are many ways in which to classify injuries to the spinal cord; one useful approach is to consider the pathology of the lesion, for this often determines the mode of management.

1. *Acute contusion with temporary neurologic deficit but complete functional recovery.* This is a rare occurrence; it usually follows sudden severe neck flexion or extension and is characterized by transitory paralysis and numbness below the lesion along with loss of sphincter function. These patients are often recovering or have recovered by the time they are examined. X-ray films of the cervical spine may indicate no fracture or dislocation but, rarely, show a congenital defect of one or more cervical vertebrae. The patient should be kept at rest for several days and wear a cervical collar for support for the following 2 months.

2. *Acute contusion with neurologic deficit and incomplete recovery.* This occurs most frequently in middle-aged and elderly patients who have cervical spondylosis. They sustain a sudden flexion or extension neck injury by tripping, falling, or some other sudden movement, or the injury may occur during the hyperextension of the neck necessary for intubation. The narrowed anterior-posterior diameter of the cervical spinal canal prevents normal spinal cord movement, the cord being compressed anteriorly by the spondylitic spurs and posteriorly by hypertrophied ligamenta flava. It is believed that the injury is sustained by the anterior spinal artery or one of its penetrating branches, with resultant ischemia and necrosis of the central gray portion of the cord so that instantaneous complete paralysis below the level of the lesion develops. Prognosis in this group of patients may be reasonably good; the clue to the diagnosis is early movement of the toes and feet, denoting that the cord damage may be localized to its most central area. Urinary and fecal retention are the rule early after the injury; the extent of return of sphincter function depends on the severity of cord damage. X-ray films of the cervical spine show cervical spondylosis but rarely any other abnormalities. These patients usually recover spontaneously and slowly, and are left with a variety of neurologic deficits. Eventually, cervical laminectomy can be considered in order to prevent further damage to the spinal cord by the spondylosis.

3. *Acute contusion and laceration or compression of the cord.* This condition is caused by fracture or fracture-dislocation of some part of one or more vertebrae, often secondary to sudden severe flexion or extension of the neck. The characteristic injury is that which occurs when diving into shallow water.

The onset of paralysis is acute, usually with associated sensory loss up to the level of the cord injury, as well as sphincter paralysis. In such cases there is no evidence of early return of function, and x-ray films of the appropriate area indicate fracture of one or both laminal arches or pedicles of one or more vertebrae, or crushing of a vertebral body, usually with significant dislocation of one vertebra on another. In this manner, the spinal cord is compressed, contused, and lacerated.

The treatment of patients with spinal cord injury has comprised mainly the patient's rehabilitation, and in this area a great deal of progress has been made stimulated by the successful results obtained during and after World War II. Unfortunately, the same type of progress has not occurred in the treatment of patients in the acute stages of spinal cord trauma. There is agreement on certain principles, the most important of which is to handle the patient in such a manner as to avoid further injury to the cord. At the scene of trauma the patient's neck must be splinted in some fashion prior to moving him. This can be accomplished by hand traction or by strapping a folded newspaper to the neck bilaterally as a splint.

Following careful neurologic evaluation to determine the level of spinal cord damage, the whole spine should be examined by x-ray. Areas of bony deformity, tenderness, or swelling serve as obvious clues to the location of the fracture. There is a difference of opinion as to the value of surgical exploration and decompression, but the majority view is that such a procedure may be beneficial, particularly during the first 48 hr, if (1) there is x-ray evidence of compressed fracture of the laminae; (2) a bone spicule compressing the cord or an acute herniated disc is suspected; or (3) the patient presents with a partial paralysis and shows signs of worsening. Otherwise the patient is placed in a special rotating frame bed and Crutchfield tongs are applied to reduce the dislocation. During the acute stage many centers use dexamethasone and hyperosmolar agents to reduce spinal cord swelling. The evidence for benefit is meager.

The chronic management of the spinal-injured patient depends directly on the location and extent of the lesion. Skin, bowel, and bladder care are essential if the patient is to survive the initial hospitalization. High cervical cord lesions causing quadriplegia cause respiratory distress. Some of these patients require a respirator, from which they may eventually be weaned.

Missile injuries to the spinal cord usually require laminectomy to remove the foreign object or bone splinters. This should be done as promptly as possible following trauma.

SUGGESTED READINGS

A Survey of Current Head Injury Research. A Report Prepared by the Subcommittee on Head Injury. National Advisory Neurological Disease and Stroke Council for the National Institute of Neurological Diseases and Stroke. National Institutes of Health, Bethesda, Maryland, 1969.

Benson VM, McLaurin RL, and Foulkes EC: Traumatic cerebral edema. *Arch Neurol* 23:179, 1970.

Blackman HA: Legal problem attendant upon the late effects of head injuries. In: *The Late Effects of Head Injuries,* edited by AE Walker, WF Caveness, and M Critchley, pp 439-446. Charles C Thomas, Springfield, Illinois, 1969.

Boshes B, Zivin I, and Tigay EI: Recent methods of management of spinal cord and cauda equina injuries: comparative study of World War II and Korean experiences. *Neurology (Minneap)* 4:690, 1954.

Boxing brains. *Lancet* 2:1064, 1973.

Boyarsky S: Recent advances in neurogenic bladder. *J Urol* 101:53, 1969.

Brink JD, Garrett AL, Hale WR, Woo-Sam J, and Nickel VL: Recovery of motor and intellectual function in children sustaining severe head injuries. *Dev Med Child Neurol* 12:565, 1970.

Brock S (ed): *Injuries of the Brain and Spinal Cord.* Williams & Wilkins, Baltimore, 1940.

Caveness WF: Onset and cessation of fits following craniocerebral trauma. *J Neurosurg* 20:570, 1963

Caveness WF, and Walker AE (ed): *Head Injury: Conference Proceedings.* Lippincott, Philadelphia, 1966.

Ciembroniewicz JE: Subdural hematoma of the posterior fossa. *J Neurosurg* 22:465, 1965.

Cooper PR, Moody S, Clark WK, Kirkpatrick J, Maravilla K, Gould AL, and Drane W: Dexamethasone and severe head injury: a prospective double-blind study. *J Neurosurg* 51:307, 1979.

Echols DH, Llewellyn R, Kirgis HD, Rehfeldt FC, and Garcia Bengochea F: Tracheotomy in the management of severe head injuries. *Surgery* 28:801, 1950.

Gallagher JP, and Browder EJ: Extradural hematoma. *J Neurosurg* 29:1, 1968.

Graham DI, and Adams JH: Ischaemic brain damage in fatal head injuries. *Lancet* 1:265, 1971.

Gudeman SK, Miller D, and Becker DP: Failure of high-dose steroid therapy to influence intracranial pressure in patients with severe head injury. *J Neurosurg* 51:301, 1979.

Gurdjian ES, and Webster JE: *Head Injuries.* Little Brown, Boston, 1958.

Guttmann L: Clinical symptomatology of spinal cord lesions. In: *Handbook of Clinical Neurology,* Vol 2, edited by PJ Vinken and GW Bruyn, p 178. Wiley, New York, 1969.

Javid M: Current concepts: head injuries. *N Engl J Med* 291:890, 1974.

Key AG, and Retief PJM: Spinal cord injuries: an analysis of 300 new lesions. *Paraplegia* 7:243, 1970.

King LR, McLaurin RL, and Knowles HC Jr: Acid-base balance and arterial and CSF lactate levels following human head injury. *J Neurosurg* 40:617, 1974.

Lindenberg R, and Freytag E: The mechanisms of cerebral contusions. *Arch Pathol* 69:440, 1960.

Lundberg N, Troupp H, and Lorin H: Continuous recording of the ventricular-fluid pressure in patients with severe acute traumatic brain injury: a preliminary report. *J Neurosurg* 22:581, 1965.

Marron JC, and Campbell RL: Subdural hematoma. *Arch Neurol* 22:234, 1970.

Marshall LF, Smith RW, and Shapiro HM: The outcome with aggressive treatment in severe head injuries. I. The significance of intracranial pressure monitoring. *J Neurosurg* 50:20, 1979.

Marshall LF, Smith RW, and Shapiro HM: The outcome with aggressive treatment in severe head injuries. II. Acute and chronic barbiturate administration in the management of head injury. *J Neurosurg* 50:26, 1979.

McKissock W, et al: Subdural hematoma. *Lancet* 1:1365, 1960.

McKissock W, et al: Extradural hematoma. *Lancet* 2:167, 1960.

Melzak J: Paraplegia among children. *Lancet* 2:45, 1969.

Meyer JS, Kondo A, Nomura F, Sakamoto K, and Teraura T: Cerebral hemodynamics and metabolism following experimental head injury. *J Neurosurg* 32:304, 1970.

Mitchell DR, and Adams JH: Primary focal impact damage to the brainstem in blunt head injuries: does it exist? *Lancet* 2:215, 1973.

Nyquist RH, and Bors E: Mortality and survival in traumatic myelopathy during nineteen years from 1946–1965. *Paraplegia* 5:22, 1967.

Ommaya AK, and Gennarelli TA: Cerebral concussion and traumatic unconsciousness: correlation of experimental and clinical observations on blunt head injuries. *Brain* 97:633, 1974.

Silver JR, and Gibbon NOK: Prognosis in tetraplegia. *Br Med J* 4:79, 1968.

Suwanwela C, and Suwanwela N: Intracranial arterial narrowing and spasm in acute head injury. *J Neurosurg* 36:314, 1972.

Suzuki J, and Takaku A: Nonsurgical treatment of chronic subdural hematoma. *J. Neurosurg* 33:533, 1970.

Symonds C: Concussion and its sequelae. *Lancet* 1:1, 1962.

Tarlov IM: Spinal cord injuries: early treatment. *Surg Clin North Am* 35:591, 1955.

Ulin AW, and Rosomoff HL: Management of airway in acute head injury. *Arch Surg* 67:765, 1953.

Walker AE, Caveness WF, and Critchley M (eds): *The Late Effects of Head Injuries.* Charles C Thomas, Springfield, Ill, 1969.

Walker AE, et al: The physiological basis of concussion. *J Neurosurg* 1:103, 1944.

Wilkins RH, and Odom GL: Intracranial arterial spasm associated with craniocerebral trauma. *J Neurosurg* 32:626, 1970.

Yen JK, Bourke RS, Nelson LR, and Popp AJ: Numerical grading of clinical neurological status after serious head injury. *J Neurology Surg Psychiatry* 41:1125, 1978.

6

Dizziness

Dizziness is a common, annoying, sometimes disabling, usually frightening symptom caused by a wide variety of disorders. Although most causes are benign, competent evaluation of the patient is important in order to avoid overlooking those which are not and, particularly, to exclude the possibility of 8th nerve tumor. Systematic localization of the origin of the dizziness by a proper history and physical examination together with certain specific laboratory diagnostic aids usually allows the physician to decide what part of the vestibular system is involved and hence how to manage the patient.

The first responsibility is to determine what the patient means when he complains of dizziness, a term frequently used to describe a variety of sensations, including faintness, weakness, vague thinking, or unsteadiness. The physician must encourage the patient to describe his symptoms as accurately as possible. The first problem then is to ascertain if the patient is describing a disturbance of vestibular function, i.e., whether the patient is complaining of true vertigo or a state of disequilibrium. Sometimes this is not easy. The complaint of "dizziness" on suddenly arising from a supine or sitting position may well be a feeling of weakness or "light-headedness" induced by orthostatic hypotension. Obviously the problem in such a case is different than if the patient has described a true vestibular disorder.

Once it has been established that the patient's complaint probably has a vestibular origin, the diagnostic problem then relates to determining which portion of the vestibular apparatus is involved.

Except in the rare instance of cortical origin, as in certain types of epilepsy, true dizziness or vertigo is the result of dysfunction of some part of the vestibular system. The end-organs of the vestibular portion of the 8th cranial nerve are the utricle, the saccule, and the three semicircular canals, each of which is located in the petrous bone immediately adjacent to the cochlea, the end-organ of hearing. These structures respond to changes in the rate of movement, particularly rotatory, of the head, which causes displacement of endolymph and stimulation of hair cells in the ampullae of the semicircular canals and of the otoliths, which are located in the utricle and the saccule. The cell bodies of the dendrites of these structures are located in the vestibular ganglion; the axons comprise the vestibular nerve, which eventually synapses with the vestibular nuclei in the medulla. Dizziness can occur from disturbance in the (1) end-organs, (2) vestibular ganglion or nerve, and (3) vestibular nuclei in the medulla. The characteristics of dizziness and accompanying symptoms and signs usually differ with each location thereby enabling the physician to decide on proper management; it is important, therefore, to learn as much as possible about the event by making specific inquiries:

1. Under what circumstances does the dizziness occur? Is it precipitated by head movement, sudden turning when walking, by changes in posture or head position?

2. What is the duration of the attack? End-organ dizziness is usually paroxysmal and brief. Chronic, persistent dizziness suggests 8th nerve tumor or brainstem disease.

3. Is there associated nausea or vomiting? Severe nausea and vomiting associated with vertigo suggests end-organ disease, although these symptoms may occur in brainstem or cerebellar lesions.

4. What are the associated, or neighborhood, signs? *Tinnitus* denotes end-organ or 8th nerve disease. It never occurs in central lesions. Deafness means an 8th nerve lesion or Meniere's syndrome. The differential diagnosis depends on other findings. Diplopia, dysphagia, dysarthria, extremity weakness, or facial numbness associated with the episode of dizziness indicate brainstem involvement.

5. Is there a disturbance of equilibrium in walking or defective extremity coordination between attacks of dizziness? An affirmative response points to 8th nerve or brainstem disease.

DIZZINESS ORGINATING FROM THE END-ORGANS

Fortunately, the most frequent origin of dizziness is in the peripheral vestibular apparatus; although unpleasant, it is not life-threatening, and treatment is usually symptomatic. Onset is sudden and the dizziness usually severe, often associated with nausea or vomiting, or both, and not infrequently with tinnitus and disturbance of hearing. Tinnitus is a strong indication of end-organ disease, although it sometimes occurs in lesions of the 8th nerve as well. The dizziness, severe at first, gradually subsides over a period of minutes or hours; it is usually worse when the head is placed in certain positions. The dizziness is often associated with sweating, pallor, and retching, so these patients are not infrequently subjected to needless gastrointestinal studies. Nystagmus, which almost invariably accompanies the vertigo, is horizontal with a rotatory component, but never vertical.

Although several specific terms are used to describe syndromes of dizziness originating in the end-organs (i.e., the labyrinths), the mechanisms whereby dysfunction in these structures causes vertigo are poorly understood.

Serous labyrinthitis and *vestibular neuronitis* are often used interchangeably to describe paroxysmal vertigo not associated with hearing loss or tinnitus. The attacks are usually self-limited. Their etiology is unknown, although viral infection has been suggested.

Middle ear disease may cause *labyrinthine inflammation* and paroxysmal vertigo. The association is usually apparent. Hearing is almost invariably temporarily impaired, and the patients complain of stuffiness in the affected ear.

Benign positional vertigo usually occurs during middle age. Dizziness appears a few seconds after the patient's head assumes a new position, and it is almost invariably associated with nystagmus. Dizziness and nystagmus are soon exhausted. The symptoms can be induced at the bedside by tilting the patient suddenly from the sitting to the supine position and extending the head below the head of the table while turning it to one side. The dizziness and nystagmus appear after a short latent period and disappear in less than 30 sec. The sequence can be repeated by suddenly moving the patient to the sitting position. Posture-induced vertigo may occur in lesions of the posterior fossa, either cerebellar or brainstem, but the nystagmus and dizziness do not have a delayed onset and they persist until the patient's position is changed. Benign positional vertigo may recur for several months but then usually subsides spontaneously. The pathology is thought to be in the otoliths, but this is not firmly established. Audiometric examination may be normal or denote cochlear disease. Caloric testing is usually normal.

Meniere's disease is characterized by recurrent attacks of vertigo and loss of hearing. Tinnitus is a frequent symptom. It is presumably caused by hydrops of the labyrinth, but the cochlea is also involved. Sensorineural hearing loss occurs, often bilaterally. The attacks may go on over a period of years, with progressive hearing decrement with each episode. Eventually there is a permanent residual of nerve deafness, tinnitus, and unsteadiness.

Posttraumatic dizziness may follow closed head injury and is thought to be secondary to trauma to the labyrinth. Vertigo, nausea, vomiting, nystagmus, loss of balance, and past-pointing appear shortly after injury and may persist for hours to weeks, but always gradually subsiding.

Treatment of vertigo of end-organ origin is symptomatic. Dimenhydrinate (Dramamine) or one of its derivatives, or meclizine (Antivert, Bonine), is used to inhibit vertigo. Dosage may be limited by the sedative action of these drugs. Section of the 8th nerve may rarely be resorted to in Meniere's disease, provided that hearing has already been lost in the affected ear.

8TH NERVE LESIONS AS A CAUSE OF DIZZINESS

Dizziness originating from the 8th nerve is usually caused by a tumor of the 8th nerve (schwannoma) or a tumor compressing the 8th nerve (meningioma). In either instance, the earlier the pathology is identified, the greater is the likelihood of successful treatment. This is particularly true since the advent of

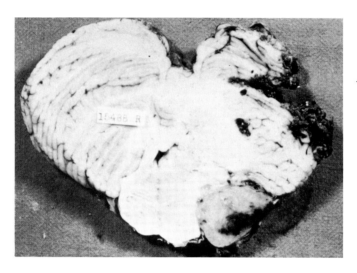

FIG. 6.1. Acoustic neuroma (schwannoma). This large extracanalicular tumor has lodged in the cerebellopontine angle and compressed both structures.

the operating microscope and surgical approach to the schwannomas through the temporal bone, for small intracanalicular tumors (i.e., confined within the acoustic canal) can be removed without sacrificing the acoustic or facial nerves. It is imperative to have a high index of suspicion for these lesions because the cost to the patient of overlooking one may be high (Fig. 6.1). Indeed most of the laboratory investigation of a patient with vertigo is primarily directed at establishing or excluding an 8th nerve tumor.

The dizziness which accompanies 8th nerve tumor usually begins insidiously and becomes slowly and progressively worse. The patients rarely describe true vertigo but, rather, complain of imbalance or disequilibrium. The sensation is practically never paroxysmal. Associated findings include horizontal jerk nystagmus precipitated by gazing to the side of the lesion, decreased hearing, decreased facial sensation and corneal reflex, facial weakness, and appendicular cerebellar ataxia, all on the same side. With the exception of hearing loss, which can also occur in peripheral lesions, these signs are unequivocal evidence of a cerebellopontine angle mass and denote that the tumor is large and is compressing the brainstem. Since 8th nerve schwannomas usually have their origin in the vestibular branch of the 8th nerve, dizziness is often the earliest sign. Prompt and appropriate diagnostic procedures permit detection of the tumor while it is still intracanalicular. Diagnostic tests are described on pages 130–131.

DIZZINESS ORIGINATING IN THE CNS

Any disease process that affects the vestibular nuclei may cause vertigo. The common etiologies are vertebrobasilar insufficiency and multiple sclerosis. Brainstem gliomas rarely produce vertigo. Cerebellar tumors and tumors of the floor of the 4th ventricle may also produce vertigo by distorting or compressing the medulla. The characteristics of centrally originating vertigo are not very distinctive. In brainstem ischemia, the onset is sudden, often with nausea and vomiting and almost invariably with nystagmus, which may be horizontal, vertical, or rotatory. Vertical nystagmus in this setting establishes the localization as central. The hallmark of vertigo originating in brainstem structures is that it is practically invariably accompanied by other signs of brainstem disease, e.g., perioral numbness, ataxia, dysarthria, double vision, extremity weakness. The longevity of these signs depends on the pathology. Central vertigo occurs rarely without accompanying signs, in which instance it is difficult to distinguish from end-organ vertigo, but tinnitus is never present and hearing is intact.

Unfortunately, it is not always easy to make such precise classifications of a patient's complaints, at least partly because the patient may be a poor observer or is incapable of describing his symptoms accurately. Furthermore, there are several causes for a sensation of dizziness that simply defy accurate anatomic localization in the manner described previously. The symptom of ataxia or unsteady gait is often described by the patient as a type of disequilibrium in standing or walking, so that cerebellar disease may closely simulate vestibular dysfunction. Midline cerebellar tumors (e.g., the medulloblastomas seen in children) may be characterized by a postural disturbance and ataxia without any evidence of extremity ataxia. Although the patient is not really dizzy, he complains of it.

A variety of drugs, particularly sedatives, tranquilizers, and anticonvulsants such as phenytoin (Dilantin), cause a sensation of dizziness, poor equilibrium, staggering gait, nystagmus, and dysarthria, all of which are usually associated with drowsiness. One of the most frequent complaints of patients with myxedema is a feeling of unsteadiness or dizziness, and examination shows that these patients do indeed appear to have a vestibular disorder. Nutritional defects such as Wernicke's encephalopathy are also characterized by, among other things, dizziness, nystagmus, and ataxia, clear evidence of vestibular nuclei disease.

EVALUATION OF PATIENT WITH DIZZINESS

1. *Careful neurologic examination.* The examiner must look particularly for evidence of early cerebellar extremity ataxia and signs of 5th, 7th, or 8th cranial nerve involvement. Testing for position-induced vertigo should be

carried out in each patient as described for benign positional vertigo (see above). Nystagmus should be carefully evaluated, for its type may be an important clue to localization.

2. *X-ray films of the skull, with particular emphasis on the petrous ridges and internal acoustic meati.* Tomograms of the internal acoustic canals should be routine if 8th nerve tumor is suspected in order to look for flaring of the acoustic meatus or evidence of bone erosion in the canal (Fig. 6.2).

3. *CAT scan.* An extra canalicular 8th nerve tumor or other posterior fossa tumors will usually be revealed by CAT scan, but intracanalicular lesions can not ordinarily be visualized (Fig. 6.3).

4. *Audiometrics.* Careful audiologic evaluation is essential if 8th nerve tumor is suspected because it usually permits distinction between cochlear and retrocochlear lesions. The classic abnormalities in retrocochlear lesions include:

A. Sensorineural deafness. This is usually characterized by a quantitatively similar decrease in bone and air conduction, as opposed to the decreased air conduction with normal bone conduction seen in middle ear disease (conductive deafness).

B. Poor speech discrimination. This is usually good in cochlear lesions.

C. Absent recruitment.

D. Tone decay.

E. Poor sensitivity to short increments.

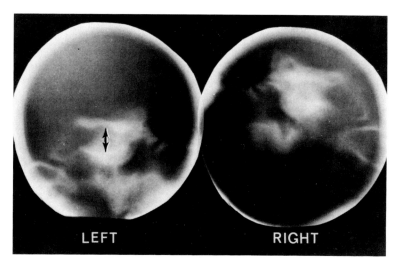

FIG. 6.2. Tomograms of internal acoustic meati. The patient had an intracanalicular schwannoma on the left. Note the flaring and slight widening of the porus on the left with thinning of the superior plate and erosion of the inferior wall of the meatus.

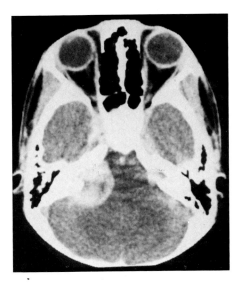

FIG. 6.3. CAT scan with contrast showing bilateral 8th nerve tumors, the left much larger than the right. The widening and asymmetry of the internal acoustic meati can also be readily appreciated.

F. More impairment in the ability to hear continuous than pulsed tones in Bekesy recordings (types III and IV Bekesy audiograms).

5. *Caloric testing.* Discriminative caloric testing is not a complicated technique. It requires only the proper positioning of the patient, ice water, and a syringe. The most relevant finding is significant unilateral reduction in caloric response (nystagmus, vertigo, or both) to ice water. Abnormal responses are obtained in about 50% of patients with Meniere's disease and 8th nerve tumor, so the test may not in itself distinguish the anatomic location of the lesion. Oculonystagmography is a more formalized recording of the eye movement responses to caloric stimulation.

6. *Thyroid function studies.*

7. *Auditory evoked responses* may be capable of distinguishing the site of auditory defect.

8. *Pantopaque contrast study of posterior fossa.* This is usually reserved for those patients in whom a strong unconfirmed suspicion of 8th nerve tumor remains despite inconclusive studies. This procedure allows visualization of intracanalicular tumors.

SUGGESTED READINGS

Etiology and Mechanisms

Bergen JJ, et al: Vascular implications of vertigo. *Arch Otolaryngol* 85:292, 1967.
Berkowitz WP, and Stroud MH: Early vascular insufficiency and the vestibular system. *Laryngoscope* 83:1084, 1973.

Carmichael EA, Dix MR, and Hallpike CS: Pathology, symptomatology and diagnosis of organic affections of the eighth nerve system. *Br Med Bull* 12:146, 1956.

Fisher CM: Vertigo in cerebrovascular disease. *Arch Otolaryngol* 85:529, 1967.

Powers WH: Symposium on Meniere's disease. II. Metabolic aspects of Meniere's disease. *Laryngoscope* 82:1716, 1972.

Pulec JL: *Meniere's Disease*. Saunders, Philadelphia, 1968.

Tyler DB, and Bard P: Motion sickness. *Physiol Rev* 29:311, 1949.

Williams D, and Wilson TG: The diagnosis of the major and minor syndromes of basilar insufficiency. *Brain* 85:741, 1962.

Types: Clinical Manifestations

Cawthorne T: Aural vertigo. In: *Modern Trends in Neurology,* edited by D Williams, Vol 2, pp 193–201. Butterworth, London, 1957.

Davey IM, and German WJ: The vestibular system and its disorders. *Annu Rev Med* 13:431, 1962.

Harrison MS: Epidemic vertigo—vestibular neuronitis. *Brain* 85:613, 1962.

Harrison MS: Benign positional vertigo. In: *The Vestibular System and Its Diseases,* edited by RJ Wolfson, pp 404–427. University of Pennsylvania Press, Philadelphia, 1966.

Harrison MS, and Ozsahinoglu C: Positional vertigo: aetiology and clinical significance. *Brain* 95:369, 1972.

Haymaker W, and Kuhlenbeck H: Disorders of the brainstem and its cranial nerves. In: *Clinical Neurology,* edited by AB Baker and LH Baker, Vol 3, pp 20–28. Harper & Row, Hagerstown, Maryland, 1973.

Koenigsberger MR, et al: Benign paroxysmal vertigo of childhood. *Neurology (Minneap)* 20:1108, 1970.

Salmon SD: Positional nystagmus: critical review and personal experiences. *Arch Otolaryngol* 90:84, 1969.

Diagnosis

Barber HO: The diagnosis and treatment of auditory and vestibular disturbances after head injury. *Clin Neurosurg* 19:355, 1972.

Berlin CI: New developments in evaluating central auditory mechanisms. *Ann Otol Rhinol Laryngol* 85:833, 1976.

Cawthorne T, Dix MR, Hallpike CS, and Hood JD: The investigation of vestibular function. *Br Med Bull* 12:131, 1956.

Clemis JD, and Mastricola PG: Special audiometric test battery in 121 proved acoustic tumors. *Arch Otolaryngol* 102:654, 1976.

Crabtree JA, and House WF: Part III. Preoperative evaluation: x-ray diagnosis of acoustic neuromas. *Arch Otolaryngol* 80:696, 1964.

Drachman DA, and Hart CW: An approach to the dizzy patient. *Neurology (Minneap)* 22:323, 1972.

Edwards CH, and Paterson JH: A review of the symptoms and signs of acoustic neurofibromata. *Brain* 74:144, 1951.

Hambley WM, Gorshenin AN, and House WF: Part III. Preoperative evaluation: the differential diagnosis of acoustic neuroma. *Arch Otolaryngol* 80:708, 1964.

Hitselberger WE, and House WF: Part III. Preoperative evaluation: other cranial nerves and cerebellar signs. *Arch Otolaryngol* 80:693, 1964.

Hitselberger WE, and House WF: Part III. Preoperative evaluation: cerebrospinal fluid protein findings. *Arch Otolaryngol* 80:706, 1964.

Hitselberger WE, and House WF: Part III. Preoperative evaluation: tumors of the cerebellopontine angle. *Arch Otolaryngol* 80:720, 1964.

Johnson EW, and House WF: Part III. Preoperative evaluation: auditory findings in 53 cases of acoustic neuromas. *Arch Otolaryngol* 80:667, 1964.

Lindsay JR: Vertigo: differential diagnosis and treatment. *Wis Med J* 49:607, 1950.

McClure JA, Lycett P, and Bicker GR: A quantitative rotational test of vestibular function. *J Otolaryngol* 5:279, 1976.

Pulec JL, and House WF: Part III. Preoperative evaluation: trigeminal nerve testing in acoustic tumors. *Arch Otolaryngol* 80:681, 1964.
Pulec JL, and House WF: Part III. Preoperative evaluation: facial nerve involvement and testing in acoustic neuromas. *Arch Otolaryngol* 80:685, 1964.
Pulec JL, House WF, and Hughes RL: Part III. Preoperative evaluation: vestibular involvement and testing in acoustic neuromas. *Arch Otolaryngol* 80:677, 1964.
Scanlan RL: Part III. Preoperative evaluation: positive contrast medium (iophendylate) in diagnosis of acoustic neuroma. *Arch Otolaryngol* 80:698, 1964.
Spector M (ed): *Dizziness and Vertigo: Diagnosis and Treatment.* Grune & Stratton, New York, 1968.
Wortzman G, Holgate RC, Sokjer H, and Noyek AM: The role of CT scanning in the diagnosis of acoustic neuromas. *J Otolaryngol* 3 (Suppl):63, 1977.

Management

Cawthorne T: The contribution of surgery to the problems of neuro-otology. *Br Med Bull* 12:143, 1956.
Fluur E: Long term postoperative results following selective section of the vestibular nerve in Meniere's disease. *Acta Otolaryngol (Stockh)* 74:425, 1972.
House HP, and House WF: Part I. Introduction and pathology: historical review and problem of acoustic neuroma. *Arch Otolaryngol* 80:601, 1964.
House WF: Part IV. Surgical technique and complications: evolution of transtemporal bone removal of acoustic tumors. *Arch Otolaryngol* 80:731, 1964.
House WF, and Hitselberger WE: Part IV. Surgical technique and complications: total versus subtotal removal of acoustic tumors. *Arch Otolaryngol* 80:751, 1964.
House WF, and Hitselberger WE: Part IV. Surgical technique and complications: morbidity and mortality of acoustic neuromas. *Arch Otolaryngol* 80:752, 1964.
Marlowe FI: Drug treatment of Meniere's disease. *Otolaryngol Clin North Am* 6:119, 1973.
Pulec JL: Symposium on Meniere's disease. I. Meniere's disease: results of a two and one half year study of etiology, natural history and results of treatment. *Laryngoscope* 82:1703, 1972.
Rubin W: Vestibular suppressant drugs. *Arch Otolaryngol* 97:135, 1973.
Schuknecht HF: Ablation therapy in Meniere's disease. *Acta Otolaryngol (Stockh)* Suppl. 132, 1957.

7

Infections of the Nervous System

There are several classes of infection of the nervous system: bacterial, viral, mycotic, protozoal, and helminthic. The protozoal and helminthic infections of the nervous system are rare in the United States, and the diagnosis is often made only by special laboratory techniques. Meningo-encephalitis of viral origin is not uncommon, and its early recognition is important in order to avoid subjecting the patient to unnecessary diagnostic procedures; moreover, there is recent evidence that drug therapy may be effective in at least one form of viral encephalitis. Modern antibiotic therapy has made it mandatory to be able to recognize bacterial meningitis, brain abscesses, and infections of the dura early. Similarly, fungal infections of the nervous system should be identified early so the patient can receive appropriate therapy, which, although not as effective as antibiotics against bacterial infections of the nervous system, may yet be life-saving.

In practice, the clinical diagnosis of meningitis is not always easy, and the identification of the offending agent may be even more difficult, requiring repeated examinations of the cerebrospinal fluid (CSF) by a wide variety of techniques including viral isolation and antibody studies. The CSF of every patient suspected of having meningitis or encephalitis must be examined even though the symptoms may be mild. The sole exception is if a brain abscess is suspected. It is far better to do an occasional normal lumbar puncture than to miss a treatable meningitis.

BACTERIAL INFECTIONS

Acute Purulent Meningitis

The clinical manifestations of the acute meningitides caused by bacteria are generally similar, although certain features are sometimes characteristic of a specific organism. The pathology of the various types of acute purulent meningitis is characterized by an inflammatory exudate in the subarachnoid space, especially over the base of the brain (Fig. 7.1). The exudate, which

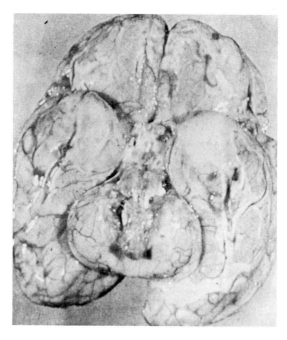

FIG. 7.1. Bacterial meningitis. Purulent exudate covers the entire surface of the brain, which is extremely edematous. The cranial nerves are bathed in pus.

early consists primarily of polymorphonuclear neutrophils (PMNs), spreads along the sheaths of the cranical nerves and into the perivascular sheaths. The inflammation usually involves the arterial and venous walls, and it is this vasculitis which is thought to be responsible for the neurologic signs that occur in the disease by causing ischemic changes in the superficial layers of the cortex, followed by brain edema. Cortical thrombophlebitis may occur late in the illness and cause areas of hemorrhagic infarction, resulting in seizures and other neurologic deficits. Occasionally the arteritis caused by the purulent material results in arterial thrombosis and brain infarction. The exudates caused by the various bacteria may have some distinguishing characteristics. The exudate of pneumococcal meningitis, for example, is thick, full of fibrin, and often loculated because of the absence of a proteolytic enzyme in the purulent material. As the exudate resolves, the arachnoidal membrane may remain thickened and scarred, with adhesions between the arachnoid and pia and arachnoid and dura. These adhesions may be responsible for the obstruction of the foramina of Luschka and Magendie and for impairment of function of the arachnoidal villi, resulting in hydrocephalus. Thus the pathology of acute purulent meningitis involves more than the meninges, as would be expected from the clinical signs of the illness.

Symptoms and Signs of Bacterial Meningitis

Many of the clinical characteristics of acute bacterial meningitis are similar regardless of the offending organism. The onset is similar to that of any acute infectious illness, with anorexia, chills, fever, weakness, and headache, but the development of a stiff and painful neck points to the presence of meningeal infection. Shortly thereafter the neck pain and stiffness become more severe, and positive Brudzinski's and Kernig's signs appear along with restlessness, photophobia, and in severe cases stupor and coma. Convulsive seizures may occur in adults but are more common in children. Cranial nerve pathology, particularly 6th nerve paresis and deafness, occur in at least one-fourth of severely ill patients. The symptoms may be mild and slowly progressive, or they may be extremely severe and catastrophically sudden.

Recognition of acute bacterial meningitis may be difficult in infants because there may be no meningeal signs. Nonlocalizing symptoms (e.g., fever, vomiting, irritability, respiratory distress) and abdominal pain are frequent, but the earliest sign of central nervous system (CNS) involvement may be convulsions or a bulging fontanelle. Infantile meningitis is most frequently caused by gram-negative bacteria, and the mortality rate in infants is several times greater than in adults.

Three organisms are responsible for approximately 80% of acute bacterial meningitis in adolescents and adults. These are Neisseria meningitidis, Diplococcus pneumoniae, and Haemophilus influenzae.

Meningococcic meningitis (Fig. 7.2) is frequently seen in epidemics, the infection being spread through respiratory passages by carriers, particularly in overcrowded barracks or schools. Nevertheless, it frequently appears sporadically. It occurs primarily during the first year of life and between the ages of 15 and 30. Bacteremia precedes the meningitis; purpura is common in meningococcemia and may produce localized skin necrosis. The presence of generalized purpura together with signs of meningitis almost invariably means that the offending organism is meningococcus (N. meningitidis). Septicemia may produce collapse and death, sometimes associated with adrenal hemorrhage (Waterhouse-Friderichsen syndrome). Neurologic sequelae are rare if the patient is treated early, but the mortality rate is still significant, mainly because of delayed diagnosis and inadequate treatment.

Pneumococcal meningitis should be suspected when there is associated infection in the middle ear or sinuses or in the presence of pneumonitis or cardiac valvular disease. Splenectomy and sickle cell disease are also reported to predispose to pneumococcal infection. Meningitis after a head trauma that causes a fracture of the skull base, in particular the cribriform plate, is often due to pneumococcus. Meningitis associated with chronic rhinorrhea is usually pneumococcal. Pneumococcal meningitis is treated successfully less often than that due to meningococcus because of the occur-

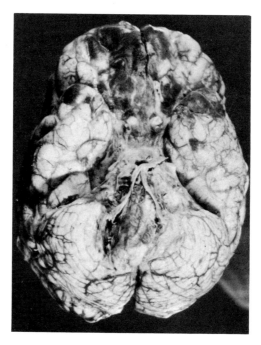

FIG. 7.2. Meningococcic meningitis. Note extensive subpial hemorrhages.

rence of loculated subarachnoid abscesses, so residual neurologic deficits are seen in about 25% of cases *of pneumococcal* .

Childhood
debilitated
adults

    Haemophilus influenzae meningitis occurs characteristically during infancy and early childhood often following ear or upper respiratory infections, but it may also occur in debilitated adults, particularly alcoholics. The clinical features are not distinctive, although subdural effusion occurs more frequently in children with *H. influenzae* meningitis than other types.

    Modern medicine has provided a setting for a variety of offending organisms to invade the subarachnoid space and CNS because patients with serious disease are kept alive longer and pharmacologic immunosuppression is a common occurrence. Meningitis in a patient with multiple furunculosis or ear, sinus, or bone infection is likely to be *Staphylococcus* or an anaerobic *Streptococcus*. Meningitis in the presence of malignancy may, of course, be due to invasion of the meninges by cancer cells, particularly in breast carcinoma, but widespread cancer and leukemia also favor infection with *Cryptococcus* or *Listeria monocytogenes*. Immunosuppressive treatment has become so frequent in the management of cancer, leukemia, multiple sclerosis, collagen vascular diseases, and in patients who have had a renal transplant that it has become necessary to recognize the increased likelihood of meningeal and CNS infection in these patients by fungi, particularly *Candida albicans* and *Cryptococcus neoformans*, and by *Listeria*, *Enterobacteriaceae*, *Pseudomonas*, and *Serratia*. Gram-negative meningitis also occurs in such patients, particularly in those with profound leukopenia.

Complications of Bacterial Meningitis

Complications occur in a significant number of patients with bacterial meningitis; proper management depends on their identification and on an understanding of their pathogenesis. The description of the pathology of bacterial meningitis given above makes it easier to understand the complications of the illness. Systemic complications are those seen with any severe infectious process and include electrolyte and fluid imbalance, shock (particularly in meningococcal infections), and disseminated intravascular coagulopathy.

Stupor and *coma* are secondary to diffuse ischemic subpial encephalopathy which results in brain swelling and increased intracranial pressure. Persistent brain swelling in the presence of evidence that the infection is responding to antibiotic therapy requires the use of steroids, specifically dexamethasone (Decadron) in doses of 24 to 36 mg intravenously daily, and/or the use of hyperosmolar agents, e.g., mannitol, urea, or glycerol. Persistent brain swelling may cause herniation and impaction of the cerebellar tonsils.

Convulsive seizures occur most frequently in children. Persistent seizures point to cortical thrombophlebitis as a cause, or they may be due to the diffuse vasculitis and ischemic encephalopathy already described. Treatment is by the methods described in Chapter 10. Persistent seizures in meningitis denote a poor prognosis for complete recovery.

Cranial nerve palsies are caused by pus bathing the cranial nerves, undoubtedly obliterating vasa nervorum and causing infarctions. Extraocular palsies, optic atrophy, and deafness are most frequently seen. There is no treatment other than vigorous control of the infection.

Hydrocephalus is a dread complication of meningitis that occurs more often in children than adults. It may be caused by inflammatory exudate obstructing the foramina of Luschka and Magendie or the Pacchionian villi. Rarely, aqueductal obstruction occurs. The clinical features include evidence of progressively increasing intracranial pressure, which in infants is accompanied by suture separation, widening of the fontanelles, and enlargement of the head. In adults the communicating hydrocephalus presumably caused by injury to the Pacchionian villi may not produce symptoms for weeks or months after the acute illness has terminated. These patients may present with the triad of gait disorder, urinary incontinence, and dementia. Recognition of hydrocephalus in the adult has been greatly facilitated by the computerized axial tomography (CAT) scan, which allows prompt identification and determination of the type of shunting procedure necessary. *Subdural effusion* is seen most frequently in infants and young children, particularly in *H. influenzae* meningitis. It may be heralded by persistent fever, anorexia, vomiting, obtundation, and seizures. The diagnosis can be made by trans-illumination and confirmed by CAT scan. Percutaneous aspiration through the lateral margin of the fontanelle is usually sufficient if the infection is under control.

Diagnosis of Bacterial Meningitis

The diagnosis of bacterial meningitis is made by examination of the CSF; there is no other way. In the great majority of instances, bacterial meningitis is a dramatic clinical event, involving an obviously seriously ill patient, so the decision to perform a lumbar puncture is a straightforward one. In infants, elderly, chronically ill, or immunosuppressed patients, the clinical picture of meningitis may be sufficiently obscure that it is not immediately considered. *It is important, therefore, to emphasize again that if meningitis enters the differential diagnosis, however peripherally, lumbar puncture is essential.* That is not to say that the diagnosis of bacterial meningitis and identification of the offending organism will be easy even after the lumbar puncture is done. Acute meningoencephalitis, fungal meningitis, tuberculous meningitis, and lues may all produce a CSF formula that is difficult to differentiate from bacterial meningitis, as may other more arcane diseases which also involve the uveal structures and the oral and urethral mucosae.

The principles involved in the diagnosis and treatment of bacterial meningitis can be stated as follows:

1. *Careful* and *complete* examination of the CSF is the key.
2. Proper treatment depends on establishing the etiology.
3. Delay in treatment may greatly increase morbidity and mortality.
4. Treatment may have to be begun without establishing a definitive etiology while CSF cultures are awaited.
5. The CSF formula (cells, protein, and glucose) is not per se diagnostic of bacterial etiology, although it clearly points to the direction of therapy while awaiting (hopefully) laboratory identification of the organism.
6. Early treatment (prior to organism identification) is based on providing adequate antibiotic coverage for the likeliest offending organisms. This means, by definition, that broad-spectrum antibiotic coverage is essential in the early stages of treatment in many patients.
7. Specific antibiotic treatment is provided as soon as the organism and its sensitivities have been identified.
8. Treatment must be continued until the fever, clinical cause, and CSF indicate recovery (sterility of CSF). This usually means a minimum of 2 weeks.

9. The principles of management of any acute systemic illness, including fluid balance, prevention of thrombophlebitis, and cardiorespiratory care must be carefully applied.

Fortunately, this system works in the majority of instances.

Lumbar Puncture and Examination

There are many myths about lumbar puncture (LP) which should be dispelled at the outset. It is basically a benign, simple procedure that should be done for a specific purpose, i.e., to look for signs of CSF infection. It is also used to look for evidence of subarachnoid bleeding in very specific circumstances but particularly when the diagnosis of primary subarachnoid hemorrhage from ruptured aneurysm is suspected. It is used much less commonly now than it once was to establish the diagnosis of intracerebral hemorrhage and dementia.

Although no procedure which requires needle puncture is entirely benign, the complications and dangers of a well-done LP are vastly overrated. Certainly LP is contraindicated in patients who clearly have a cerebral hemispheric or cerebellar mass lesion, for such lesions increase the likelihood of transtentorial uncal or cerebellar tonsillar herniation. Nevertheless the numbers of *documented* episodes of herniation caused by LP must be extremely small, even in patients with posterior fossa tumors. It is, notwithstanding, important to dispel the notion that an LP is part of a "routine" neurologic work-up. First of all, there is no such thing as a "routine" work-up; hopefully, each is individualized. The LP should not be done because the doctor does not know what else to do, and certainly it should not be done in hospital emergency rooms to clarify a problem of stupor or coma or to "see if a patient has had a stroke." Extant diagnostic sophistication obviates the necessity for such an outmoded practice, particularly since the information obtained from the majority of LPs done in those circumstances is not just incomplete but downright confusing. The consultant is often left to struggle with the question of whether the bloody CSF was caused by disease or the LP needle.

Post-LP headache does occur in a small number of patients—ironically it is usually in those individuals for whom the original indication of the procedure was questionable. Even this can be avoided or greatly reduced by two simple steps:

1. Use a 20- or 21-gauge LP needle. Make as small a dural hole as possible.

2. Immediately after the LP, place the patient in the prone position with his head 6 inches below the LP site for 2 hr. This prevents immediate CSF leak from the dural hole and allows a fibrin plug to form.

Since post-LP headache is caused by continuous leakage of CSF from the dural hole and not by the amount of CSF removed at the time of the examination, the above measures are logical and helpful.

As soon as the physician has decided that the patient may have meningitis, LP is mandatory, the sole exception being the strong suspicion of a brain abscess. Because brain abscess can now be diagnosed or at least strongly suspected by CAT scan, this caveat becomes easy to deal with. With the exception of the above points, the actual technique of the LP is not discussed further here.

Treatment of Bacterial Meningitis

The whole purpose of the CSF examination is to help determine what antibiotic or other therapeutic agent to use. As was previously mentioned, *no CSF formula is absolutely diagnostic* so that specific treatment depends ultimately on identification of the organism. There is, however, a reasonable correlation between the CSF formula and the etiology of the meningitis; and it is this correlation, imperfect as it is, which directs immediate therapy.

Although the types of CSF abnormalities are almost limitless, a few groups of patterns can be described.

1. *Frankly purulent CSF.* Usually this fluid is under very high pressure. The white blood cell (WBC) count varies from 500 to $> 20,000/mm^3$, with 85 to 95% PMNs; protein is usually > 100 mg% and may be over 2,000 mg%; glucose is less than 40 mg% but may be too low to measure. The usual ratio between blood and CSF sugar is 3:2, so blood to determine the glucose level is drawn within 15 min of the time of the LP in order to exclude the possibility that low CSF glucose was due to hypoglycemia or that a CSF glucose within a normal range (i.e., 50 mg or greater) was not caused by hyperglycemia. It is important to remember that in acute bacterial meningitis even hyperglycemia may not elevate CSF glucose significantly because of impairment of carrier-mediated glucose transport across the blood-brain barrier, together with the glycolytic action of the bacteria and WBCs in the CSF.

The above CSF picture is "classic" for acute bacterial meningitis and usually denotes that appropriate antibiotic therapy can be started. A similar CSF picture may obtain in rare instances of acute viral meningoencephalitis, early tuberculous (TBC) meningitis, and parameningeal infections. Other entities (e.g., Molleret's recurrent meningitis or Behçet's syndrome) have clinical pictures that are not likely to be confused with bacterial meningitis, although the CSF formula may resemble it.

2. *CSF pleocytosis with lymphocytic predominance.* Inadequately treated bacterial meningitis (the patient may have received one or two doses of antibiotics prior to the lumbar puncture), TBC or fungal meningitis, and rare instances of viral meningoencephalitis must all be considered in the differential diagnosis if the CSF shows a predominantly lymphocytic pleocytosis along with elevated protein and low glucose. Usually CSF glucose in these circumstances is somewhat higher than that seen in frankly purulent CSF.

Carcinomatous and sarcoid meningitis may produce a similar CSF formula, but the history of the illness and the clinical findings are usually quite different from those seen in bacterial meningitis. Lymphocytic predominance in the CSF, together with increased protein and normal glucose, is typical of viral meningoencephalitis, but TBC or fungal meningitis, brain abscess, or parasitic infections of the CNS must also be included in the differential diagnosis, along with postinfectious encephalomyelitis.

In addition to cell count, protein, and sugar, the CSF examination must include the following:

1. *Gram stain of the CSF sediment.* This frequently permits immediate identification of the organism, particularly pneumococcus or *H. influenzae*. Meningococci are more difficult to find. Artifacts from precipitated dye in the gram stain may confuse the issue.

2. *CSF culture.* These are positive in about 75% of patients with untreated bacterial meningitis. Often growth of the organisms can be seen within 24 hr, and identification and sensitivities are reported after an additional 12 hr.

3. If no organism can be seen by gram stain, a *stain for acid-fast bacilli* (TBC) is performed and a TBC culture set up. Similarly an India ink preparation and a wet smear for fungi and parasites is performed and fungal cultures (Sabaraud's medium) begun. Serologic studies for fungi and viral antibody studies are also ordered on the CSF specimen. CSF serology for lues (VDRL or FTA) should always be included, although meningovascular or parenchymatous lues is unlikely to be confused clinically with acute bacterial meningitis.

It is understood, of course, that the laboratory evaluation of the patient includes a hemogram, serum electrolytes, and blood culture, looking for any clue which will contribute to the diagnosis.

As has been repeatedly emphasized, the treatment of bacterial meningitis is a true emergency because of the dire consequences of delay. If the clinical picture and CSF formula suggest the diagnosis of bacterial meningitis, treatment must be initiated even though the infecting organism has not been identified.

If the organism is unknown, the following regimens should be instituted:

1. *Adults:* Because *H. influenzae* is unlikely in adolescents or adults, treatment is directed mainly at meningococci or pneumococci. Drugs of choice are: penicillin G (2 million units i.v. every 2 hr) or ampicillin (2 g i.v. every 4 hr). An alternative approach is the combination of erythromycin (1 g i.v. q.i.d.) plus chloramphenicol (1 g i.v. q.i.d.).

2. *Young children:* Combination of chloramphenicol (20 to 25 mg/kg i.v. q.i.d.) plus ampicillin (100 mg/kg i.v. q.i.d.).

3. *Neonates:* Ampicillin (40 mg/kg i.v. b.i.d.) plus gentamicin (2.5 mg/kg i.v. t.i.d.).

Upon identification of the infecting organism with its sensitivities, the antibiotic is appropriately changed. *H. influenzae* meningitis can usually be successfully treated with ampicillin; but if the organism is insensitive to ampicillin, chloramphenicol is used. Further principles of antibiotic therapy are beyond the scope of this book.

In addition to the proper adjunctive medical therapy, patients with severe meningococcal septicemia may require adrenal cortical therapy. Management of common complications has already been remarked.

Tuberculous Meningitis

Despite the progressive decrease in the incidence of tuberculosis in western countries, TBC meningitis still occurs with sufficient frequency that pediatricians, generalists, internists, and neurologists should be sensitive to its special problems in diagnosis and management. It usually develops subacutely rather than dramatically, but the clinical signs are similar to those described for purulent meningitis except more chronic and protracted. The exudate is mainly at the base of the brain, although tubercles may be scattered everywhere in the brain including the ependymal surfaces of the ventricles. Arteritis with resulting cerebral infarction is not uncommon, and hydrocephalus and cranial nerve palsies are frequent complications of the poorly treated disease. Other foci of tuberculosis can be found in 75 to 80% of patients with TBC meningitis, and the tuberculin skin test is positive in over 90%.

The CSF formula has been previously described and is quite variable. Usually mononuclear cells predominate (50 to 1,000 cells/mm^3), the protein is quite elevated, and the glucose around 25 to 40 mg%. When the CSF is centrifuged, a pellicle forms; this pellicle should be stained for acid-fast organisms and meticulously examined. Microscopic identification may obviate a wait of 4 to 6 weeks for the growth of the organism *in vitro*.

In most instances treatment must be begun before there is positive identification of the organism; such a decision is therefore a clinical one. Once begun, the patient is committed to treatment until its completion 18 to 24 months later, even though no organism is ever positively identified and the patient appears clinically well. The relapse rate in incompletely treated TBC meningitis is substantial.

The following medications are used:

1. INH (isoniazid) 15 mg/kg/day. Pyridoxine 50 mg daily accompanies this to prevent INH-induced neuropathy or encephalopathy.
2. Rifampin 600 mg/day.
3. Ethambutol 20 mg/kg/day.
4. In severe, critically ill patients, streptomycin 20 mg/kg/day for 4 to 6 weeks.

Other Intracranial Purulent Infections

Brain Abscess

Despite the benefits which have resulted from a combination of antibiotic therapy and surgery, brain abscess remains a serious problem, with significant mortality and morbidity in the form of residual neurologic deficit in about 25% of patients. About 60% of brain abscesses are caused by contiguous spread from infections in the middle ear and mastoid (40%) or from the paranasal sinuses or nasal cavity (20%). The remaining 40% are either metastatic from infections in the lung, skin, teeth, or long bones, or from an acute ulcerative endocarditis; or the source is never found. Patients with congenital heart disease with a right-to-left shunt (viz., tetrology of Fallot) are susceptible to brain abscess because of the absence of the pulmonary filter, so the occurrence of any signs of focal brain disease in a child or adult with a known congenital heart lesion should immediately raise the suspicion of abscess.

The mechanisms responsible for brain invasion by an infection in a contiguous cranial site are not perfectly understood. It is thought that local osteomyelitis is followed by a track of infection which somehow penetrates the brain substance rather than the parameningeal spaces. As is described below, occasionally frontal sinus infection spreads to the subdural space rather than involving the brain parenchyma. The bacterial invasion of the brain at first causes a local "cerebritis" consisting of necrotic tissue and inflammatory exudate, with indistinct margins and surrounding edema. Fibroblastic proliferation begins to form a capsule around the center of the infected area within a few days. The wall of the capsule is eventually comprised of collagenous connective tissue, but infection may still extend from the center of the abscess to contiguous brain, and it is this extension and eventual rupture into the ventricular system which is responsible for a fatal termination in some instances (Fig. 7.3).

The signs of an abscess depend, of course, on its localization. Ear and mastoid infections cause abscesses in the adjacent inferior temporal lobe or cerebellar hemisphere, whereas sinus and nasal infections spread to the frontal or anterior temporal lobes. The resulting neurologic deficits are appropriate to the anatomic location in the brain. In addition, headache, fever, subacute systemic illness, obtundation, and seizures may be present. The *absence of evidence of infection [no fever, low WBCs, low erythrocyte sedimentation rate (ESR)] does not exclude abscess, and the origin of the infection may not be immediately obvious or easily discovered.*

The diagnosis is based on the chemical signs and the CAT scan, which is usually characterized by a ring of increased density, with adjacent brain edema (Fig. 7.4). Mass effect from the abscess is common. Angiography confirms the presence of an avascular mass lesion. If there is an obvious

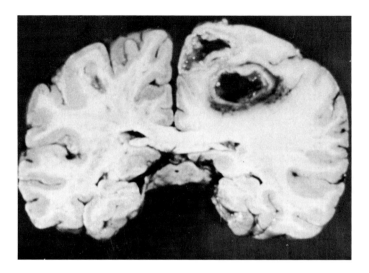

FIG. 7.3. Multiple brain abscesses. Note encapsulation and massive adjacent edema.

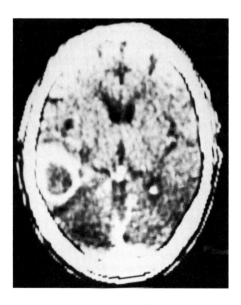

FIG. 7.4. Large left temporoparietal lobe abscess with heavily enhancing ring which probably represents the capsule. Note that there appears to be little or no adjacent edema and no mass effect as evidenced by ventricular shift. One reason for this may have been that there was another large abscess in the right middle fossa (temporal lobe).

source of infection, the diagnosis can be made with assurance, but otherwise direct examination of the tissue may be required.

If an abscess is suspected, LP should be avoided because of the proved increased risk of herniation. In the first stages of abscess formation, the CSF usually shows pleocytosis (PMNs and mononuclear cells), mildly increased protein, and normal glucose. Following encapsulation, the CSF may be normal.

The theory behind modern therapy is to delay surgical excision or drainage of the abscess until the most favorable time, which is when the encapsulation is complete and the infection and edema best controlled. If a source of infection (ear, mastoid, sinus, blood) can be identified, it is possible to deduce the identity of the organism causing the abscess and to use the appropriate antibiotic at once. If this information is not available, initial therapy is begun with penicillin and chloramphenicol as described under *Treatment of Bacterial Meningitis*, above, but it is essential to use every clue derived from a careful evaluation of the patient to provide the best antibiotic coverage. Control of edema is by dexamethasone in doses of 24 to 30 mg i.v. daily, with progressive and judicious reductions.

The best time for surgical intervention is when the clinical picture and CAT scan indicate encapsulation and decreased edema, but it should not be delayed if there is evidence of a poor response to antibiotics.

Subdural Empyema

Typically, subdural empyema occurs in boys or young men with acute frontal or maxillary sinusitis, and less commonly from aural infection. These patients usually have severe pain localized to the area of the infected sinus followed by generalized headache, nausea, vomiting, and dehydration leading to stupor and coma. Focal hemispheric signs (seizure, hemiparesis, aphasia, etc.) are common, and the patient invariably shows systemic signs of infection.

The subdural collection of pus may migrate over the entire hemisphere, even extending to the interhemispheric fissure. Spread is partially determined by gravity. The damage to brain tissue is secondary to septic thrombophlebitis and arteritis.

Diagnosis is made from the clinical picture as described. CAT scan may not be specifically diagnostic, although a space-occupying nonenhancing subdural lesion can usually be seen. Angiography may be helpful by showing the characteristic medial displacement of cortical vessels.

Treatment is by immediate surgical drainage, preceded by at least one massive dose of antibiotic (ampicillin or penicillin and chloramphenicol) and followed by antibiotic therapy dictated by the organism found in the pus. Prompt treatment of the infected sinus or ear is also essential. This is a life-threatening illness which requires immediate and aggressive management.

Epidural Spinal Abscess

Fortunately epidural spinal abscesses are uncommon lesions. The clinical presentation may be no different from that which occurs in metastatic disease of the spine: (1) local back pain not always accompanied by nerve root pain; (2) signs (of varying rapidity) of spinal cord compression (viz., weakness of the legs, numbness, and sensory abnormalities below the site of the lesion), and (3) usually last, sphincter disturbances, which may be urinary urgency and incontinence or urinary retention with or without fecal incontinence. The actual physical findings depend on the vertical localization of the abscess—which level of the spinal cord or cauda equina is compressed. The syndromes associated with pathology at various levels of the spinal cord or cauda equina are discussed in some detail in Chapter 15.

Unless there is clear evidence of an infectious etiology, spinal epidural abscess may be mistaken for metastatic disease. The evidence includes the presence of furunculosis, recent septicemia, fever, elevated WBC count in the hemogram, and elevated ESR. X-ray films of the area suspected may show osteomyelitis of a vertebral body. It is nevertheless important to point out that all of the above can also occur with metastatic disease or lymphomas, which are the commoner causes of this syndrome.

Spinal epidural abscesses constitute emergencies. The location of the block must be established by myelography. The lower and upper margins of the lesion should be identified. The CSF usually has a few PMNs, increased protein, and normal glucose. Great care must be taken not to pass the LP needle through the abscess into the subarachnoid space. If an abscess is suspected, an effort can be made to aspirate a few milliliters of pus by needle for gram stain and culture. The commonest organisms are *Staphylococcus aureus* or *Staph. pyogenes*.

Once the diagnosis is established, high-dose penicillin and gentamicin are started and the abscess drained surgically. Subsequent antibiotic therapy depends on the results of cultures of the pus obtained at operation. The value of high-dose dexamethasone (24 to 40 mg daily i.v.) to minimize spinal cord edema has not been clearly established, but it probably should be used in patients whose symptoms and signs denote severe cord or cauda equina compression.

Cavernous Sinus Thrombosis

Cavernous sinus thrombosis is a dramatic clinical event usually caused by infection in the nose or the paranasal sinuses, particularly the ethmoid and sphenoid. The patient appears toxic and has a severe headache. These are followed or accompanied by periorbital swelling on the involved side, chemosis, proptosis, ophthalmoplegia, papilledema, and retinal edema and hemorrhages. Numbness over the first division of the 5th cranial nerve is common (cranial nerves III, IV, V, and VI all lie in the lateral wall of the cavernous sinus). Thrombosis of the intracavernous portion of the internal carotid artery has been reported.

The differential diagnosis includes nasopharyngeal carcinoma and mucormycosis or other fungus infections. The CSF may be normal. The diagnosis is not difficult to make clinically; unfortunately, therapy is not uniformly effective. The choice of antibiotic depends on the offending organism; until it is identified, penicillin and gentamicin are the drugs of choice.

MYCOTIC INFECTIONS

Fungal meningitis and CNS abscesses have increased strikingly during the past 10 years *pari passu* with the increased use of immunosuppressive agents and powerful cell toxins used in the treatment of cancer, as well as the aggressive use of immunosuppressants in the management of patients with organ transplants, and in the treatment of a variety of diseases, including collagen vascular diseases, polymyositis, myasthenia gravis, and multiple sclerosis. Suppression of immunologic protection against infection by drugs or disease allows other types of opportunistic infection in additon to fungi, particularly gram-negative rods, toxoplasmosis, and certain viruses, viz., papovavirus and herpes simplex and zoster. Specific types of cancer appear to be accompanied by specific CNS infections. Patients with lymphoma, leukemia, or tumor of the head or spine have the largest percentage of CNS infections. The responsible organisms vary from hospital to hospital and from time to time within the same hospital.

The clinical picture of fungal infection of the nervous system is indistinguishable from chronic meningitis or brain abscess. Fungal etiology is suspected because of the presence of predisposing illness or treatment (systemic cancer, immunosuppressant therapy, debilitation, drug addiction, liver disease, diabetes). Some CNS fungal infections occur without obvious predisposing cause, specifically coccidiomycosis and histoplasmosis. The former occurs mainly in the southwestern part of the United States and ordinarily produces a benign pneumonitis; invasion of the CNS, however, is fatal in at least 50% of patients, even with prompt treatment with amphotericin B.

Cryptococcal meningitis is the commonest fungal infection of the nervous system. It is often associated with a predisposing illness as described above. It may run a fulminant course or be quite indolent. The clinical picture resembles TBC meningitis.

Other fungi which invade the nervous system in a setting of altered immunologic responses include *Candida*, *Asperigillus*, and *Nocardia*. Of these, *Candida* is probably the most frequent, particularly in severely burned patients and individuals with prolonged intravenous alimentation. Mucormycosis is a particularly destructive fungus invasion which begins in the nose and paranasal sinuses and spreads to the retro-orbital soft tissue and thence to the brain. It causes a severe vasculopathy with arterial and venous occlusion and cerebral infarction. It occurs mainly in the setting of severe diabetes, usually in a patient in diabetic ketosis, although it has also been reported in patients with lymphoma or those who have been immunosuppressed. Diabetic control and amphotericin B comprise the treatment of choice. The prognosis is extremely grave.

Diagnosis of Mycotic Infections

The diagnosis of fungal meningitis may be difficult. All of the above clinical characteristics are taken into consideration, but there may be nothing distinctive about the illness. The temporal profile may be subacute to chronic; signs include malaise, weight loss, cranial nerve pathology, headache, and indications of hydrocephalus. Coccidiomycosis can sometimes be diagnosed by biopsy of a skin lesion or lymph node. Mucormycosis may be identified by direct nasal smear. Diagnosis of fungal infection depends, of course, on examination of the CSF, which always shows an abnormality consisting of mononuclear pleocytosis (usually less than 1,000/ml³), increased protein, and (not invariably) decreased glucose. This CSF formula does not establish fungal etiology, however. That depends on further examination of the CSF, including gram stain, India ink preparation, culture on Sabaraud's medium,

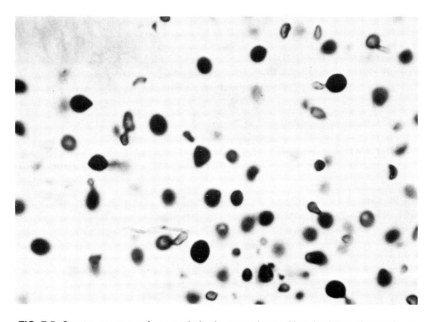

FIG. 7.5. *Cryptococcus neoformans* in brain parenchyma. Note budding of organisms.

and testing for fungal antigens. *Cryptococcus neoformans* may be identified by gram stain or India ink preparation, allowing early presumptive diagnosis (Fig. 7.5).

Treatment of Mycotic Infections

The treatment of fungal invasion of the CNS is fraught with toxicity and complications. Therefore before treatment is begun, the diagnosis should either be established absolutely or be so strongly presumptive that the risks of treatment can be accepted. Amphotericin B is the only drug of proved therapeutic value for any of the fungi. It is given intravenously in doses beginning at 0.5 mg/kg/day in patients with *Cryptococcus* infection to as much as 1.5 mg/kg/day for patients with *Aspergillus* infection. Subarachnoid injection of the drug is utilized if there is no evidence of response to intravenous injection; intraventricular administration through an Ommaya reservoir is recommended in coccidiomycosis. The major complications of amphotericin treatment are nausea, vomiting, chills, fever, headache, and faintness, but the most serious toxicity is renal. Renal impairment is permanent in a significant number of otherwise successfully treated patients, and evidence of progressing renal toxicity [rising blood urea nitrogen level (BUN)] requires careful reevaluation of dosage and consideration of temporary cessation of therapy. Hypokalemia is a common complication of amphotericin therapy, requiring supplementary potassium replacement.

NEUROSYPHILIS

The ubiquitous use of antibiotics is probably responsible for the modification of the classic clinical picture of neurosyphilis that was so familiar to physicians 30 years ago. The flagrant syndromes of paresis or tabes dorsalis are rare in the United States today. These included progressive psychotic behavior with a strong delusional system and poor judgment, and eventually progressive erosion of motor and language functions, as was consistent with the pathology of cerebral vasculopathy and parenchymatous invasion of brain tissue by the spirochete. The classic features of tabes dorsalis were lightning pains around the trunk, impotence, urinary retention, loss of proprioceptive functions in the lower extremities with resultant gait abnormalities, Charcot joints, Argyll-Robertson pupils, and primary optic atrophy. Syphilitic meningitis was seen during the septicemia which characterized secondary lues.

These caricatures are uncommon. Neurosyphilis should be suspected in individuals with otherwise unexplained central or peripheral nervous system disorders, unexplained dementia, or pupils that react more briskly to accommodation than to light. Additional suspicious symptoms and signs include severe impairment of vibration and position sensibilities in the lower extremities with absent deep tendon reflexes, urinary retention and diminished bladder sensitivity, painless joint deformities in the lower extremities, progressive unexplained visual loss, and unexplained orthostatic hypotension.

The Venereal Disease Research Laboratory serology test (VDRL) is not an effective screening test for neurosyphilis, whether in blood or CSF. If CNS lues is suspected, the fluorescent treponema antibody test (FTA) on the patient's blood is indicated; it is particularly sensitive in the detection of late seronegative lues. Preferred treatment is benzathine penicillin G, 2.4 million units i.m. weekly for 4 weeks. Tetracycline or erythromycin in doses of 500 mg orally q.i.d. for 20 days can be used in patients who are allergic to penicillin.

VIRAL DISEASES OF THE NERVOUS SYSTEM

Meningoencephalitis

The clinical picture of meningoencephalitis ranges from innocuous to devastating, depending on the viral etiology. Mild cases may be characterized by only headache, stiff neck, fever and mild systemic symptoms, e.g., aching, anorexia, nausea, diarrhea, and rash. In these cases the illness is usually brief (less than 14 days) and recovery complete. The diagnosis is made by examination of the CSF, which reveals a modest mononuclear pleocytosis, with little or no elevation of protein and normal glucose. No organisms can be found by smear or culture. The diagnosis of viral infection is usually inferred because the illness is self-limited; occasionally, associated symptoms or signs suggest the etiologic agent. These include parotitis, orchitis, and oophoritis of mumps or the associated lymphadenopathy and positive serum heterophile antibody test of infectious mononucleosis. Otherwise diagnosis is made by serologic tests and viral isolations, all of which are negative in at least one-third of cases. The commonest causes are probably the enteroviruses, Coxsackie virus, echovirus, and nonparalytic poliomyelitis virus, but mumps virus, lymphocytic choriomeningitis virus, adenoviruses, and herpes simplex are also offenders. Each of these organisms is capable of producing a virulent infection.

Since no treatment is indicated or available, the diagnosis is academic so long as the patient is improving. It must be remembered that the clinical syndrome and CSF formula described above are no guarantee of virus etiology, and the possibility of TBC or fungal meningitis, carcinomatous meningitis, inadequately treated bacterial meningitis, or sarcoid must always be included in the differential diagnosis.

Severer cases show clear and definite signs of nervous system involvement, the extent and type depending on the virus. The common causes are the arbo (arthropod-borne) viruses, all of which have seasonal incidence and therefore tend to occur in clusters, and herpes simplex encephalitis, a sporadic form of encephalitis which is extremely serious and for which there is thought to be effective drug therapy. The mode of transmission is from infected host (bird or animal) to man by mosquitoes; the more frequent types include St. Louis encephalitis, Japanese B encephalitis, Western equine encephalitis, and, probably least common, eastern equine encephalitis. The clinical picture includes fever, headache, nuchal rigidity, confusion, seizures, delirium, corticospinal tract signs, cranial nerve palsies, cerebellar signs, myoclonus, and coma. These occur in various combinations and with varying severity. Residual defects—specifically dementia, seizures, blindness, deafness, aphasia, and motor abnormalities—occur in 5 to 50% of patients. Overall mortality for viral encephalitis is at least 10%. Diagnosis depends on the clinical picture, the CSF formula (which is similar to that described above), and serologic and special viral isolation tests. There is no effective treatment.

Herpes Simplex Encephalitis

Herpes simplex encephalitis merits special mention because it is the most frequent form of sporadic severe meningoencephalitis, occurring in all ages. It is caused by type 1 herpes simplex virus, which is also responsible for the oral mucosal lesions, although no association between the two locations of infection has been found. The clinical picture is similar to that of the other viral encephalitides, but there is the added feature of temporal lobe signs, e.g., gustatory or olfactory hallucinations, psychotic behavior, temporal lobe seizures with automatisms, and memory disturbance. Aphasias and hemiparesis are frequent. The CSF is often under increased pressure and differs from the usual findings in viral encephalitis because of the presence of red blood cells, increased protein, and infrequently decreased glucose.

The lesions appear to be localized mainly to the medial portions of the temporal lobes and inferior portions of the frontal lobes, which are hemorrhagic, necrotic, and edematous. Uncal herniation is a common cause of death. The CAT scan may be helpful by revealing the temporal lobe location of the lesions (enhancing areas of decreased density with mass effect). The electroencephalogram (EEG) may show high-voltage spike wave forms in the temporal regions. Angiography may reveal a temporal lobe mass indistinguishable from a tumor.

Diagnosis can be made only by fluorescent antibody staining and viral culture from tissue obtained at brain biopsy.

The mortality is high, probably about 50%. Survivors have a high incidence of neurologic sequelae, particularly Korsakoff's syndrome and seizures. Because (1) early symptoms may be nonspecific, (2) there is evidence that to be effective treatment must be initiated early, and (3) the drug appears to have few serious toxic effects, treatment with adenine arabinoside together with dexamethasone should be initiated at once in patients with sporadic meningoencephalitis that fits the general picture described above. Seizure control with phenytoin or other anticonvulsants is also usually necessary in the acute stage of the illness.

Herpes Zoster

Herpes zoster is believed to be a reactivation of a latent varicella virus infection. It occurs sporadically and in patients in whom there is almost always a history of chickenpox. It is contagious only to a person who has not had chickenpox. The virus has a predilection for the cells of the dorsal root ganglia and specific cranial nerve ganglia. The most frequent area of involvement is between D5 and D10. In the cranial nerves, the first division of the sensory portion of the 5th nerve (herpes ophthalmicus) and the facial nerve (geniculate herpes) are most commonly involved, but the sensory ganglia of cranial nerves 9 and 10 may also be the site of infection, although much less frequently.

The virus appears to migrate from its site of infestation in the dorsal root ganglion to the skin, resulting in an eruption of vesicles on an erythematous base. The eruption is often preceded by itching and radicular pain, and is usually accompanied by intense pain and dysesthesia. During the acute stage the virus can often be recovered from the vesicles. The rash usually lasts 10 to 14 days and commonly leaves sensitive pigmented scars. Involvement of the cornea in herpes ophthalmicus may cause scarring. In geniculate herpes the vesicles are seen on the eardrum and in the external canal, and are accompanied by facial palsy (Ramsey-Hunt syndrome). In the majority of instances only one dermatome is involved in the infection, but involvement of two or more adjacent dermatomes is not uncommon.

There is no specific treatment for the infection. The association of symptomatic herpes zoster with lymphoma, particularly in patients who have had radiation therapy and splenectomy, is well recognized. Lymphoma should be suspected in an otherwise well patient who develops herpes zoster. There is not complete accord about the role of steroids in the management of acute herpes; some consider that they increase the possibility of more extensive spread of the infection.

Posthepatic pain is a major problem, occurring in various degrees in about 50% of elderly patients. The spontaneous burning pain is associated with dysesthesia of the skin at the site of the vesicles; it may persist for months, resulting in severe depression, which should be treated pharmacologically. Drugs which have proved most successful in the management of this particular chronic pain problem include phenytoin, carbamazepine, and amitriptyline HCl. Surgical treatment should be eschewed because it is seldom effective.

Poliomyelitis

Poliomyelitis has become extremely rare in the United States since the introduction of the Salk and Sabin vaccines. It is a highly communicable disease caused by an enterovirus which produces only minor flu-like symptoms in 95% of infected persons. In paralytic polio the clinical picture is that of an acute febrile illness accompanied by muscle aching and asymmetrical paralyses of the lower motor neuron type. Signs of meningitis are common, and the CSF shows pleocytosis (up to 500 cells) with PMNs predominating early and mononuclear cells later, elevated protein, and normal glucose. The virus attacks the anterior horn cells of the spinal cord and the bulbar nuclei in a scattered distribution. Although there is no specific treatment, involvement of the bulbar nuclei, the nuclei which innervate the respiratory muscles, requires early tracheostomy and respiratory care. Care to details of nursing and medical problems is important during the early stage of the disease because the extent of recovery is unpredictable.

Rabies

Rabies is a uniformly fatal viral disease of the brain which is extremely rare in Western countries. It is caused by the bite of a rabid animal (e.g., dogs, cats, squirrels, bats, skunks, foxes), which innoculates the victim with the virus; the virus eventually gains access to the brain by spread along the peripheral nerves. The incubation period varies from 7 days to 3 months, and the clinical picture is that of a period of headache and fever, followed by psychomotor hyperactivity, confusion, severe dysphagia characterized by laryngeal spasm when attempting to swallow liquids, spasms of the facial muscles, and eventually coma and death. The pathology is distinctive and diagnostic; aside from perivascular cuffing and other signs of inflammation, there are Negri bodies and eosinophilic cytoplasmic inclusion bodies, mainly in the hippocampus but to a lesser extent in all cerebral neurons.

Animal bites are extremely common in the United States, but proper precautions against rabies infection are infrequently taken. The animal should be quarantined for 10 days. If signs of illness appear, it should be killed and the refrigerated brain sent for appropriate laboratory tests, particularly fluorescent antibody determinations. If the animal is found to be rabid or if it was a wild animal that escaped, the patient should receive human rabies immune globulin, one-half intravascularly and one-half infiltrated around the wound. This generates passive immunity long enough for the patient to receive active immunization with duck embryo vaccine.

Slow Viral Infections

The identification of a viral etiology for chronic, progressive neurologic disorders has been a major scientific advance, broadening our concept of the pathogenesis of neurologic disease and stimulating research into the possible viral etiology of a number of neurologic diseases. The prototypes of slow viral infections are scrapie and visna, transmissible diseases of sheep, with known incubation periods of up to 4 years and with different pathologies. Scrapie causes neuronal degeneration without evidence of inflammation, and the causative agent cannot be identified as a true virus. Visna, on the other hand, is a disease of white matter with extensive demyelinization and evidence of inflammation, and its etiologic agent is readily identifiable as a virus.

Of the five chronic human neurologic disorders which have been identified as being caused by transmissible agents and are called slow viral infections, two—Jakob-Creutzfeldt disease (subacute transmissible spongioform encephalopathy) and kuru—are caused by agents which do not have the characteristics of typical viruses in that they do not cause immune responses, cannot be visualized by electron microscopy, and are not affected by physical-chemical manipulations which inactivate ordinary viruses. In this sense they resemble scrapie.

Jakob-Creutzfeldt disease is characterized by rapidly developing dementia, myoclonus, stupor, and coma. It is worldwide in distribution and sporadic, with a positive family history in 5 to 10% of cases. The disease is of short duration. The patient may progress from essentially normal function to death within 6 weeks. The EEG shows periodic high-voltage spikes on a diffusely slow background. The CAT scan shows no typical changes, and the CSF is normal. The pathology is characteristic, consisting of cytoplasmic vacuolation of neurons and astrocytes with neuronal loss; the overall appearance is that of spongy gray matter without evidence of inflammation (Fig. 7.6). The

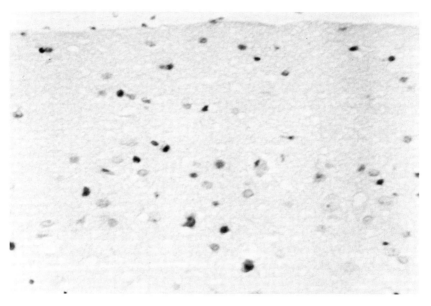

FIG. 7.6. Subacute transmissible spongioform encephalopathy (Jakob-Creutzfeldt syndrome). Note areas of vacuolation and neuronal destruction. The spongioform appearance is typical.

disease has been transmitted to chimpanzees, cats, and guinea pigs; the clinical picture in the chimpanzee is similar to that seen in humans.

The mode of transmission of the disease is not understood, although it is now clear that tissue transmission occurs in humans as evidenced by at least one corneal transplant and following stereotactic recording in two patients, the electrodes having previously been used on a patient with Jakob-Creutzfeldt disease. The transmissibility of the agent has caused concern about the hospital management of the patients, but respiratory or enteric isolation procedures are not recommended. All needles or instruments which have had contact with the patient's tissues must be autoclaved for 1 hr at 121°C and 15 psi or soaked in 5% hypochloride, 0.3% permanganate, phenolic, or iodine solutions. If the patient is autopsied, all tissues must be handled and disposed of with care because they are potentially infectious and the autopsy table and instruments specially treated with hypochloride solution.

Kuru is now mainly of historic interest because it is confined to the Fore group of highland New Guinea natives; moreover, since the suppression of ritual cannibalism, the mode by which kuru was believed to be transmitted, the incidence of the disease has greatly decreased. It is presumed to have an incubation period of 4 to 25 years, and the clinical syndrome is mainly that of severe cerebellar ataxia followed by mental status changes. The pathology is not dissimilar from that of Jakob-Creutzfeldt disease, with severe vacuolation in the cytoplasm of neurons, neuronal loss, and secondary gliosis. No virus-like particles have been seen in electron microscope studies. Transmission to primates has been successfully carried out many times. The transmissible agent has, as described above, the characteristics of that seen in scrapie.

Progressive multifocal leukoencephalopathy is seen almost exclusively in patients with lymphoma, leukemia, or sarcoid, or following immunosuppression for any reason. The clinical picture is that of relentlessly progressing dementia, visual loss, paralysis, and ataxia, leading to death in less than 1 year. The CSF is normal. The CAT scan characteristically shows nonenhancing areas of decreased density in the white matter of both hemispheres. The EEG changes are not specific.

The disease is caused by an opportunistic papovavirus infection in the brain and is characterized pathologically by extensive multifocal demyelinization; oligodendroglia adjacent to the lesions contain intranuclear inclusion bodies, and the astrocytes within the lesions are huge and show mitoses. The inclusion bodies consist of aggregates of viral particles, and JC virus and SV-40 virus have been recovered from the brains of affected patients. JC virus, which is the more frequently encountered, is ubiquitous in humans but is not known to be associated with any other disease process.

Subacute sclerosing panencephalitis (SSPE) is an uncommon, slowly progressive inflammatory disease that occurs mainly during childhood; it is caused by rubeola virus. The clinical picture is typically that of behavior alterations, deterioration of school work, myoclonus, seizures, spastic paralysis, cerebellar ataxia, dystonia, and finally blindness, coma, and decerebation. The disease usually runs its course in about 18 to 36 months, although much shorter and longer, chronic courses have also been described. Chorioretinitis, papilledema, and optic atrophy are not uncommonly seen.

The EEG shows a fairly typical pattern of high-voltage slow waves followed by a brief period of isoelectric activity. The CSF is normal except for elevated immunoglobulin G (IgG), which is oligoclonal and thought to be an antibody against measles virus. Measles antibodies are always elevated in the serum and CSF of these patients. Brain pathology consists of perivascular cuffing, mononuclear cell infiltration into the gray and white matter, and intranuclear eosinophilic inclusion bodies in neurons, oligodendroglia, and astrocytes.

Although the etiology of SSPE is the measles virus, the reason this common agent causes SSPE is not known. It has been suggested that mutations of M protein determinants occur during the replication of standard measles virus, and that early infection provides factors which encourage the mutation or somehow enhance the expression of the latent virus.

Progressive rubella panencephalitis is a rare slow virus invasion of the brain by rubella virus. Clinically it simulates SSPE, but the patients have a history or some stigmata of congenital rubella infection. Symptoms of encephalitis begin during adolescence. No inclusion bodies are seen in the brain; otherwise the pathology is similar to that of SSPE.

There is no effective treatment for any of the slow virus infections of the brain.

LESS FREQUENT CAUSES OF MENINGOENCEPHALITIS IN THE U.S.

The frequency of international travel and the continued immigration to the United States of students and political refugees from all parts of the world increase the likelihood that American physicians may encounter one of the less frequent meningoencephalitides.

The two helminthic diseases which merit mention are *trichinosis* and *cysticercosis*. The former is indigenous, and the latter is more commonly seen in South Americans. Trichinosis is the result of infestation by the organism *Trichinella spiralis* via consumption of inadequately cooked pork. The organism causes an acute illness characterized by fever, rash, subcutaneous and muscular nodules (which contain the encysted *Trichinella*), conjunctivitis, and eosinophilia. In rare instances the trichina may metastasize to the CNS, producing signs dependent on their eventual localization. Treatment is with thiabendazole and prednisone.

Cysticercosis is caused by *Taenia folium*, the pork tapeworm. The ova of this organism are ingested, and the embryos penetrate the intestinal wall from which they are carried to all organs of the body. They encyst in the brain and other organs. Neurologic signs include seizures, cranial nerve palsies, and signs of an expanding intracranial mass. Usually multiple calcified lesions are seen by x-ray in the skull and thigh muscles. CAT scan of the brain reveals the cysts. Treatment of the cerebral lesion is surgical.

Toxoplasmosis occurs in infants to whom it has been transferred *in utero*. The clinical picture includes chorioretinitis, cerebral calcifications, hydrocephalus, and psychomotor retardation, all of which may appear immediately after birth or after several months. Most infected infants die; survivors usually have a residual defect.

Acquired toxoplasmosis occurs primarily in patients who have undergone prolonged immunosuppression. The signs of a fulminant meningoencephalitis are present; the diagnosis can be presumed if there is a rising toxoplasma titer or if there is a positive fluorescent antibody test. Treatment is sulfadiazine and pyrimethamine.

Cerebral malaria is still encountered in tropical countries. It occurs in a small percentage of patients infected with *Plasmodium falciparum*. It is a dramatic, malignant disease caused by invasion of cerebral capillaries by the malarial parasites. Two rickettsial diseases are still encountered with some frequency in the United States, viz., murine typhus and Rocky Mountain spotted fever; meningoencephalitis may occur in both. Presumptive diagnosis is made by the Felix-Weil reaction; treatment is with chloramphenicol or tetracycline.

POSTINFECTIOUS ENCEPHALOMYELITIS

Some systemic viral infections, particularly rubeola and varicella, are accompanied or immediately followed by signs of encephalomyelitis, which vary in severity but which are clinically indistinguishable from viral encephalomyelitis. The mortality rate is about 25%, and there are permanent neurologic sequelae in a significant percentage of the survivors. A similar illness may follow smallpox or rabies innoculation. It is thought to be an acute myelinoclastic process caused by an immune reaction between myelin and a virus-induced antibody. In addition to perivascular foci of demyelinization, the pathology is also characterized by perivascular inflammatory cell cuffing. The CSF usually shows mononuclear pleocytosis, moderately increased protein, and normal glucose. The CSF IgG may be elevated. Treatment is with intravenous ACTH or oral prednisone.

TETANUS

Tetanus is caused by *Clostridium tetani*, an anaerobic organism that produces a powerful exotoxin that is responsible for the symptoms of the disease. The organisms are commonly found in the feces of many animals, including man, but particularly in horses. Following soil contamination, spores of the organism may remain dormant for years and are converted into the active vegetative form when they contaminate a wound, particularly when accompanied by a foreign body. Because of the ubiquity of the organism, wound contamination is probably frequent, and the decreased incidence of the disease is therefore due only to immunization. Unfortunately immunization against tetanus is not yet universal, even in industrialized Western societies, so that sporadic cases are seen in the United States and there is a substantial incidence in undeveloped countries.

The organism thrives in an anaerobic environment, generating the exotoxin tetanospasmin which is thought to ascend by way of the axis cylinder or perineural sheaths of the peripheral nerves or by hematogenous and lymphatic spread. The clinical effect of the toxin simulates that of strychnine, and its mechanism of action is thought to be by blocking the action of glycine, the putative neurotransmitter responsible for mediating most forms of postsynaptic inhibition in the spinal cord, the locus most likely being the interneurons in the central gray.

The clinical picture of the generalized form of tetanus usually begins with trismus after an incubation period which may vary from a day to 2 months. The patient complains of a sensation of stiffness and muscle spasms which shortly progresses to severe persistent muscle extensor rigidity, soon to be followed by tetanic contractions or spasms of all muscles that are precipitated by the slightest stimuli. Laryngeal and respiratory muscle spasms may cause severe hypoxia and death. The patients may die from pneumonitis, cardiovascular collapse, or asphyxia. Despite improvements in management the death rate still approaches 60%.

Local tetanus is infrequent and relatively benign. It appears after a long incubation period and is characterized by tightness and stiffness in the involved muscles with interspersed brief spasms. Recruitment spasm is characteristic. The symptoms may persist for weeks or months before disappearing spontaneously.

Delay in therapy can be fatal. A high index of suspicion early in the disease is essential. The modern intensive care unit is the proper setting for treatment. Surgical debridement of the wound; initiation of penicillin therapy for the associated bacterial infection in the wound; administration of 6,000 to 12,000 units of tetanus-immune globulin, the presently preferred form of antitoxin; and infiltration around the wound with the antitoxin are all carried out as soon as possible.

Early establishment of an airway is essential. An endotracheal tube can be utilized up to 15 days and then, if necessary, a tracheostomy performed. Blood gases should be checked frequently to prevent hypoxia or carbon dioxide retention or disturbances of acid-base balance. The room should be as dark and quiet as possible. Various regimens of sedation have been utilized, including chlorpromazine in combination with short-acting barbiturates or diazepam (Valium), to prevent or minimize the severe spasms. Tracheal toilet is painstakingly watched and mechanical respiration used if necessary. If the above measures fail to control the tetanic spasms, *d*-tubocurarine should be utilized as needed, usually in doses of 12 to 15 mg hourly intramuscularly, with the patient on a positive pressure respirator.

SELECTED READINGS

Bacterial and Tuberculous Meningitis

Appelbaum E, and Abler C: Advances in the diagnosis and treatment of acute pyogenic meningitis. I. *NY J Med* 58:204, 1958.

Appelbaum E, and Abler C: Advances in the diagnosis and treatment of acute pyogenic meningitis. II. *NY J Med* 58:363, 1958.

Ashby M, and Grant H: Tuberculous meningitis treated with cortisone. *Lancet* 1:65, 1955.

Barber M, and Waterworth PM: Activity of gentamicin against Pseudomonas and hospital staphylococci. *Br Med J* 1:203, 1966.

Barrett FF, Eardley WA, Yow MD, and Leverett HA: Ampicillin in the treatment of acute suppurative meningitis. *J Pediatr* 69:343, 1966.

Buchan GC, and Alvord EC Jr: Diffuse necrosis of subcortical white matter associated with meningitis. *Neurology (Minneap)* 19:1, 1969.

Carpenter RR, and Petersdorf RG: The clinical spectrum of bacterial meningitis. *Am J Med* 33:262, 1962.

Defuccio P, and Dresner EE: Meningococcemia with meningitis accompanied by bilateral gangrene of the lower extremities (Waterhouse-Friderichsen syndrome). *Pediatrics* 3:837, 1947.

Desmit EM: A follow-up study of 110 patients treated for purulent meningitis. *Arch Dis Child* 30:415, 1955.

Dodge PR, and Swartz MN: Bacterial meningitis—a review of selected aspects. II. Special neurologic problems, postmeningitic complications and clinicopathological correlations. *N Engl J Med* 272:954–960, 1003–1010, 1965.

Donald G, and McKendrick W: The treatment of pyogenic meningitis. *J Neurol Neurosurg Psychiatry* 31:528, 1968.

Eigler JO, Wellman WE, Rooke ED, Keith HM, and Svien HJ: Bacterial meningitis. I. General review (294 cases). *Mayo Clin Proc* 36:357, 1961.

Erickson TC, Masten MG, and Suckle HM: Complications of intrathecal use of penicillin. *JAMA* 132:561, 1946.

Feigin RD, and Dodge PR: Bacterial meningitis: newer concepts of pathophysiology and neurologic sequelae. *Pediatr Clin North Am* 23:541, 1976.

Feigin RD, and Shackelford PG: Value of repeat lumbar puncture in differential diagnosis of meningitis. *N Engl J Med* 289:571, 1973.

Fox HA, Hagen PA, Turner DJ, Glasgow LA, and Connor JD: Immunofluorescence in the diagnosis of acute bacterial meningitis: a cooperative evaluation of the technique in a clinical laboratory setting. *Pediatrics* 43:44, 1969.

Fox MJ, Kuzma JF, and Washam WT: Transitory diabetic syndrome associated with meningococcic meningitis. *Arch Intern Med* 79:614, 1947.

Graber CD, Higgins LS, and Davis JS: Seldom-encountered agents of bacterial meningitis. *JAMA* 192:956, 1965.

Hardman JM, and Earle KM: Meningococcal infections: a review of 200 fatal cases. *J Neuropathol Exp Neurol* 26:119, 1967.

Heycock JB, and Noble TC: Pyogenic meningitis in infancy and childhood. *Br Med J* 1:658, 1964.

Hosfield WB: Management and complications of acute bacterial meningitis. *Postgrad Med* 50:100, 1971.

Levin S, and Painter MB: The treatment of acute meningococcic infection in adults: a reappraisal. *Ann Intern Med* 64:1049, 1966.

Nelson E, Blinzinger K, and Hager H: An electron-microscopic study of bacterial meningitis. *Arch Neurol* 6:390, 1962.

Nyhan WL, and Richardson F: Complications of meningitis. *Annu Rev Med* 14:243, 1963.

Petersdorf RG, and Harter DH: The fall in cerebrospinal fluid sugar in meningitis. *Arch Neurol* 4:21, 1961.

Quaade F, and Kristensen KP: Purulent meningitis: a review of 658 cases. *Acta Med Scand* 171:543, 1962.

Rahal JJ Jr, Hyams PJ, Simberkoff MS, et al: Combined intrathecal and intramuscular gentamicin for gram-negative meningitis. *N Engl J Med* 290:1394, 1974.

Rahal JJ Jr, and Simberkoff MS: Bactericidal and bacteriostatic action of chloramphenicol against meningeal pathogens. *Antimicrob Agents Chemother* 16:13, 1979.

Smith JF, and Landing BH: Mechanisms of brain damage in H. influenzae meningitis. *J Neuropathol Exp Neurol* 19:248, 1960.

Swartz MN, and Dodge PR: Bacterial meningitis—a review of selected aspects. I. General clinical features, special problems and unusual meningeal reactions mimicking bacterial meningitis. *N Engl J Med* 272:725, 779, 842, 898, 1965.

Tyler R: Botulism. *Arch Neurol* 9:652, 1963.

Winkelstein A, Songster CL, Caras TS, Berman HH, and West WL: Fulminant meningococcemia and disseminated intravascular coagulation. *Arch Intern Med* 124:55, 1969.

Brain Abscess

Berg B, Franklin G, Cuneo R, Boldrey E, and Strimling B: Nonsurgical cure of brain abscess: early diagnosis and follow-up with computerized tomography. *Ann Neurol* 3:474, 1978.

Calkins RA, and Bell WE: Cerebral abscess and cyanotic congenital heart disease. *Lancet* 87:403, 1967.

Carey ME, Chou SN, and French LA: Experience with brain abscesses. *J Neurosurg* 36:1, 1972.

Duffy GP: Lumbar puncture in the presence of raised intracranial pressure. *Br Med J* 1:407, 1969.

Eberhard SJ: Diagnosis of brain abscess in infants and children: a retrospective study of twenty-six cases. *NC Med J* 30:301, 1969.

Eberhard SJ: Diagnosis of brain abscess in infants and children: a retrospective study of twenty-six cases (conclusion). *NC Med J* 30:363, 1969.

Garfield J: Management of supratentorial intracranial abscess: a review of 200 cases. *Br Med J* 1:7, 1969.

Jefferson AA, and Keogh AJ: Intracranial abscesses: a review of treated patients over 20 years. *Q J Med* 183:389 1977.

Victor M, et al: Brain abscess. *Med Clin North Am* 47:1355, 1963.

Viral Encephalitis

Adams JS: Clinical pathology of measles and sequelae. *Neurology (Minneap)* 18:52, 1968.

Appelman PH: Treatment of herpes zoster with ACTH. *N Engl J Med* 253:693, 1955.

Athanassiades T, and Nicolopoulos D: Complications of varicella. *Lancet* 2:403, 1968.

Carmon A, Behar A, and Beller AJ: Acute necrotizing haemorrhagic encephalitis presenting clinically as a space-occupying lesion: a clinico-pathological study of six cases. *J Neurol Sci* 2:328, 1965.

Cooney FD: The herpes simplex virus and the nervous system: review of the literature. *Med Am DC* 37:266, 1968.

Davis LE, and Johnson RT: An explanation for the localization of herpes simplex encephalitis. *Ann Neurol* 5:1, 1979.

Elian M: Herpes simplex encephalitis: prognosis and long term follow-up. *Arch Neurol* 32:39, 1975.

Johnson RT, and Mims CA: Pathogenesis of viral infections of the nervous system. *N Engl J Med* 278:23, 1968.

Juel-Jensen BE: Clinical spectrum of herpes simplex virus infections. *Postgrad Med J* 49:375, 1973.

Levine DP, Lauter CB, and Lerner AM: Simultaneous serum and CSF antibodies in herpes simplex virus encephalitis. *JAMA* 240:356, 1978.

McAllister RM: Viral encephalitides. *Annu Rev Med* 13:389, 1962.

Meyer HM, et al: Central nervous system syndromes of "viral" etiology. *Am J Med* 29:334, 1960.

Miller JK, Hesser F, and Tompkins VN: Herpes simplex encephalitis: report of 20 cases. *Ann Intern Med* 64:92, 1966.

Phillips CA: Inclusion bodies in measles encephalitis. *JAMA* 195:307, 1966.

Ross CAC, et al: herpes simplex meningoencephalitis. *Lancet* 2:682, 1961.

Stadler H, Oxman MN, Dawson DM, and Levin MJ: Herpes simplex meningitis: isolation of herpes simplex virus type 2 from cerebrospinal fluid. *N Engl J Med* 289:1296, 1973.

Whitley RJ, et al: *N Engl J Med* 297:289, 1977.

Zeman W, and Sever JL: Measles virus and subacute sclerosing panencephalitis. *Science* 159:451, 1968.

Slow Viruses

Gajdusek DC: Slow-virus infections of the nervous system. *N Engl J Med* 276:392, 1967.

Gajdusek DC: Unconventional viruses and the origin and disappearance of kuru. *Science* 197:943, 1977.

Gajdusek DC, Gibbs CJ Jr, Asher DM, Brown NP, Diwan A, Hoffman D, Nemo G, Rohwer R, and White L: Precautions in medical care of, and in handling materials from, patients with transmissible virus dementia (Creutzfeldt-Jakob disease). *N Engl J Med* 297:1253, 1977.

Johnson RT, and Herndon RM: Virologic studies of multiple sclerosis and other chronic and relapsing neurological diseases. *Prog Med Virol* 18:214, 1974.

Johnson RT, and ter Meulen V: Slow infections of the nervous system. *Adv Intern Med* 23:353, 1978.

Lampert PW, Gajdusek DC, and Gibbs CJ Jr: Subacute spongiform virus encephalopathies. *Am J Pathol* 68:626, 1972.

Narayan O, Penney JB Jr, Johnson RT, Herndon RM, and Weiner LP: Etiology of progressive multifocal leukoencephalopathy: identification of papovavirus. *N Engl J Med* 289:1278, 1973.

Padgett BL, Walker DL, ZuRhein GM, Hodach AE, and Chou SM: JC papovavirus in progressive multifocal leukoencephalopathy. *J Infect Dis* 133:686, 1976.

Roos R, Gajdusek DC, and Gibbs CJ Jr: The clinical characteristics of transmissible Creutzfeldt-Jakob disease. *Brain* 96:1, 1973.

Wolinsky J: Progressive rubella panencephalitis. In: *Handbook of Clinical Neurology*, Vol 34, edited by PJ Vinken and GW Bruyn. North-Holland, Amsterdam, 1978.

Viral Meningitis

Adair CV, Gauld RL, and Samdel JE: Aseptic meningitis, a disease of diverse etiology: clinical and etiologic studies on 854 cases. *Ann Intern Med* 39:675, 1953.

Hopkins AP, and Harvey PKP: Chronic benign lymphocytic meningitis. *J Neurol Sci* 18:443, 1973.

Fungal Meningitis

Appelbaum E, and Shtokalko S: Cryptococcus meningitis arrested with amphotericin B. *Ann Intern Med* 47:346, 1957.

Fitzpatrick MJ, Rubin H, and Poser CM: The treatment of cryptococcal meningitis with amphotericin B, a new fungicidal agent. *Ann Intern Med* 49:249, 1958.

Williams TW: Treatment of mycotic meningitis. *Mod Treatm* 4:951, 1967.

Subdural Empyema

Hitchcock E, et al: Subdural empyema: a review of 29 cases. *J Neurol Neurosurg Psychiatry* 27:422, 1964.

8

Multiple Sclerosis

Multiple sclerosis and related diseases characterized by demyelinization are responsible for a great deal of neurologic disability in young and middle-aged adults. The illness is worldwide in distribution, but epidemiologic evidence suggests that it is much more prevalent in colder climates. For example, prevalence in North America is approximately 40 to 60 per 100,000 population in Canada and the northern United States, as compared to 6 to 14 per 100,000 in the southern states. Studies in South Africa and Israel have shown that individuals who migrated from a high-risk to a low-risk latitude prior to age 15 have the same incidence of multiple sclerosis as the native population to which they migrated, whereas if migration took place after age 15 their incidence is the same as that in the parent country. One inference is that multiple sclerosis may be due to a delayed immune reaction to a virus infection commoner in cold climates, but this is certainly not proved. Furthermore the risk of developing multiple sclerosis is 12 to 15 times as great in a sibling of a patient with multiple sclerosis as it is in the general population, whereas there is little or no evidence of increased incidence in spouses.

Recent studies indicate an increased incidence of multiple sclerosis in families which own dogs, and another recent study supports a transmissible etiology by pointing to a cycle of increased multiple sclerosis incidence in the population of a small island off the Scottish coast coincident to the housing of British soldiers there during the war. Recently certain histocompatibility antigens have been found to be more common in patients with multiple sclerosis and their families than in control subjects.

The data suggest, but do not confirm, that a specific virus infection occurring before the age of 15 sets the stage for later development of multiple sclerosis by some type of autoimmune reaction, a reaction between myelin basic protein antibodies and an antigen that may be a viral agent.

Multiple sclerosis is usually classified as a disorder of central nervous system (CNS) myelin, for there is no doubt that the lesions in the brain and the spinal cord are confined to the white matter, and the initial primary target appears to be the myelin sheath of the axons. The tendency for dramatic

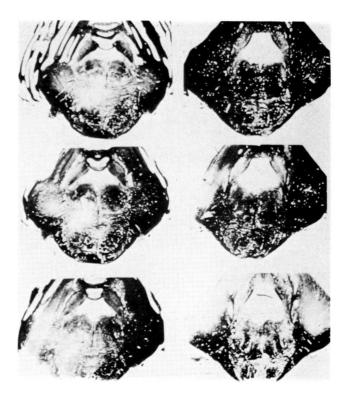

FIG. 8.1. Multiple sclerosis. Brainstem sections with myelin stain. Intact myelin stains black. The plaques are pale. Patient had internuclear ophthalmoplegia from involvement of medial longitudinal fasciculi.

improvement to occur even after severe neurologic disability is a reflection of the pathology, for the initial confinement of the pathology to the myelin spares the axons and allows recovery to take place (Figs. 8.1–8.3). Eventually, the axons themselves are destroyed, and the neurologic deficit no longer remits. In its pure form, this illness does not involve the peripheral nervous system, which has its own set of myelinopathic disorders. The sharp distinction between the diseases that attack the central and peripheral myelin sheaths speaks for the differences in the biologic structures of each and their capacities for immunologic responses. Some of the morphologic differences between central and peripheral myelin are well known, particularly that central myelin seems to be a part of the cell membrane of the oligodendroglia and that the Schwann cell is its counterpart in the peripheral nervous system.

A great deal of confusion has arisen about the term demyelinating diseases, for it may legitimately apply to any process that attacks the CNS or peripheral nervous system, ultimately resulting in a loss of the myelin sheath of the axon. In fact, demyelinization is a nonspecific process, occurring after neuronal

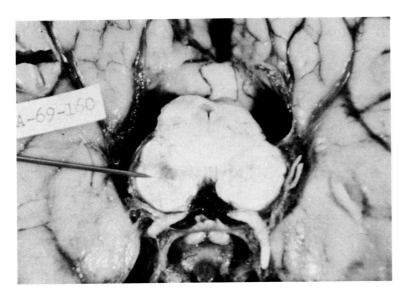

FIG. 8.2. Multiple sclerosis. Fresh plaque in cerebral peduncle.

injury, injury to the axis cylinder with subsequent Wallerian degeneration, ischemia, hypoxia, intoxication, and a host of other processes, including specific enzymatic disorders in the CNS and peripheral nervous system (e.g., cerebral lipidoses and the diffuse scleroses). Nevertheless, the term demyelinating disease has come to be associated with multiple sclerosis and related disorders and is part of the neurologist's vocabulary.

THE CLINICAL PROBLEM

As mentioned above, multiple sclerosis is primarily a disease of young adults, some 50 to 70% of patients experiencing the onset of symptoms between the ages of 20 and 40 years. Onset prior to 10 years is extremely rare; adolescent onset accounts for 10 to 15% of total cases, and onset after age 40 accounts for about 25%. The initial symptoms may reflect involvement of any part of the brain or spinal cord, but the hallmark of the disease in its early stages is that these symptoms usually cannot be explained on the basis of a single lesion. The onset is often progressive over a period of days to weeks, and the initial attack is almost invariably followed by complete remission. It was once believed that optic neuritis, characterized clinically by monocular visual loss developing over a period of hours, frequently associated with pain in the orbit and with no abnormality of the optic disc or retina initially visible to the examining physician, was a sure sign of early multiple sclerosis, but it is now recognized that other signs of multiple sclerosis follow such a lesion in fewer than half the instances.

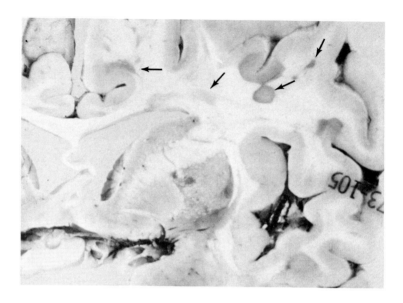

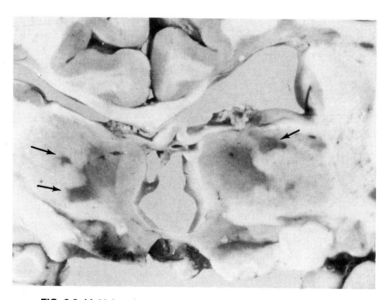

FIG. 8.3. Multiple sclerosis. Note multiple plaques (*arrows*).

Classically, then, the neurologic dysfunction consists of scattered sensory and motor defects in the head, limbs, and trunk, sphincter disturbances, special sensory defects, and occasionally defects in personality and mentation. Initially, the signs are usually asymmetrical, but in the later stages of the disease there may be extensive bilateral involvement. The patients may complain of dysesthesia, numbness and weakness of an extremity, ataxia of gait or loss of coordination, sphincter incontinence, and cranial nerve involvement resulting in slurred speech, vertigo, and double vision. The diplopia is frequently the result of a lesion involving the medial longitudinal fasciculus in the brainstem, producing internuclear ophthalmoplegia. The occurrence of this neuro-ophthalmologic syndrome in young adults is practically pathognomonic of multiple sclerosis. It consists of failure of adduction of one or both eyes on horizontal conjugate gaze. Cerebellar involvement is characterized by ataxia of gait and of one or more extremities, and by scanning speech (slow syllable pronouncing, slurring), which is caused by incoordinate articulation resulting from involvement of cerebellar pathways.

Vision defects are frequent, particularly monocular visual loss. Optic atrophy is a common finding in multiple sclerosis. Rarely, generalized or focal Jacksonian seizures may occur, and these may be confusing in the absence of other neurologic deficits pointing to the correct diagnosis.

Ordinarily, therefore, the diagnosis is suggested by the multifocal involvement of the nervous system and is strengthened by the course of the illness— which is erratic, associated with partial or complete remission—or with long quiescent intervals during which previously developed neurologic dysfunction persists.

Disturbances of mental function are rare early in the course of multiple sclerosis. Most patients are anxious and depressed over the uncertainty and potential significance of their symptomatology, but true alterations in mental function usually occur only after a number of attacks during which there has been extensive cerebral white matter involvement. Under these circumstances, there is clear evidence of disturbance of judgment and affect, and these patients sometimes appear to be inappropriately stoic in the presence of significant neurologic disorder.

A few clinical symptoms and signs common to multiple sclerosis merit comment. Facial myokymia is diagnostic of brainstem disease and is practically diagnostic of multiple sclerosis or brainstem tumor. Neuralgic pain in the distribution of the trigeminal nerve occurring in a young person should lead the examiner to consider multiple sclerosis, as should the unique buzzing, electric-like sensation which extends from the cervical spine down the back or into the upper extremities upon neck flexion or extension (Lhermitte's sign). Any lesion of the dorsal funiculi of the cervical cord may produce this dysesthesia, but it is strongly suggestive of a plaque or tumor.

The onset of multiple sclerosis may be abrupt, with neurologic symptoms and signs developing within a few hours, or it may be slowly progressive over a period of months. The course of the illness is characteristically marked by remissions and exacerbations, but in some instances progression is persistent, so that the temporal nature of the illness is suggestive of a tumor. It is difficult to predict a patient's prognosis early in the course of the disease, at a time when the patient and the patient's family most wishes to have this information. About one-half have an exacerbation within 2 years after the first attack, but another one-third may not relapse for 5 to 25 years. At least 10% are progressive, without evidence of remission. Overall statistics indicate that about one-third of surviving patients are still able to work 25 years after the onset of their illness, and that at least one-half are still ambulatory. At least three-fourths survive 25 years from the time of the first attack.

There is a clinical impression that the severity of the disease is roughly proportional to the youth of the patient at onset; early onset usually means a severer course, whereas middle-aged onset is frequently associated with an indolent nonincapacitating illness.

The relationship between the onset or exacerbation of multiple sclerosis and other factors is still debated. Pregnancy and parturition are said to increase the risk of exacerbation, but there is no consistent pattern. It is clear that exacerbations may be provoked by infectious illnesses, but the relationship to trauma is unconvincing, in the judgment of this observer. There is no doubt that exacerbations of multiple sclerosis may occur following injury, but of course they also occur in the absence of trauma, and injuries to multiple sclerosis patients frequently are not followed by exacerbations. The issue of relationship of onset of the disease or exacerbation to trauma is not an uncommon legal one; the patient's treating physician has an obligation to react responsibly and objectively.

On the other hand, there is clearly a consistent relationship in some patients between worsening of symptoms and signs and increased body temperature. Many patients report increased weakness, ataxia, diplopia, or loss of vision in a hot shower or while sunbathing, and this well-known phenomenon is sometimes used in the form of a warm water bath to aid in the diagnosis in questionable cases. The cable conductive properties of the bare, demyelinated axonal sheath are further impaired by increased temperature (and improved by decreased temperature). There have been a few reports of a sustained exacerbation following the warm bath test, so it is not without risk.

Two other conditions, each uncommon but pathologically similar to multiple sclerosis, should be included in any discussion of demyelinating disorders. *Schilder's disease (diffuse cerebral sclerosis)* occurs in children or young adults and is characterized by a slow, progressive or saltatory course of visual disturbances (cortical blindness), dementia, spastic paralysis, pseudobulbar palsy, coma, and death within 3 months to 6 years. It is nonfamilial. The pathology is that of extensive myelin destruction involving an entire lobe or hemisphere or both hemispheres. The cerebrospinal fluid (CSF) in these patients is usually normal save for elevated immunoglobulin G (IgG). Computerized axial tomography (CAT) scans show extensive white matter destruction. Schilder's disease is almost certainly a different entity from the leukodystrophies, which have a similar clinical course, occur almost exclusively in children, have a strong familial history, and in which there are almost certainly genetically determined enzymatic defects affecting the pro-teolipids of myelin.

Neuromyelitis optica (Devic's disease) is even more uncommon, also oc-curs mainly in children, and is characterized by unilateral or bilateral optic neuritis, followed or accompanied by signs of transverse myelitis. The pathol-ogy is that of spinal cord necrosis, somewhat more than simple demyeliniza-tion. There is often no clinical improvement; or if there is, recurrence is rare.

DIFFERENTIAL DIAGNOSIS

The diagnosis of multiple sclerosis is usually straightforward when it occurs in its classic form; on the other hand, other types of lesion may simulate multiple sclerosis, and specific forms of therapy may be available for some of these. Spinal cord compression, either by tumor or cervical spondylosis, may produce intermittent symptoms and changing signs, although the differential diagnosis is usually not difficult. Intrinsic cervical cord lesions, in particular ependymoma, astrocytoma, or angioma, may also simulate spinal multiple sclerosis, as may meningioma of the posterior rim of the foramen magnum. Intracranial tumors which may be diagnostically confusing include brainstem glioma, chordoma, middle fossa meningioma, or cerebellar tumor. Early symptoms of a hereditary spinocerebellar degeneration (Friedreich's ataxia) may also resemble those of multiple sclerosis, as may collagen vascular disease and sarcoid. Arnold-Chiari malformation and/or platybasia may pro-duce a clinical picture which suggests localized multiple sclerosis.

DIAGNOSIS

In this disease there is no substitute for a careful probing history and detailed physical examination. These will provide or strongly suggest the diagnosis in the majority of instances. CSF examination, as previously men-tioned, shows an elevation of the gamma globulin (above 12% of the total protein) in about 70% of patients in exacerbation or with a smoldering, subacute course; CAT scans may show scattered areas of nonenhancing decreased density in the hemispheres (Fig. 8.4). The warm bath test, as previously described, may be helpful in diagnosis but requires careful inter-pretation. Cortical evoked responses from visual, auditory, or peripheral sensory stimuli may show characteristic patterns of delay or alteration in wave form as a consequence of lesions in the spinal cord, brainstem, or optic nerve. These diagnostic procedures are still being elaborated technically, but it is already evident that they are useful diagnostic tools.

In instances of spinal cord multiple sclerosis in which there is no evidence of pathology above the foramen magnum, myelography may be required to exclude spinal cord neoplasm or other compressive pathology. This should be

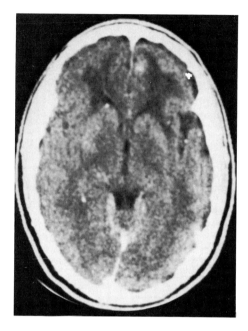

FIG. 8.4. CAT scan of brain in patient with multiple sclerosis. Note periventricular areas of decreased density, nonenhancing, particularly in frontal poles. These are throught to represent plaque formation.

done if there is a serious question about the diagnosis, even though symptoms and signs have been reported to worsen after myelography. The use of metrizamide contrast medium is less likely to aggravate the disease process.

TREATMENT

Although there is still argument as to whether steroids are effective in the treatment of multiple sclerosis, it is our belief that acute symptomatology of this illness can occasionally be improved by the administration of large doses of steroids. Whereas many physicians prefer the use of ACTH by intravenous injection followed by outpatient intramuscular injection, we use large doses of oral steroids (e.g., prednisone) beginning with a dose of 100 to 120 mg daily for 5 to 7 days. If there is no improvement during that time, it is unlikely that further such therapy will be helpful, and it is therefore discontinued. If the patient has immproved significantly, he is then placed on a dosage of 100 mg prednisone every other day, thereby avoiding some of the cushingoid effects of steroids. Treatment with steroids must be accompanied by measures to avoid such complications as hypokalemia, peptic ulcer exacerbation or bleeding, and possible spread of tuberculosis. For that reason, these patients are treated with supplementary potassium, a mild ulcer regimen, and if the treatment is to be prolonged isoniazid. In any event, steroids should not be continued indefinitely and must be discontinued if they are not shown to be effective. Statistical verification of the value of such treatment is still lacking.

Evidence has begun to accumulate which supports the concept that long-term immunosuppression favorably modifies the long-term course of the disease; it inhibits exacerbations and maintains useful neurologic function longer than is the case in controls. Azothioprine in doses of 50 mg twice daily was utilized and the dosage adjusted to maintain the white blood cell (WBC) count at about 3,500 mm³ and/or a differential count of less than 20% lymphocytes. The hematocrit was kept above 35%, serum glutamic acid transaminase below 75 international units/liter, and blood urea nitrogen (BUN) below 250 mmoles/liter. The usual daily dose of azothioprine was between 100 and 200 mg. Despite the apparent effectiveness of this drug in one study, it should be emphasized that many authorities consider long-term immunosuppressive therapy in multiple sclerosis to be experimental.

Other modalities of therapy may modify the patient's symptoms or improve his attitude about his illness. Dantrolene sodium (Dantrium) and baclofen (Lioresal) have been used to ameliorate spasticity, which may be so severe as to prevent ambulation by virtue of repeated clonic spasms of the legs when the patient attempts to walk. Both of these drugs are helpful in some patients, but their value is unpredictable in any given individual, and they not infrequently cause weakness of the extremities along with diminished spasticity.

Urinary sphincter problems are particularly troublesome. Evaluation of the patient's bladder function is essential to sensible pharmacologic intervention in these circumstances. A spastic, contracted, small-volume, poorly inhibited bladder usually causes extreme urgency and incontinence. An anticholinergic agent such as propantheline bromide (Pro-banthine) 15 mg twice daily or an hour prior to an anticipated social engagement may be helpful. In the presence of urinary retention or sufficiently poor detrusor function to empty the bladder, usually associated with detrusor-sphincter asynergy, bethanechol chloride (Urecholine) in doses of 25 mg t.i.d. may be helpful in decreasing the residual and lessening the likelihood of urinary tract infection. A urinary antiseptic such as trimethoprim (Septra) should be given daily. Female patients with significant urinary retention can readily learn to catheterize themselves three times daily. Male patients may eventually require an indwelling cathether.

Other supportive measures are important to the well-being of the patient and his family. Productive work should be continued as long as possible, even from a wheelchair if necessary. Rehabilitative measures are appropriate if they are realistically applied. Excessive therapy can be fatiguing and disheartening. Occupational therapy is often useful.

It is very important for the physician to recognize the anxiety and depression produced by multiple sclerosis, particularly in a young wage earner, and with sympathetic willingness to provide counsel for the patient and the family.

Divorces are common when one partner develops the disease. Often the divorce results because of a misunderstanding on the part of the unaffected partner about the prognosis of the disease or because of the frustration, anxiety, and depression of the affected partner. Skilled counseling can save these marriages. Pharmacologic management of anxiety and depression is also frequently extremely helpful.

SUGGESTED READINGS

Etiology and Pathogenesis

Adams J: Measles antibodies in patients with multiple sclerosis. *Neurology (Minneap)* 17:707, 1967.

Altrocchi P: Acute transverse myelopathy. *Acta Neurol* 9:111, 1963.

Bartfield H, and Atoynatan T: Lymphocyte transformation in multiple sclerosis. *Br Med J* 2:91, 1970.

Bernsohn J, and Stephanides T: Aetiology of multiple sclerosis. *Nature* 215:821, 1967.

Bornstein M, and Appel S: The application of tissue culture to the study of experimental "allergic" encephalomyelitis. I. Patterns of demyelination. *J Neuropathol Exp Neurol* 20:141, 1961.

Caron G: Lymphocyte transformation in multiple sclerosis. *N Engl J Med* 276:699, 1966.

Hughes D, Caspary E, and Field E: Lymphocyte transformation induced by encephalitogenic factor in multiple sclerosis and other neurological diseases. *Lancet* 2:1205, 1968.

Laterre EC, Callewaert A, Heremans JF, and Sfaello Z: Electrophoretic morphology of gamma globulins in cerebrospinal fluid of multiple sclerosis and other diseases of the nervous system. *Neurology (Minneap)* 20:982, 1970.

Lisak RP, and Zweiman B: In vitro cell-mediated immunity of cerebrospinal fluid lymphocytes to myelin basic protein in primary demyelinating diseases. *N Engl J Med* 297:850, 1977.

Poser CM: Disseminated vasculomyelinopathy: a review of the clinical and pathologic reactions of the nervous system in hyperergic diseases. *Acta Neurol Scand [Suppl 37]* 45:1, 1969.

Raine CS, Hummelgard A, Swanson E, and Bornstein MB: Multiple sclerosis: serum-induced demyelination in vitro; a light and electron microscope study. *J Neurol Sci* 20:127, 1973.

Seil FJ: Tissue culture studies of demyelinating disease: a critical review. *Ann Neurol* 2:345, 1977.

Van den Noort S, and Stjernholm RL: Lymphotoxic activity in multiple sclerosis serum. *Neurology (Minneap)* 21:783, 1971.

Waxman SG: Conduction in myelinated, unmyelinated, and demyelinated fibers. *Arch Neurol* 34:585, 1977.

Pathology

Courville C: Acute lesions of multiple sclerosis: possible significance of vascular changes. *J Neuropathol Exp Neurol* 27:159, 1968.

McDonald WI: Pathophysiology in multiple sclerosis. *Brain* 97:179, 1974.

Epidemiology

Alter M, and Kurtzke JF (eds): *Epidemiology of Multiple Sclerosis.* Charles C Thomas, Springfield, Illinois, 1968.

Kurtzke JF: An epidemiologic approach to multiple sclerosis. *Arch Neurol* 14:213, 1966.

Kurtzke JF, Beebe GW, Nagler B, Auth TL, Kurland LT, and Nefzger MD: Studies on natural history of multiple sclerosis. 4. Clinical features of the onset bout. *Acta Neurol Scand* 44:467, 1968.

Kurtzke JF, Beebe GW, Nagler B, Nefzger MD, Auth TL, and Kurland LT: Studies on the natural history of multiple sclerosis. V. Long-term survival in young men. *Arch Neurol* 22:215, 1970.

Leibowitz U, Sharon D, and Alter M: Geographical considerations in multiple sclerosis. *Brain* 90:871, 1967.

Clinical Course

Adams CWM: The onset and progression of the lesion in multiple sclerosis. *J Neurol Sci* 25:165, 1975.

Aldes J: Rehabilitation of multiple sclerosis patients. *J Rehabil* 33:10, 1967.

Bradley W, and Whitty C: Acute optic neuritis: prognosis for development of multiple sclerosis. *J Neurol Neurosurg Psychiatry* 31:10, 1968.

Chokravorty B: Association of trigeminal neuralgia with multiple sclerosis. *Arch Neurol* 14:95, 1966.

Collis W: Acute unilateral retrobulbar neuritis. *Arch Neurol* 13:409, 1965.

Fog T: The course of multiple sclerosis. *Acta Neurol Scand* 42:608, 1966.

Guthman L, Thompson H Jr, and Martin J: Transient facial myokymia: an uncommon manifestation of multiple sclerosis. *JAMA* 209:389, 1969.

Hutchinson WM: Acute optic neuritis and the prognosis for multiple sclerosis. *J Neurol Neurosurg Psychiatry* 39:283, 1976.

Kahana E, Leibowitz U, and Alter M: Brainstem and cranial nerve involvement in multiple sclerosis. *Acta Neurol Scand* 49:269, 1973.

Matthews WB: Tonic seizures in disseminated sclerosis. *Brain* 81:193, 1958.

Miller H: Trauma and multiple sclerosis. *Lancet* 1:848, 1964.

Namerow NS: A discussion concerning physical trauma in multiple sclerosis. *Bull Los Angeles Neurol Sci* 32:117, 1967.

Namerow NS, and Thompson LR: Plaques, symptoms, and the remitting course of multiple sclerosis. *Neurology (Minneap)* 19:765, 1969.

Scheinberg LC, and Korey SR: Multiple sclerosis. *Annu Rev Med* 13:411, 1962.

Schumacher GA: Demyelinating diseases. *N Engl J Med* 262:969, 1019, 1119, 1960.

Sever JL: Perspectives in multiple sclerosis—1975: introduction. *Neurology (Minneap)* 25:486, 1975.

Shibasaki H, and Kuroiwa Y: Painful tonic seizure in multiple sclerosis. *Arch Neurol* 30:47, 1974.

Diagnosis

Asselman P, Chadwick DW, and Marsden CD: Visual evoked responses in the diagnosis and management of patients suspected of multiple sclerosis. *Brain* 98:261, 1975.

Cala LA, Mastaglia FL, and Black JL: Computerized tomography of brain and optic nerve in multiple sclerosis. *J Neurol Sci* 36:411, 1978.

Davis F: The hot bath test in the diagnosis of multiple sclerosis. *J Mt Sinai Hosp NY* 33:280, 1966.

Ivers R, McKenzie B, McGuckin W, and Goldstein N: Spinal fluid gamma globulin in multiple sclerosis and other neurologic diseases. *JAMA* 176:137, 1961.

Mastaglia FL, Black JL, and Collins DWK: Visual spinal evoked potentials in the diagnosis of multiple sclerosis. *Br Med J* 2:732, 1976.

Michael JA, and Davis FA: Effects of induced hyperthermia in multiple sclerosis: differences in visual acuity during heating and recovery phases. *Acta Neurol Scand* 49:141, 1973.

Shahrokhi E, Chiappa KH, and Young RR: Pattern shift visual evoked responses in two hundred patients with optic neuritis and/or multiple sclerosis. *Arch Neurol* 35:65, 1978.

Treatment

Cendrowski WS: Therapeutic trial of Imuran (azathioprine) in multiple sclerosis. *Acta Neurol Scand* 47:254, 1971.

Miller H, et al: Multiple sclerosis: treatment of acute exacerbation with corticotrophin (ACTH). *Lancet* 2:1120, 1961.

Miller J, Vas C, Norouha M, Liversedge L, and Rawson M: Long-term treatment of multiple sclerosis with corticotrophin. *Lancet* 2:429, 1967.

Nelson DA, Vates TS Jr, and Thomas RB Jr: Complications from intrathecal steroid therapy in patients with multiple sclerosis. *Acta Neurol Scand* 49:176, 1973.

Ring J, Lob G, Angstwurm H, et al: Intensive immunosuppression in the treatment of multiple sclerosis. *Lancet* Nov. 9:1093, 1974.

Rinne UK, Sonninen V, and Tuovinen T: Corticotrophin treatment in multiple sclerosis. *Acta Neurol Scand* 44:207, 1968.

Rose A, Kuzma J, Kurtzke J, Namerow N, Sibley W, and Tourtellotte W: Cooperative study in the evaluation of therapy in multiple sclerosis: ACTH versus placebo. *Neurology (Minneap)* 20:1, 1970.

Rosen JA: Prolonged azathioprine treatment of non-remitting multiple sclerosis. *J Neurol Neurosurg Psychiatry* 42:338, 1979.

Schumacher GA, Beebe G, Kibler RF, Kurland LT, et al: Problems of experimental trials of therapy in multiple sclerosis: report by the panel on the evaluation of experimental trials of therapy in multiple sclerosis. *Ann NY Acad Sci* 122:552, 1965.

Swank RL: Multiple sclerosis: twenty years on low fat diet. *Arch Neurol* 23:460, 1970.

Tourtellotte WW, and Haerer AF: Use of an oral corticosteroid in the treatment of multiple sclerosis. *Arch Neurol* 12:536, 1965.

Related Diseases

Berry K, and Olszewski J: Central pontine myelinolysis: a case report. *Neurology (Minneap)* 13:531, 1963.

9

Headache

Because headaches are probably the most frequent of all human ailments, it behooves all physicians to understand the mechanisms of head pain and to feel comfortable and confident when handling patients with headaches. Headaches can be frightening to the patient and the physician, for they frequently conjure up visions of brain trumor, intracranial bleeding, and other serious neurologic disorders. The fortunate fact is that very few headaches, particularly chronically recurrent ones, have a serious or threatening etiology; rather, well over 90% of headache problems do not have a provable etiology and fall into the general categories of muscle tension or vascular headaches, terms descriptive of the presumed site of origin of the pain and implying an emotional or psychogenic basis. Nevertheless, such headaches can be serious in the sense that they are unpleasant, debilitating, result in decreased efficiency in work, and generally diminish the quality of life. The treating physician must have an effective system for evaluating and managing such patients so as to reduce their anxiety, provide appropriate medical management, and at the same time avoiding lengthy, expensive, and inappropriate work-ups.

The key to diagnosis and management of headaches is that the type of head pain is almost always indicative of which structures or tissues of the head are responsible for the pain, thereby giving meaningful insight into the etiology of the headache. First, then, the treating physician must be familiar with the pain-sensitive structures of the head. These include:

1. Skin and its blood vessels
2. Muscles of the head and neck
3. Arteries of the dura and arteries at the base of the brain
4. Dura at the base of the skull only
5. Intracranial venous sinuses and some intracranial veins
6. The 5th, 9th, and 10th cranial nerves and upper two cervical nerves
7. Periosteum of the skull

It is important to remember that the brain parenchyma is itself pain-insensitive. Of the pain-sensitive structures, by far the most important in the evaluation of a headache problem are the muscles of the head and neck and the blood vessels, intracranial and extracranial. Pain originating in the muscles is usually of a special type (i.e., dull, squeezing, pressing, or aching), whereas headache of vascular origin tends to be throbbing and is often made worse by head movement or coughing. It is apparent, then, that the first step in the evaluation of any headache problem is to obtain a careful history, insisting that the patient describe the quality of pain. This is remarkably difficult for most patients to do accurately. They can rarely find the appropriate adjectives to describe the pain, other than "severe" or "like a toothache" unless the examiner offers a shopping list of terms and encourages the patient to choose one. The list should include: throbbing, squeezing, pressing, sharp, and sticking. Despite the most articulate description, it may still be difficult for the examiner to deduce the anatomic structure involved. The history must also include the following additional clues:

1. *Duration of the headache problem.* Obviously, a story of headache that began recently, without prior history, has a different significance than one of chronic recurrent headaches of many years' duration. In the former instance, one must have a high index of suspicion about an organic etiology, whereas longstanding chronic headache problems rarely have such a basis and require a different type of management. Just as important as the duration of the problem is the question of whether there has been a recent change in the type of severity of the headache, for this also should alert the examiner to look for organic disease.

2. *Location of the headache.* Recurrent hemicranias are typical of the classic migraine syndrome. Occipital, posterior cervical, and vertex headaches are strongly suggestive of muscle tension origin. Highly localized head pains require a careful inspection of the area in question to look for localized scalp, bone, or sinus infection, almost all of which are usually accompanied by local tenderness and frequently evidence of the pathology. Headaches caused by compression of or traction on cranial nerves 5, 9, and 10 and the first two cervical nerves are located in the distribution of the involved nerve. Involvement of the 5th cranial nerve usually causes intermittent facial pain similar to that seen in trigeminal neuralgia. Posterior fossa tumors may compress or stretch cranial nerves 9 and 10 and C-1 and C-2, producing high cervical and occipital pain. Temporal arteritis may cause pain localized to a tender superficial temporal artery but may also produce generalized headache.

3. *Association of the headache with other symptoms and signs.* Headaches of a vascular character preceded by contralateral neurologic symptoms— usually visual (e.g., scintillating scotomas, field defects), as well as occasional dysesthesias of a hand or one side of the face, and rarely temporary hemiparesis or even transient aphasia—are the hallmarks of the classic migraine syndrome. Obviously, one must be certain that such dramatic neurologic phenomena are not caused by a focal cerebral lesion, e.g., tumor or vascular

anomaly. Occasionally, the transient neurologic phenomena (particularly the visual ones) occur without a subsequent headache. Such patients require careful evaluation even though this may be consistent with a migraine syndrome.

Autonomic phenomena accompanying headache are also useful in the differential diagnosis and management of the problem. Unilateral lacrimation, miosis, and nasal stuffiness accompanying hemicrania speak for cluster headache. Nausea and vomiting may accompany any type of headache but are most frequent in severe vascular headaches. Sudden, precipitate, recurrent vomiting without prior nausea, and in association with occipital or unilateral nuchal pain, demands careful investigation to exclude posterior fossa brain tumors.

Special relationships are obvious to any observant physician. For example, acute headache accompanied by fever and stiff neck suggests meningitis, just as acute headache, stiff neck, and drowsiness in the absence of fever suggest primary subarachnoid hemorrhage.

4. *Circumstantial association of the headache.* Headaches that routinely occur following or during periods of special emotional stress are almost invariably benign, and such a relationship gives the physician a therapeutic handle by urging the patient to cushion such stressful situations pharmacologically. Rarely, vascular headaches seem to occur after ingestion of specific types of food (e.g., cheeses or seafoods) and particularly after certain varieties of wines. Our experience has been, however, that truly "allergic" headaches are extremely rare, and that individuals whose headaches seem to correlate with foods not infrequently also have headaches with which no such correlation can be made. The important point is that good headache management requires utilization of all clues, no matter how trivial.

In addition to a careful history, giving the patient time to explore all of the above-mentioned correlations, the work-up for headache includes routine general and neurologic examinations. Patients found to be hypertensive must be treated, but in our experience hypertension is not a common cause of headache; patients who are hypertensive not infrequently have a personality structure that is conducive to having headaches as well. Therefore the physician cannot assume that he has discovered the cause of the patient's headache when he finds him to be hypertensive.

There is no doubt that acute sinusitis may be associated with headache, often fairly localized and associated with tenderness; the mechanism is probably obstruction of the ostia of the sinus and failure of pressure within the sinus to equalize with the atmospheric pressure. Decongestants usually stop this type of headache quickly. On the other hand, "chronic sinus headache" is probably unrelated to sinus disease in the majority of instances. Eye strain may also cause headaches, usually of muscle tension origin and occasionally associated with soreness of the eyes. The setting is usually prolonged study or following a movie, and the mechanism is refractive error. Eye pain and periorbital pain in the presence of visual blurring suggests optic neuritis or glaucoma. Patients with cerebral angiomas may also have headaches but as many do not, and a true causative relation between the angioma and headache can rarely be established in the absence of an intracranial bleed.

EVALUATION OF THE PATIENT WITH HEADACHE

The factors described above are all taken into account when determining the extent of the diagnostic work-up of a patient with headache. The headache characteristics are probably the most important part of the evaluation. Physical examination rarely clarifies the mechanism of the patient's pain unless the patient has an intracranial mass lesion. It is understood that each patient must have a complete neurologic examination. The extent of the laboratory evaluation depends on the particular problem, but routine chronic vascular or muscle tension headaches do not require more than a regular medical work-up. Computerized axial tomography (CAT) scanning has largely replaced skull X-rays, isotope brain scans, and electroencephalograms (EEGs) in headache evaluation, but certainly should not be done routinely; rather, it should be reserved for those cases which, because of history or physical findings, provoke suspicion of an intracranial lesion. Routine CAT scanning in the evaluation of simple headache cannot be justified on a cost-efficiency basis.

TYPES OF HEADACHE AND THEIR MANAGEMENT

Muscle Tension, or Contraction, Headaches

Muscle tension, or contraction, headaches have their origin in the muscles of the scalp and neck and are usually described as "squeezing," "pressing," "aching," "like a band or vise around the head," or "a pressure on top of the head." They are not throbbing and are often benefited by gentle massage or neck stretching. They frequently occur after a "long, hard day" or following any stressful situation, or they may occur in response to a generally unsatisfactory life. The pain may last several hours to several days, is not usually accompanied by nausea or vomiting, and may be relieved by simple analgesics, tranquilizers, or an alcoholic beverage. Physical examination shows no neurologic abnormalities, but the cervical and scalp muscles are often tender and in sustained contraction. Most important, these patients are frequently observed to be mildly depressed.

Although the differential diagnosis of such a headache problem must include cervical osteoarthritis, spondylosis, or some rare bony anomaly of the junction of the cervical spine and skull, the fact is that these are rarely found to be the cause of the patient's problem.

Helpful management of these patients requires a firm, assured, affirmative approach on the part of the physician. He must help the patient understand the relationship between his pain and life's vicissitudes, eliminate the element of fear about the cause of the pain, and then deal with the problem symptomatically. Our custom is to begin vigorously by prescribing antidepressant and tranquilizing drugs to be taken *regularly* in small doses, and to encourage the patient to use adequate quantities of the analgesics which he tolerates best at the onset of the headache (acetylsalicylic acid, plain, buffered, or in combination with caffeine or barbiturates), prescribe the use of heat to the neck and lower occiput regularly for 15 min twice daily, and be available for suggestions, support, or change in therapy.

Vascular Headaches

Vascular headaches include migraine, migraine-like headaches, and cluster headaches. The common characteristic is that the type of pain is throbbing, often worsened by position or movement, unilateral or generalized, and frequently associated with other symptoms.

The classic textbook features of migraine probably occur in fewer than one-fifth of patients with the migraine syndrome. These characteristics include the migraine prodrome, described earlier; strict hemicrania, periodic and recurrent; familial history; and a so-called compulsive, rigid passive-aggressive personality. Nausea and vomiting are the rule. Occurrence is not uncommonly on weekends or after a period of emotional stress. The headaches may last several hours to several days and, in severe cases, may be prostrating and have a less definable endpoint than in the true migraine syndrome.

Cluster headaches are so named because of their propensity to occur in clusters, i.e., regularly for several weeks, followed by a respite, followed by return, with gradually increasing frequency. In addition, they have specific characteristics. The pain usually occurs suddenly, often awakening the patient at night; it is unilateral, often periorbital, and throbbing or aching, and is associated with lacrimation, nasal stuffiness, and frequently homolateral miosis and ptosis. It is usually of short duration, i.e., 1.5 to 2 hr. It may occur twice during a 24-hr period and often occurs at the same time daily. It is much more common in men. We do not understand the mechanism of this peculiar syndrome which seems so ominous but which often subsides spontaneously.

All the above-mentioned types of vascular headaches have a common pharmacologic basis for therapy: the use of ergot preparations which presumably act by constricting the dilated tender cranial arteries responsible for the pain. The theoretical basis for this therapy is that the arteries first constrict, sometimes producing the migraine prodromes described earlier, and then become dilated and edematous, so that the systolic thrust is painful. The biochemical basis for these phenomena is not well understood, although abnormalities of polypeptides and catecholamines in the vascular walls have been described.

Patients with vascular headaches should be managed as well as treated. By this is meant that every effort must be made to find a means of reducing or eliminating the attacks, as well as treating them when they occur. It is essential that these patients be given support by their physician and that the relationship between their illness and emotional stress or personality structure be explained to them, if such a relationship exists. They may benefit from a course of antidepressants or regular use of a mild sedative as tranquilizing agent. Experience indicates that the most effective antidepressants are amitriptyline HCl (Elavil) and imipramine HCl (Tofranil), the former in doses of 50 to 150 mg daily, the latter in doses of 75 mg daily. Methysergide maleate (Sansert) in doses of 6 mg daily has proved effective in prophylaxis of migraine in some patients; however, this drug, a potent serotonin antagonist, cannot be used longer than 6 months during any period of treatment because of a variety of complications, the most serious of which is retroperitoneal fibrosis. It has no value in the treatment of an acute attack.

Propranolol HCl (Inderal) has been reported to be useful in the prophylaxis of vascular headaches, particularly migraine. It is a β-adrenergic blocking agent, and its presumed action is on receptor sites in the arterial walls. Initial dosage is 10 mg q.i.d., but this can be increased to 160 mg daily if necessary. A significant complication of propranolol is easy fatigability. Personal experience with this drug has been disappointing.

There is some evidence that oral contraceptives increase the frequency and severity of migraine attacks, and we urge that they be avoided if possible in young women with problem headaches.

Ergotamines are the pharmacologic basis for the treatment of the acute migraine attack, and a lengthy list of these preparations with appropriate dosage instructions is available in the *Physician's Desk Reference* under "Anti-Migraine Preparations." As previously mentioned, ergotamine tartrate acts on smooth muscle and causes constriction of arteries, including the presumably dilated tender cranial arteries. If the patient is able to tolerate oral medication, he should be instructed to take 2 mg ergotamine tartrate in the form of Cafergot-PB (two tablets), which includes caffeine, bellafoline, and pentobarbital, *immediately* at the onset of the headache, followed by another two tablets every hour until the headache ceases or until a total of 10 mg ergotamine tartrate has been ingested. If nausea prevents oral ingestion, ergotamine tartrate alone can be given sublingually, or Cafergot-PB suppositories (each containing 2 mg ergotamine) can be used. The suppositories can also be repeated hourly times four if necessary. If the patient is seen by the physician after the attack has fully developed, a preparation called D.H.E. 45 (dihydroergotamine methanesulfonate) can be given in a single 0.5 mg dose intramuscularly or intravenously.

Every physician is aware that serious complications can result from the use of ergot drugs, so these are not described in detail here. It is worthwhile to mention, however, that the greatest danger is from severe vasoconstriction and gangrene, which occurs with long-term use. Nevertheless, great caution must be exercised with patients with any type of vascular disease, even for short-term use.

Patients usually learn their own dosage tolerance quickly. Many prefer the rectal route, believing it produces less nausea and vomiting. Failure of this type of therapy can often be attributed to inappropriate use of the drug, which must be given as early as possible in the course of the headache and in sufficiently large doses. Sometimes a combination of the ergotamine tartrate preparations and oral analgesics is effective. The important thing is to continue to seek a proper combination of drugs, hopefully without resorting to narcotics.

The management of cluster headaches is a special situation. Our preference is to prescribe one Cafergot-PB suppository every 12 hr, one of which is applied at bedtime, for 5 to 6 days in an effort to prevent the attacks. This regimen frequently allows the patient to enter into a remission, and the drug can then be discontinued gradually during the next 2 to 3 days.

Temporal arteritis is a special cause of headache already discussed briefly in Chapter 2. It is important because it requires a special treatment (i.e., steroids) and because failure to identify and treat it may result in occlusion of retinal or cerebral vessels. The clinical characteristics are that such patients are almost invariably over 60 years of age; have had a preceding illness of weakness, fatigue, aching, fever, and weight loss (polymyalgia rheumatica); and often complain of recurrent fever even between the episodes of headache. Examination may show a tender, tortuous, superficial temporal artery, and the erythrocyte sedimentation rate (ESR) may be elevated. Just as important is the fact that neither of these findings may be present. If arteritis is suspected, temporal artery biopsy should be done and the patient given a trial on steroids. We recommend beginning therapy with 100 mg prednisone daily. If true arteritis is present the response is dramatic.

The emphasis in this discussion of headaches has been on muscle tension and vascular headaches, neither of which often have a provable etiology and both of which are frequently vaguely ascribed to psychogenic causes. The reason for this emphasis is that these comprise well over 90% of headache problems. This in no way diminishes the importance of the fact that any intracranial pathology may also be the cause of headaches. It is just that headaches *alone* are an infrequent mode of presentation of brain tumors. By the time a brain tumor produces headache, which it does by displacement of intracranial structures and traction on the pain-sensitive arteries or nerves, other neurologic signs (e.g., motor weakness, gait disturbances, visual abnormalities, or seizures) are also fairly obvious. Although the physician must always suspect brain tumor as a cause for headache, his approach to the problem should be systematic, as outlined earlier; moreover, particularly in the instance of long-standing headaches, he must not add to the patient's anxiety by showing inappropriate concern. Unfortunately, pains from brain tumors do not have any readily identifiable characteristics unless it is the concurrence of neurologic dysfunction. The type of pain, however, is rarely distinguishable from other causes of headache. The most important clues should be: (1) recent onset of headache; (2) change in the pattern of a chronic headache problem; (3) absolute persistence of localized head pain; (4) any neurologic deficit.

Finally, it should be emphasized that the vast majority of patients with headache can be helped, and some may be permanently relieved. Failure is usually the result of poor understanding of head pain mechanisms by the physician, inadequate history, and lack of real diligence or imagination in trials of various therapeutic regimes.

FACIAL PAIN

Facial pain was alluded to previously, but the frequency of recurrent, paroxysmal facial pain in middle-aged and elderly individuals is justification for additional comments. Trigeminal neuralgia (tic doloreaux) is a very unpleasant disorder in which the patient experiences flashes of severe pain in the distribution of one of the branches of the trigeminal nerve on one side. Although of brief (several seconds' to minutes') duration, the pain is of such intensity that the patient actually lives in fear of the next one. It is often provoked by certain facial movements, talking, chewing, brushing the teeth, or washing the face. The paroxysms seem to occur in a cyclic pattern. They may gradually increase in intensity and frequency, until they are occurring as often as 50 times daily, and then gradually subside, only to recur months or years later. Careful neurologic examination reveals no deficit. If there is evidence of hypalgesia or 5th nerve motor involvement, the examiner must be suspicious of a structural lesion involving the 5th nerve, in particular nasopharyngeal carcinoma. X-rays of the skull should include views of the skull base so as to visualize the foramina rotundum and ovale in order to be certain that no bone destruction exists.

The etiology of trigeminal neuralgia is rarely discovered. When it occurs in young patients, multiple sclerosis should be suspected, as previously mentioned. One school of thought has it that the nerve root or ganglion is partially entrapped by an aberrant blood vessel or dural scar, and that surgical decompression of the nerve root is an effective form of treatment. Convincing evidence that this theory is correct is still lacking. Usual management is by the use of phenytoin (Dilantin) in doses of 200 to 400 mg daily or carbamazepine (Tegretol) 400 to 1,200 mg daily. Both of these drugs may produce drowsiness and ataxia, and the latter may cause thrombocytopenia and leukopenia, necessitating monthly blood counts during treatment. Many of these patients become discouraged and depressed, and require antidepressant medications.

PSEUDOTUMOR CEREBRI

Pseudotumor cerebri is an interesting disorder which classically occurs in young, obese, amenorrheic women; it usually presents with headache as the major complaint and hence its consideration here. The only abnormality on neurologic examination is papilledema, which is the major cause for alarm in this otherwise benign and self-limited syndrome. The papilledema may eventually cause damage to the optic nerves and secondary optic atrophy, so visual acuity must be closely monitored. The pathogenesis is not completely understood. In the majority of instances the increased brain volume is secondary to increased intra- and extracellular water, but the cause for this diffuse edema is not known. The same syndrome may be caused by thrombosis of a lateral (transverse) venous sinus (optic hydrocephalus), which is seen in children with recurrent middle ear infections or sagittal sinus thrombosis. Pseudotumor cerebri is associated with vitamin A administration, steroids, urea withdrawal, tetracyclines, and adrenal insufficiency.

Diagnosis is made by noting the presence of above findings plus a computerized axial tomography (CAT) scan, which usually shows small ventricles and no other abnormality. Treatment is with acetazolamide (Diamox) in doses of 250 mg three or four times daily. This drug decreases the rate of cerebrospinal fluid (CSF) production. Dexamethasone (Decadron) 6 to 24 mg daily is also helpful in cases with severe papilledema and in which early changes in visual acuity occur. Repeated (daily) lumbar puncture, using an 18-gauge needle so the dural hole will be sizable, is utilized by some. CSF pressure is gradually reduced to half its initial value by CSF removal. Replacement of CSF is at the rate of 0.3 ml/min so that the continued leakage of CSF from the dural hole may be an important factor in maintaining decreased introcranical pressure.

With the above management subtemporal decompression should never be necessary to prevent visual loss.

SUGGESTED READINGS

Etiology and Mechanics
Amines and migraine. *Br Med J* 2:1340, 1966.
Amines and migraine. *Br Med J* 4:693, 1967.
Anthony M, and Lance JW: Histamine and serotonin in cluster headaches. *Arch Neurol* 25:225, 1971.
Basser LS: Relation of migraine and epilepsy. *Brain* 92:285, 1969.
Blau JN: Migraine research. *Br Med J* 2:751, 1971.
Dalsgaard-Nielsen T: Migraine and heredity. *Acta Neurol Scand* 41:287, 1965.
Hanington E, and Harper AM: The role of tyramine in the aetiology of migraine, related studies on the cerebral and extracerebral circulation. *Headache* 8:84, 1968.

Kangasniemi P, Sonnien V, and Rinne UK: Excretion of free and conjugated 5-HIAA and VMA in the urine and concentration of 5-HIAA and HVA in CSF during migraine attacks and free intervals. *Headache* 12:62, 1972.

Kunkle E, Charles R, Bronson S, and Wolff HG: Studies on headache: the mechanisms and significance of the headache associated with brain tumor. *Bull NY Acad Med* 18:400, 1942.

Lance JW: Headaches related to sexual activity. *J Neurol Neurosurg Psychiatry* 39:1226, 1976.

Ray BS, and Wolff HG: Experimental studies on headache: pain-sensitive structures of the head and their significance in headache. *Arch Surg* 41:813, 1940.

Types and Clinical Characteristcs

Aring CD: The migrainous scintillating scotoma. *JAMA* 220:519, 1972.

Bickerstaff ER: Basilar artery migraine. *Lancet* 1:15, 1961.

Bradshaw P: Hemiplegic migraine. *Q J Med* 34:65, 1965.

Bradshaw P, and Parsons M: Hemiplegic migraine, a clinical study. *Q J Med* 34:65, 1965.

Callaghan N: The migraine syndrome in pregnancy. *Neurology (Minneap)* 18:197, 1968.

Friedman AP, Pool NS, and von Storch TJC: Tension headache. *JAMA* 151:174, 1953.

Friedman AP: The migraine syndrome. *Bull NY Acad Med* 44:45, 1968.

Friedman AP: Migraine headaches. *JAMA* 222:1399, 1972.

Friedman AP, and Mikropoulos HE: Cluster headaches. *Neurology (Minneap)* 8:653, 1958.

Friedman AP, Harter DH, and Merritt HH: Ophthalmoplegic migraine. *Arch Neurol* 7:320, 1962.

Guest IA, and Woolf AL: Fatal infarction of brain in migraine. *Br Med J* 1:225, 1964.

Simard D, and Paulson OB: Cerebral vasomotor paralysis during migraine attack. *Arch Neurol* 29:207, 1973.

Von Knorring J, Erma M, and Lindstrom B: The clinical manifestations of temporal arteritis. *Acta Med Scand* 179:691, 1966.

Whitty CWM: Migraine without headache. *Lancet* 2:283, 1967.

Wolff HG: *Headache and Other Head Pain.* Oxford University Press, New York, New York, 1963.

Management

Anthony M, and Lance JW: Current concepts in the pathogenesis and interval treatment of migraine. *Drugs* 3:153, 1972.

Carroll JD: Migraine—general management. *Br Med J* 2:756, 1971.

Friedman AP: Treatment of headache. *JAMA* 184:124, 1963.

Graham JR: Methysergide for prevention of headache. *N Engl J Med* 270:67, 1964.

Kerbel NC: Retroperitoneal fibrosis secondary to methysergide bimaleate. *Can Med Assoc J* 96:1420, 1967.

Southwell N: Methysergide in the prophylaxis of migraine. *Lancet* 1:523, 1964.

Special Reviews

Special issue—headache: its diagnosis and management. *Headache* 19:1113, 1979.

10

Epilepsy

Convulsive seizures are among the most dramatic and impressive of all neurologic signs. They may occur during the course of or following almost any disease (structural or metabolic) or injury to the brain, and may also occur in the absence of other demonstrable brain dysfunction. Many acute brain lesions—particularly metabolic encephalopathies (e.g., hypoglycemia, electrolyte abnormalities, or hypoxia), meningoencephalitis, cerebral ischemia, drug intoxication or withdrawal, and acute cerebral contusion—may cause focal or generalized cerebral seizures that are part of the acute illness but which do not recur on recovery from that illness.

The prevalence of epilepsy, in the sense of recurrent seizures, is probably greater than 400 per 100,000 population, or in the neighborhood of a million people in the United States. If all who have had a single convulsive seizure were considered, the figure would probably be at least 10 to 15 times as great. The significance of these statistics is that seizures are so common that all practicing physicians are confronted with the problem and should be capable of making appropriate decisions *a propos* differential diagnosis and management. Although epilepsy itself is a complex disorder whose mechanisms are still poorly understood, the diagnosis and management of the great majority of patients with epilepsy is actually not complicated and requires the application of only a few principles and the use of a few drugs. This chapter is concerned with the practical aspects of the clinical problem of epilepsy and does not undertake to review in depth the burgeoning knowledge which pertains to its pathophysiology.

DEFINITION

By common usage the term *epilepsy* is usually reserved for convulsive seizures that recur chronically, although the underlying physiologic mechanism may be the same in all types of seizure.

It is difficult to define epilepsy in simple terms because there is a great variety of seizure types that do not have a single clinical common manifestation. Probably the most frequent manifestation of epilepsy is alteration of consciousness; but this is by no means a universal sign, for some epileptic seizures may consist of motor, sensory, or psychic phenomena without loss of consciousness. Epilepsy is the clinical phenomenon that occurs because a group of cerebral neurons discharge abnormally in recurrent paroxysms. It produces a variety of disturbances of brain function, and the cause may be biochemical, genetic, or structural.

The classifications of epilepsy are useful if the physician uses them to decide how to manage a given patient. A classification of seizures according to clinical symptomatology does not have to be exhaustive to be helpful, but it is nevertheless essential in order to evaluate the patient properly.

The first issue to be decided is whether the patient has had a true cerebral seizure. The phenomenon most frequently confused with a seizure is the simple faint, vasodepressor syncope. Such a differential is usually simple, but not always. No one would confuse a major motor (grand mal) seizure with a faint; nor would one confuse a classic syncopal attack associated with the typical feeling of faintness, sweating, pallor, and a brief period of flaccid unconsciousness followed by immediate recovery with no confusion or drowsiness, with a true convulsive seizure; but intermediate clinical syndromes may be difficult to diagnose. It is essential to obtain from a witness an accurate picture of what occurred. Did the patient have convulsive movements? Was there tongue-biting or incontinence? Was there a period of postictal confusion and drowsiness? These are the characteristics of seizure activity and essentially exclude the diagnosis of syncope.

What type of seizure occurred? The actual clinical symptomatology of the seizure is of the greatest diagnostic and therapeutic importance because it determines to a considerable extent the nature of the neurologic investigation into the cause of the seizure and the type of treatment to be used, as well as frequently helping to identify the area of the brain involved.

In this regard various classifications of epilepsy have been used over the years, each having an underlying theme which had practical application to the management of the patient. One such generic classification divided epilepsy into two groups: *idiopathic* and *symptomatic*. These were, in fact, diagnoses of exclusion and were recognized to be incomplete, but seizures for which no structural or biochemical cause could be found were termed idiopathic, which further implied that additional diagnostic investigation was not needed. The paradigms of idiopathic epilepsy were petit mal and unlocalized generalized convulsions (grand mal); all others were believed to have a structural basis even though no lesion could be demonstrated by conventional means. The fallacy of this concept is evident.

The International League Against Epilepsy has formulated a classification which, even if it does little more to explain pathophysiologic principles, at least permits accurate communication among interested physicians. This classification is as follows:

I. Partial seizures beginning locally
  A. Partial seizures with elementary symptoms generally without impairment of consciousness
    1. With motor symptoms (includes Jacksonian)
    2. With special or somatosensory symptoms
    3. With autonomic symptoms
    4. Compound (or mixed) forms
  B. Partial seizures with complex symptomatology, generally with impairment of consciousness awareness (includes psychomotor)
    1. With impaired consciousness only
    2. With cognitive symptoms
    3. With mood (affective) symptoms
    4. With psychosensory symptoms
    5. With psychomotor automatisms*
    6. With compound (mixed) symptoms of the above
  C. Partial seizures which generalize secondarily*
II. Generalized seizures (i.e., those which are bilateral, symmetrical, and without clinical evidence of focal or lateralized onset)
  A. Absences (so-called petit mal)*
  B. Bilateral massive epileptic myoclonus
  C. Infantile spasms
  D. Tonic seizures
  E. Clonic seizures
  F. Mixed tonic-clonic seizures*
  G. Atonic seizures
  H. Akinetic seizures
III. Unilateral seizures (predominantly)
IV. Unclassified epileptic seizures (usually so classified because of incomplete historical data)

Those indicated with an asterisk(*) are by far the commonest, comprising together over 95% of patients with epilepsy.

PARTIAL SEIZURES

The term *partial* is used in the context that the seizure is not generalized; that is, the seizure is not a "complete" one. The term itself has built-in contradictions. Some occur without impairing consciousness or memory for the event. The symptomatic expression of such seizures runs the gamut of clinical cortical physiology. *Focal motor seizures* begin with a repetitive slow jerking of some part of the body (a finger, hand, corner of the mouth). The jerking usually increases in tempo and may spread to involve the entire side of the body. *Focal sensory seizures* are far less frequent. The patient feels dysesthesias or an unusual sensation on the side opposite the discharging lesion, or has visual, auditory, or olfactory experiences. *Autonomic* seizures are usually characterized by nausea, vomiting, abdominal cramps, diarrhea, sweating, pallor, and faintness.

Partial seizures with complex symptomatology are termed *psychomotor seizures* or *temporal lobe seizures*, indicating their origin from a lesion within one or both temporal lobes. They may begin with an olfactory or gustatory aura, during which the patient smells or tastes something peculiar or unpleasant; this is followed by automatic, stereotyped, well-coordinated semi-purposeful behavior, for which the patient has no recall and during which he appears to be confused. The typical seizure lasts 1 to 5 min during which the patient appears preoccupied and exhibits chewing movements and rubbing, patting, or picking movements of the hands. Less frequently the attack may be more complex and prolonged. The patient may behave abnormally and strangely, moving about freely. Many customary acts (e.g., eating, dressing, combing the hair, or even driving a car) may be performed, but more complex actions requiring appropriate interaction with others cannot. *Deja vu* states, in which the patient feels that he is reliving a familiar scene or a sense of unwarranted familiarity are another manifestation of temporal lobe epilepsy (Fig. 10.1).

Partial seizures which generalize secondarily may well be the most frequent type of epileptic seizure. Basically these are focal at onset and then become generalized. Often the focal portion of the seizure is extremely brief, as manifested by sudden adversive movements of the eyes and head to one side, tingling of an extremity, or a sensation of lights flashing, but it provides highly valuable information about the location of the initial abnormal cortical discharge and therefore the location of the cerebral pathology responsible for the seizure. This particular point requires emphasis; the focal parts of a seizure,

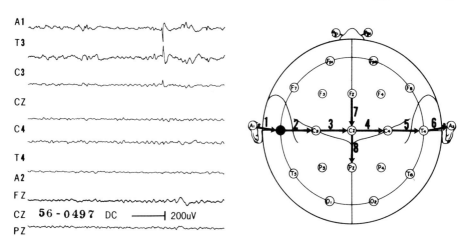

FIG. 10.1. T3 (left temporal lobe) epileptic focus. Pathology was arteriovenous malformation.

which include the aura, are relevant to the localization of the offending lesion. It is for this reason that details of the *onset* of the seizure, including a description of the aura from the patient, are especially important.

GENERALIZED SEIZURES

Generalized seizures have no clinical focalization at onset; and although there may be a local discharging focus, the bihemispheric diffusely projecting neuronal systems of the reticular activating system are immediately involved and the patient loses consciousness.

Absences (petit mal epilepsy) often begin with the patient suddenly stopping normal activity and staring vacantly with mouth open and eyes slightly turned up. The eyes may blink and the head nod; and it has been shown recently that the majority of these children have some movement during the attack and do not necessarily stop their ongoing activity during the seizure. *Short kids (<18 years old)* The seizure usually lasts 2 to 10 sec, but much longer attacks (petit mal status) may occur; recovery is instantaneous, and the patient may continue preictal activity without being aware that a seizure has occurred. This type of epilepsy begins during childhood and practically never persists into adult life, although it may be accompanied or replaced by generalized motor seizures.

The electroencephalography (EEG) pattern consists of an excitatory discharge (spike) followed by a slower high-voltage slow wave repeated at the *spike and wave 3cps* rate of 3 per sec (Fig. 10.2). The history is classic, and the neurologic examination shows no special abnormality. If the diagnosis is suspected, an attack may be provoked by having the patient hyperventilate. The history plus the EEG pattern are sufficient evidence on which to initiate therapy. No

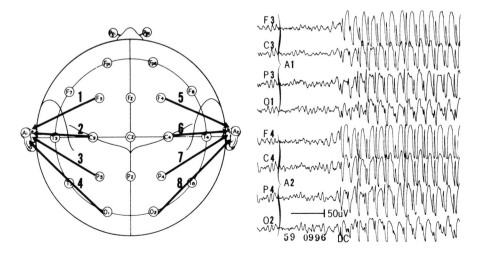

FIG. 10.2. Petit mal. Three-per-second spike and wave, generalized.

further diagnostic studies are required because petit mal seizures never have a proved structural basis.

The other seizure types usually classified as part of the petit mal triad are much rarer, probably have no common etiologic basis, and are usually more refractory to treatment. In fact, the major characteristic in common with absence attacks is their brevity. These are akinetic and myoclonic seizures. The former are brief (1 to 2 sec) episodes of sudden loss of postural tone, during which the patient may stumble or fall without cause and immediately regain normal posture. Myoclonic seizures are sudden episodes of trunk flexion associated usually with an upward jerking of the arms, occurring so rapidly that it is difficult to know that consciousness has been lost. Akinetic and myoclonic seizures show a characteristic EEG pattern of brief paroxysms of symmetrical spike activity (Fig. 10.3), and both are often associated with mental retardation and other signs of diffuse brain disease.

GRAND MAL OR MAJOR MOTOR ATTACKS

In unlocalized grand mal the onset is without aura, *the aura being considered part of the attack and frequently having localizing value*. The patient loses consciousness and has a generalized symmetrical convulsion, often characterized just by tonic extension of the extremities and trunk followed by clonic jerks. Urinary incontinence and tongue-biting are common. The attacks usually last 2 to 3 min, after which the patient relaxes, breathes regularly, and is then unresponsive for several minutes. Upon awakening, he is confused, unaware of what has happened, and if left undisturbed often sleeps

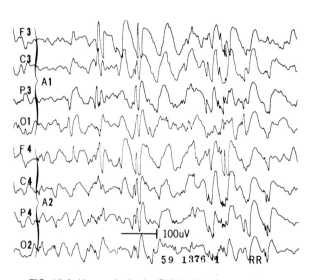

FIG. 10.3. Hypsarrhythmia. Child with salaam epilepsy.

postictal depression

for several hours. Injuries caused by the fall are frequent. The frequency is extremely variable, for they may occur at less than yearly intervals or several times weekly. In some patients they occur only during sleep.

Unlocalized grand mal convulsions may be idiopathic or symptomatic. When they begin during childhood or occur in conjunction with petit mal attacks, they are usually idiopathic. A focal EEG abnormality denotes that they are symptomatic, and investigation into the cause is in order. The EEG during a grand mal seizure goes through several stages, beginning with a generalized burst of high-voltage sharp waves (multiple spikes) which correlates with the tonic phase of the seizure. During the clonic phase there are bilaterally synchronous spikes and slow waves, and during the quiet period of unconsciousness there are diffuse moderate- to high-voltage slow waves. The EEG may not return to normal for 18 to 24 hr. During the interictal period the EEG may be normal or show random sharp waves and high-voltage slow activity, which is accentuated during hyperventilation.

The *mechanisms* responsible for the initiation and cessation of an epileptic seizure are only partially understood. Probably some biochemical event triggers the excitatory discharges from one or more neurons, and the seizure ends when the cells have exhausted their high-energy substrates or when hyperpolarization of surrounding cells contain and quench the discharge. The energy consequences of the seizure are of interest because local metabolic rate is greatly increased along with acceleration of all cellular metabolic processes. The increased metabolic demand cannot be met by production of high-energy phosphates; consequently ATP in brain tissue diminishes and there is local tissue acidosis, which likely is responsible for the increased blood flow to the discharging areas. Much of the above may be attributed to the hypoxemia which accompanies the tonic phase of the seizure, during which respiration is ineffective and arterial PaO_2 decreases and $PaCO_2$ increases. The tenuous metabolic balance that exists during a seizure may be further disturbed by repeated seizures, which may therefore cause neuronal destruction.

SEIZURE WORK-UP

The work-up of a patient with epilepsy is comprised first and foremost of a careful history and physical examination, with special attention to the neurologic examination. The types of questions asked and the significance of the responses have been discussed; in addition, the careful physician looks for any clue that may help to explain the seizure. The presence of adenoma sebaceum, previously overlooked, may suggest tuberous sclerosis, which is known to produce seizures that may not begin until adolescence or adulthood. An old scalp scar or skull depression may incriminate trauma. Auscultation of the eyeballs is important to detect the bruit of a cerebral arteriovenous anomaly. Of course any neurologic deficit calls attention to the likelihood that

infant + child: congenital malformation, birth injury, idiopathic, infections, trauma
adolescent: idiopathic, trauma
young adult: trauma, EtOH, neoplasm
middle age: neoplasm, EtOH, vascular disease, trauma
late life (>65) vascular disease, neoplasm

the seizure has a structural basis. Seizures having their onset during a patient's hospitalization for other causes present a different type of diagnostic problem. Many of these are manifestations of a metabolic or toxic encephalopathy, which must be examined for carefully. Serum electrolytes, blood sugar, and serum calcium, phosphorus, and magnesium must be evaluated promptly.

The extent of work-up of a seizure problem obviously depends on how old it is, whether there has been a problem controlling the seizures, and the age of the patient. The incidence of previously asymptomatic, unsuspected tumors, with no evidence of associated neurologic deficit in patients who present to the physician with a recent single seizure and no history of seizures, increases with age. Extremely uncommon in children, they are sufficiently common during late adolescence and early adult life that these patients should all have computerized axial tomography (CAT) scans of the brain as a part of the work-up, which of course, also includes the usual blood work, X-ray film of the chest, and EEG. The EEG is an essential part of the evaluation of any patient with seizures, not only as a diagnostic tool to help define the possible etiology and localization of a lesion, but also to help in planning pharmacologic therapy. Our experience has been that the CAT scan may detect a totally unsuspected mass lesion in patients who have had only one seizure and who are without abnormal signs. It is an invaluable aid. If it is negative, the patients may be begun on anticonvulsants and then followed carefully during the next 2 years; *during this time, the possibility that the seizure was caused by a tumor or other mass lesion must always be kept in mind.*

Although most seizures are readily diagnosable, others may be subtle, confusing, and suggestive of hysteria or other psychogenic disease. These may be quite difficult to diagnose, particularly if the interictal EEG is normal. More sophisticated diagnostic techniques have recently evolved, but they are available in only a few centers. Patients may be kept under closed circuit television monitoring and EEG recording for periods up to 36 or 48 hr, allowing correlation of the observed clinical event and brain electrical activity.

Invasive neuroradiologic procedures are rarely indicated in the modern diagnosis of epilepsy. Angiography may be necessary to explain an unusual CAT finding or if an arteriovenous anomaly is suspected. There is virtually no indication for pneumoencephalography in the work-up of a patient with epilepsy.

TREATMENT

The ideal objective of therapy in epilepsy is to prevent seizures without producing any complications from the treating drug. Except for those rare instances in which surgical removal of a brain lesion that has been causing seizures actually results in a cure of the patient, the management of the patient with epilepsy is usually a long-term contract between the patient and physician based on the regular use of anticonvulsant drugs. The patient must understand that therapy is directed toward suppressing the abnormal cerebral neuronal activity and that the price of success is regularity of drug administration. The physician must be prepared to adjust medication dosage depending on the patient's needs, varying between continuing seizures and drug intoxication, and to utilize other anticonvulsant drugs should one prove unsuccessful, even if pushed to toxicity. The availability of gas chromatographic means of measuring blood levels of the most common anticonvulsant drugs has been a powerful weapon for the clinician, who can now adjust dosage much more scientifically and accurately.

It is clear that exploitation of a few basic principles permits excellent if not perfect seizure control, with a minimum of disability from drug toxicity, in about 85% of patients with uncomplicated grand mal epilepsy. Mixed and complex seizure patterns are considerably more difficult to control, and those children with severe myoclonic seizures or infantile spasms (hypsarrhythmia) are the least effectively managed, particularly so because they usually have progressively worsening brain disease. The basic management principles are as follows:

1. The proper drug should be chosen for the seizure type.
2. Keep therapy simple by avoiding drug combinations if possible.
3. Exploit one drug thoroughly (i.e., to the point of toxicity) before changing.
4. Changes of drugs should be accomplished gradually, except in the instance of an acute drug reaction. Sudden discontinuation of a drug may precipitate status epilepticus.
5. Failure to take medication is the most frequent cause of seizure recurrence in a patient who has been previously well controlled.
6. Drug toxicity must be anticipated by regular physical examinations and blood counts.
7. Proper use must be made of anticonvulsant blood levels.

Seizure Type and Drug Choice

Petit Mal Absences

Ethosuximide (Zarontin)

The dosage of ethosuximide (Zarontin) is 20 to 30 mg/kg. Begin therapy with 250 mg daily and increase by 250 mg at weekly intervals until seizures are controlled or the patient becomes somnolent. Drug reactions are rare. This is the advantage of this drug over trimethadione (Tridione), which results in a much higher incidence of bone marrow depression and hepatic and renal toxicity. However, even with ethosuximide these complications must be looked for regularly. Plasma levels of 35 to 60 μg/ml are therapeutic and usually do not produce somnolence, but the levels may be increased to 100 μg/ml if necessary to control seizures.

Sodium valproate

Sodium valproate, or valproic acid, has been used for several years in Europe in the management of petit mal or myoclonus, and observations in the United States have now confirmed its effectiveness in these two seizure disorders. The dose is 15 mg/kg, increasing slowly to 30 mg/kg; and the therapeutic serum level range is 40 to 100 μg/ml. The major complications are gastrointestinal upset (nausea, vomiting, cramps, diarrhea) and hepato-toxicity. Clinical follow-up must take the latter into account. Valproate reduces the phenytoin level by half and increases the phenobarbital level by 50%.

Major Motor Seizures, Focal and Generalized

Carbamazepine (Tegretol)

Carbamazepine is now considered the drug of first choice in all generalized and focal major motor seizures. A major reason is that it produces fewer complications than phenytoin and is just as effective. Treatment must be begun slowly, building to an effective blood level of 4 to 12 μg/ml within 5 to 7 days; otherwise the patient will become drowsy and unsteady. Begin with 200 mg t.i.d. and increase up to a maximum of 2 g daily. Carbamazepine may cause bone marrow depression, particularly leukopenia. Blood counts should be done every 2 weeks for 2 months, then monthly.

Phenytoin (diphenylhydantoin; Dilantin)

The therapeutic blood level for phenytoin (diphenylhydantoin; Dilantin) is 10 to 20 μg/ml. The dosage (usually 400 mg daily) may be divided into three or four equal parts during the day or the entire dosage taken at bedtime. Nystagmus usually accompanies a therapeutic dose. Toxicity includes drowsiness, unsteadiness, gingival hypertrophy, and increased facial hair. *Permanent cerebellar damage may occur after prolonged use.* Allergic effects include blood dyscrasia, hepatitis, and various rashes.

Phenobarbital

Phenobarbital may be effective but usually causes excessive sedation in adequate doses. In addition, it has been reported to cause hyperactivity in children. The required dosage may be 90 to 360 mg daily. Phenobarbital is often used with phenytoin if the former alone has not controlled the seizures. The therapeutic serum range is 20 to 50 μg/ml.

Primidone (Mysoline)

Primidone has been at least partially replaced by carbamazepine, but it is the most effective drug in psychomotor seizures and generalized or focal motor seizures in some patients. Dosage must be initiated slowly because the drug may produce intolerable somnolence until the patient acclimates to it. It is available in 250 and 50 mg tablets; the maximum dose is 750 to 1,000 mg daily. Mysoline is converted to phenobarbital, and so the two should never be given together. The therapeutic serum range is 4 to 10 μg/ml.

Myoclonic Seizures

Clonazepam (Clonopin) is the drug of choice for myoclonic seizures in doses of 0.01 to 0.03 mg/kg increasing to 0.2 mg/kg daily. Drowsiness is the major complication.

Infantile Spasms

The treatment of choice for infantile spasms is ACTH or steroids.

Status Epilepticus

The seizures of status epilepticus occur without recovery between attacks. It is a life-threatening situation, requiring immediate attention. The treatment of status actually depends on its cause, and this may not be immediately evident. In the epileptic patient, status may be the result of rapid withdrawal of medications, and the treatment is therefore directed at raising the blood level of the anticonvulsant to a therapeutic range as rapidly as possible. Status usually requires at least a two-drug treatment: diazepam (Valium) plus a major anticonvulsant. Diazepam is started immediately and given intravenously in a single 10-mg dose over a period of 5 to 10 min. The patient should be observed carefully to prevent airway obstruction. This is followed by phenytoin, 50 to 75 mg/min up to 10 to 20 mg/kg total dosage. The same dosage schedule may be followed for phenobarbital if it is preferred or if phenytoin proves to be ineffective, so long as the patient is assured of a patent airway and assistive respiration.

Simultaneous with anticonvulsant therapy, the patient in status should receive oxygen, intravenous glucose, and, according to some authorities, $NaHCO_3$. Dexamethasone (Decadron) in doses up to 24 mg during the first 12 hr may be helpful, but convincing proof is lacking.

Part of the management of the patient with status epilepticus is the search for its cause. In a known epileptic, anticonvulsant blood levels may be demonstrated to be inadequate. Metabolic disturbances of all sorts, including hyponatremia, hypoglycemia, hypoxia, and uremia, must be considered, and recent head injury or subdural hematomas may also be responsible.

If the usual measures described above do not control the seizures, other measures must be taken. Intravenous paraldehyde may be useful, particularly in children, in a 5% solution in saline intravenously by *slow drip* up to 2.5 mg/kg. It may cause a painful abscess if given intramuscularly and can dissolve plastic tubing and syringes.

The services of an anesthesiologist may be required if status persists despite treatment. Pancuronium (Pavulon) may be used to paralyze the patient if the persistent muscle contractions caused by the seizures impair respiration significantly. The patient must, of course, be intubated and on a respirator. General anesthesia may be used as a last resort.

Surgical Treatment

Medically uncontrolled seizures, focal and generalized or psychomotor, are sometimes helped by surgical excision of the discharging focus. The operation should be done only if electrocorticography is available. The electrophysiologist must locate the electrical focus for the surgeon.

Miscellaneous

It is important to re-emphasize the principles of drug management for epilepsy as outlined earlier in this section. A drug must be tried to the point of toxicity before abandoning it for another. Most patients do not require more than one anticonvulsant, or two at the most. It is essential to monitor the anticonvulsant blood levels. Alcohol increases the likelihood of seizures. Phenytoin effect is depressed by carbamazepine and folic acid, and enhanced by bishydroxycoumarin (dicumarol), chloramphenicol, paraamino salicylic acid, and isoniazid.

The proper management of a patient with chronic seizures requires not only a knowledge of drug choices and dosages, but also a great deal of patience and common sense. Seizure is a disorder in which the physician and patient literally must enter a partnership to achieve proper control and to allow the patient to live a normal life. The patient's activities should not be restricted more than is absolutely necessary, but questions about driving, swimming, or other hazardous pursuits must be handled firmly. There is a great deal of job discrimination against epileptics; hence the physician must be prepared to deal with his patient's disappointments and, most important, serve as an educational resource for his community.

SUGGESTED READINGS

Classification

Ajmone-Marsan C: A newly prepared classification of epileptic seizures: neurophysiological bases. *Epilepsia* 6:275, 1965.

Types

Caveness WF, Meirowsky AM, Rish BL, Mohr JP, Kistler JP, Dillon JD, and Weiss GH: The nature of post-traumatic epilepsy. *J Neurosurg* 50:545, 1979.

Chen R-C, and Forster FM: Cursive epilepsy and gelastic epilepsy. *Neurology (Minneap)* 23:1019, 1973.

Evans JH: Post-traumatic epilepsy. *Neurology (Minneap)* 12:665, 1962.

Neidermeyer E, and Khalifeh R: Petit mal status ("spike wave stupor"). *Epilepsia* 6:250, 1965.

Sumi SM, and Teasdall RD: Focal seizures: a review of 150 cases. *Neurology (Minneap)* 13:582, 1963.

Physiology and Pathogenesis

Beresford HR, Posner JB, and Plum F: Changes in brain lactate during induced cerebral seizures. *Arch Neurol* 20:243, 1969.

Blennow G, Brierley JB, Meldrum BS, and Siesjö BK: Epileptic brain damage: the role of systemic factors that modify cerebral energy metabolism. *Brain* 101:687, 1978.

Brazier MAB: The search for the neuronal mechanisms in epilepsy: an overview. *Neurology (Minneap)* 24:903, 1974.

Falconer MA, et al: The etiology and pathogenesis of temporal lobe epilepsy. *Arch Neurol* 10:233, 1964.

Rosenblatt DE, Lauter CJ, and Trams EG: Deficiency of a Ca^{2+}-ATPase in brains of seizure prone mice. *J Neurochem* 27:1299, 1976.

Wasterlain CG: Effects of epileptic seizures on brain ribosomes: mechanism and relationship to cerebral energy metabolism. *J Neurochem* 29:707, 1977.

Clinical

Cole M, and Zangwell OL: Deja vu in temporal lobe epilepsy. *J Neurol Neurosurg Psychiatry* 26:37, 1963.

Currie S, Heathfield KWG, Henson RA, and Scott DF: Clinical course and prognosis of temporal lobe epilepsy: a survey of 666 patients. *Brain* 94:173, 1971.

Currier RD, Kooi KA, and Saidman LJ: Prognosis of "pure" petit mal: a follow-up study. *Neurology (Minneap)* 13:959, 1963.

Eisner V: Hereditary aspects of epilepsy. *Bull Johns Hopkins Hosp* 105:245, 1959.

Epilepsia (special issue): Symposium on epilepsy and heredity. 10:100, 1969.

Glaser FH: The problem of psychosis in psychomotor temporal lobe epileptics. *Epilepsia* 5:271, 1968.

Jennett W: Predicting epilepsy after blunt head injury. *Br Med J* 1:1215, 1965.

Jensen I, and Larsen JK: Mental aspects of temporal lobe epilepsy: follow-up of 74 patients after resection of a temporal lobe. *J Neurol Neurosurg Psychiatry* 42:256, 1979.

Jensen I, and Klinken L: Temporal lobe epilepsy and neuropathology. *Acta Neurol Scand* 54:391, 1976.

Kristensen O, and Sindrup EH: Psychomotor epilepsy and psychosis. I. Physical aspects. *Acta Neurol Scand* 57:361, 1978.

Oxbury JM, and Whitty CWM: Causes and consequences of status epilepticus in adults: a study of 86 cases. *Brain* 94:733, 1971.

Porter RJ, Penry JK, and Lacy JR: Diagnostic and therapeutic re-evaluation of patients with intractable epilepsy. *Neurology (Minneap)* 27:1006, 1977.

Radin EA: *The Prognosis of Patients with Epilepsy.* Charles C Thomas, Springfield, Illinois, 1968.

Schmidt RP, and Wilder BJ: *Epilepsy.* Davis, Philadelphia, 1968.

Williams D: The border-land of epilepsy revisited. *Brain* 98:1, 1975.

Diagnosis

Brazier MAB, and Crandall PH: Tests of the predictive value of EEG recording from within the brain in the partial epilepsies. *Contemp Clin Neurophysiol* 34:83, 1978.

Management

Adams DJ, Luders H, and Pippenger C: Sodium valproate in the treatment of intractable seizure disorders: a clinical and electroencephalographic study. *Neurology (Minneap)* 28:152, 1978.

Bailey DW, and Fenichel GM: The treatment of prolonged seizure activity with intravenous diazepam. *Pediatr Pharmacol Ther* 73:923, 1968.

Bruni J, and Wilder BJ: Valproic acid: review of a new antiepileptic drug. *Arch Neurol* 36:393, 1979.

Costeff H: Convulsions in childhood: their natural history and indications for treatment. *N Engl J Med* 273:1410, 1965.

Falconer MA: Significance of surgery for temporal lobe epilepsy in childhood and adolescence. *J Neurol Neurosurg Psychiatry* 33:233, 1970.

Gastaut H, Naquet R, Poire R, and Tassinari CA: Treatment of status epilepticus with diazepam (Valium). *Epilepsia* 6:167, 1965.

Goldring S: A method for surgical management of focal epilepsy, especially as it relates to children. *J Neurosurg* 49:344, 1978.

Holcomb R, Lynn R, Harvey B Jr, Sweetman BJ, and Gerber N: Intoxication with 5,5-diphenylhydantoin (Dilantin). *J Pediatr* 80:627, 1972.

Jensen I, and Larsen JK: Mental aspects of temporal lobe epilepsy: follow-up of 74 patients after resection of a temporal lobe. *J Neurol Neurosurg Psychiatry* 42:256, 1979.

Kutt H, and McDowell F: Management of epilepsy with diphenylhydantoin sodium: dosage regulation for problem patients. *JAMA* 203:969, 1968.

Pincus JH, Grove I, Marion BB, and Glaser GE: Studies on the mechanism of action of diphenylhydantoin. *Arch Neurol* 22:566, 1970.

Pippenger CE, Penry JK, White BG, Daly DD, and Buddington R: Interlaboratory variability in determination of plasma antiepileptic drug concentrations. *Arch Neurol* 33:351, 1976.

Ruuskanen I, Kilpelainen O, and Riekkinen PJ: Side effects of sodium valproate during long-term treatment in epilepsy. *Acta Neurol Scand* 60:125, 1979.

Toman JEP: Drugs effective in convulsive disorders. In: *Pharmacological Basis of Therapeutics,* edited by L Goodman and A Gilman, pp 215–236, 3rd ed. Macmillan, New York, 1965.

Wilder BJ, Willmore LJ, Bruni J, and Villarreal HJ: Valproic acid: interaction with other anticonvulsant drugs. *Neurology (Minneap)* 28:892, 1978.

Wolf SM: Controversies in the treatment of febrile convulsions. *Neurology (Minneap)* 29:287, 1979.

Social: Legal

Barrow RL, and Fabing HD: *Epilepsy and the Law*, 2nd edition. Hoeber, New York, 1966.

11

Management of the Unconscious Patient

Disturbance of consciousness is a medical emergency, requiring that the physician immediately institute measures to determine the cause and begin proper management. Failure to do so may result in the patient's death, either from the causative lesion or the secondary effects of coma, i.e., aspiration and asphyxiation or pneumonitis. As the primary care physician is usually the first called on to deal with the problem, he should be familiar with the basic concepts and approaches that will enable him to evaluate the unconscious patient competently and thereafter either institute proper therapy or call for appropriate consultative assistance. This chapter is a discussion of the types and locations of the lesions resulting in disturbed consciousness and how to proceed in the evaluation and management of a comatose patient.

TYPES AND LOCATIONS OF LESIONS THAT CAUSE
DISTURBANCES OF CONSCIOUSNESS

Any true disturbance of consciousness is an indication of a disorder of brain function, and the responsible mechanisms are the same, regardless of the degree to which consciousness is impaired. This is an important point because the treating physician must be adept at recognizing the early stages of alterations of consciousness if treatment is to be effective. By the time a patient becomes comatose the responsible pathology will be much more advanced and therefore difficult to treat. *The quantitative assessment of consciousness by the physician is entirely for the purpose of following a patient's progress; the mildest state of consciousness impairment is an indication of pathology and requires evaluation and management.*

Although there are variations, the clinical quantitation of consciousness is usually as follows: alert, lethargic, stupor, and coma. The discussion of what comprises the alert state can be complex and philosophic; it obviously varies among individuals. Each physician must have a standard by which he measures the normal state of alertness if he is to identify the earliest evidence of impaired consciousness which we arbitrarily designate *lethargy*. Lethargy must be distinguished from disorders of attention, which occur in otherwise alert individuals with certain types of focal hemispheric disease (viz., right parietal lesions) and in patients with specific forms of psychiatric disease (schizophrenia).

Lethargy is a mild blunting of consciousness, drowsiness, slowness in reaction. The patient may have difficulty following instructions, and he may appear confused. Unless there is associated delirium or agitation, the patient shows little spontaneity and does not initiate conversation. He may be disoriented and demonstrate defects in memory and incoherent thinking. A characteristic of lethargy then is that the patient shows mental status defects of dementia in addition to blunting of consciousness. An important distinction is that a patient may be demented but show none of the signs of lethargy.

Stupor is a state of severe drowsiness requiring vigorous stimuli to arouse the patient. The response to spoken commands is either absent, incorrect, or slowed. The patient appears to be shielded from external stimuli but is still capable of being roused.

The comatose patient does not respond meaningfully or appropriately to any type of stimulus, although reflex activity may be intact or even exaggerated. It is pointless to argue whether a patient who moves or groans following a painful stimulus is comatose or stuporous; the physiologic significance is the same. In deep coma there is no reaction of any type to any stimulus. *The intensity and characteristics of the coma state are often determined by its etiology* (described below).

It is generally accepted that consciousness depends on the integrity of the reticular activating system (RAS), a morphologically varied group of neurons extending, together with their axons, from the medulla to the thalami, which in turn have diffuse projections to the cortical mantle of both hemispheres. Clinicopathologic correlations have shown that relatively small lesions of the midbrain and pons result in coma, for here the fibers of the RAS are compact, whereas a widespread diffuse lesion of both cerebral hemispheres is necessary to cause coma.

Thus *the anatomy of the RAS is such that discrete structural lesions of the cerebral hemispheres (e.g., infarction, tumor, or abscess) do not cause coma unless the increased volume of the hemisphere caused by the lesion (e.g., edema in infarction, tumor mass) secondarily affects the structures responsible for maintenance of consciousness in the hypothalamus, midbrain, and upper pons.* For example, an expanding mass lesion in one cerebral hemisphere exerts a caudal and lateral pressure on the hypothalamus and may also cause the most medial portion of the temporal lobe (uncus) to be squeezed medially and caudally so that it herniates beneath the tentorium, the dural shelf that separates the middle and posterior cerebral fossae. This herniated brain acts as a foreign body in the crowded space adjacent to the cerebral peduncles, squeezing the midbrain against the opposite sharp rim of the tentorium. The RAS in this part of the midbrain is damaged by the pressure, and the patient becomes unconscious.

The structural cerebral hemisphere lesions which cause coma all do so, therefore, by secondary effect on the hypothalamus or brainstem. This applies even to the comatose state that accompanies a massive intracerebral hemorrhage, which usually causes coma by the sudden rupture of blood into the lateral ventricles, allowing it to spread rapidly throughout the ventricular system and subarachnoid space. In many such instances it is felt that consciousness is lost because of the concussive effects of the blood on the midbrain and pons as it flows into and engorges the 3rd ventricle, aqueduct of Sylvius, and 4th ventricle.

Thus any type of supratentorial (cerebral hemisphere) structural lesion may cause coma by virtue of the effects described above. Such lesions include *tumor, intracerebral hemorrhage, subdural or epidural hemotomas, abscess, infarction with edema, and brain injury and swelling.* In all instances, the damage caused to the brainstem structures may be permanent, preventing

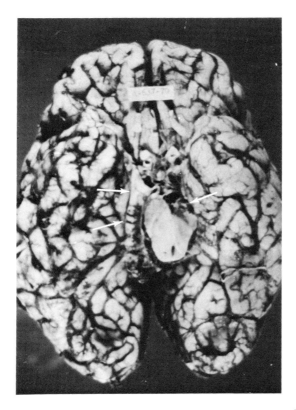

FIG. 11.1. Right uncal herniation from increased intrahemispheric pressure. A massive intra-cerebral hemorrhage caused the medial portion of the hippocampus to herniate beneath the tentorial shelf (removed), which has grooved the inferior surface of the uncus (*arrows*). Note how the midbrain has been pushed to the left, and that the left cerebral peduncle (*arrow*) has been crushed against the opposite tentorial shelf (Kernohan's notch).

recovery, even though the primary lesion in the hemisphere is successfully treated (Fig. 11.1).

The clinical sequence of events which accompanies the expansion of an intracranial mass does not always follow a rigid or textbook pattern. As a rule, rapidly expanding mass lesions (intracerebral clot, epidural hemotoma, brain swelling after trauma) produce greater neurologic deficits and more disturbance of consciousness for the amount of brain distortion and displacement they cause than do more slowly developing mass lesions (slow-growing brain tumors, chronic subdural hematomas). The reason for this is not understood; it is speculated that there is time for an adjustment of the blood supply in the latter instance. As the hemispheric mass lesion expands and stretches, and displaces the 3rd ventricle and hypothalamus, the patient becomes increasingly lethargic and sometimes displays restlessness, agitation, and variations in pulse rate and blood pressure, followed by dilatation and poor light response of the pupil and drooping eyelid on the homolateral side. These signs denote stretching of the blood supply to the hypothalamus and mesencephalon as the midline structures are displaced laterally and caudally, and pressure on the homolateral oculomotor nerve by the herniating uncus. The oculomotor nerve is trapped between the posterior cerebral artery and superior cerebellar artery as both of these vessels encircle the cerebral peduncle. All of these structures are distorted by the downward thrust of the brainstem.

Subsequent signs usually follow in rapid sequence or *pari passu*: complete homolateral oculomotor nerve paralysis, stupor and coma, decorticate and then decerebrate posturing (Fig. 11.2), disturbances of conjugate ocular movement, and abnormalities of respiratory patterns. The herniating uncus and caudal compression of the brainstem cause coma and the other described signs by damaging the midbrain, the damage being in the form of scattered, but mainly midline, venous hemorrhages (Duret's hemorrhages); but it is also caused by ischemia and infarction due to the vascular distortion. Compression of the posterior cerebral artery against the hard tentorial shelf during herniation may result in infarction of the homolateral occipital pole.

Another syndrome associated with transtentorial herniation and coma may cause confusion in the lateralization of the hemisphere lesion. It is referred to as the syndrome of Kernohan's notch. When the uncus herniates beneath the tentorium, it may displace the midbrain sharply to the opposite side, compressing the contralateral cerebral peduncle against the adjacent sharp, unyielding tentorial edge and injuring the corticobulbar and corticospinal tract fibers in that peduncle. This results in hemiparesis or hemiplegia on the side opposite the injured peduncle, thereby causing a clinical syndrome in which the hemiparesis is on the same side as the original cerebral hemisphere mass lesion and homolateral to the oculomotor palsy. Because surgical treatment must be directed to the hemisphere mass lesion, the possibility of such a syndrome must always be taken into account when planning surgery. The localizing clue is the oculomotor palsy. Fortunately, computerized axial to-

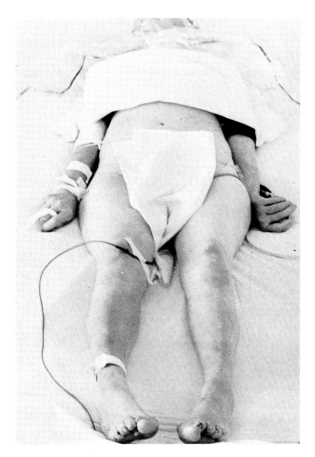

FIG. 11.2. Decerebrate posturing. Arms extended at sides with palms externally rotated, legs extended and adducted, neck and back extended. Diagnosis: high pontine infarction.

mography (CAT) scanning has practically eliminated the uncertainty of localizing hemisphere mass lesions, so the likelihood of an error in localization is negligible.

It follows that only a small lesion of the midbrain or pons is required to cause coma, and this may occur in conjunction with brainstem hemorrhage or infarction, whereas diffuse bihemispheric dysfunction, as is seen in metabolic or toxic encephalopathies, is necessary to cause unconsciousness. Examples of this are anoxia, hypoglycemia, or barbiturate poisoning. Such metabolic abnormalities may produce neurologic abnormalities in addition to coma and therefore present a diagnostic challenge.

In contrast, metabolic and toxic causes of coma develop gradually, often without lateralizing neurologic signs, and most often in the setting of previously recognized illness, e.g., hepatic or renal disease, diabetes, or endocrine disorders. The diagnosis of the cause of coma is more difficult, of course, if no historical data are available, as is often true when a patient is brought unconscious to a hospital emergency room. In that condition, the attending physician must exert his powers of observation and deduction, and look for the telltale signs that denote the cause of the coma.

METHOD OF MANAGEMENT

The paramount issues in taking care of an unconscious patient are to protect the patient from the consequences of coma (e.g., aspiration) and to determine as quickly as possible the cause of the coma in order to institute correct treatment. As much historical information as is available should be obtained, for this may indicate the etiology of the problem. A history of a preceding convulsion may explain the patient's unconsciousness and stertorous breathing. The history of diabetes leads to consideration of diabetic acidosis or hypoglycemia, which are usually readily distinguishable. The sudden onset of headache, hemiparesis, followed by collapse and coma usually denotes intracerebral hemorrhage with intraventricular or subarachnoid extension. The sudden onset of coma without a history of trauma or convulsion in a previously well person almost invariably means an intracranial hemorrhage of some sort.

Management is best accomplished following a set procedure:

1. *Establish an airway.* No matter the cause of the coma, known or not, the first responsibility is to be certain that the patient has a patent airway and that he is protected against aspiration. This may require nothing more than positioning the head or, at the other extreme, a tracheostomy. The rule is that, no matter what is necessary to establish and maintain a clear airway, it must be done at once.

2. *Look for shock and treat immediately.* Severe hypotension, if prolonged, will cause cerebral ischemia.

3. If the cause of the coma is in doubt, draw blood immediately for glucose determination and, through the same needle, *give 100 ml of 50% glucose (50 g).* If the patient is comatose due to hypoglycemia (usually secondary to insulin overdose), he will probably awaken. No matter what the cause of the coma, even if caused by diabetic acidosis, the intravenous glucose will not harm the patient, and the blood sugar determination may establish the diagnosis for proper management. It should be remembered that the hypoglycemia may be so profound that as much as 150 g glucose is necessary to wake the patient, so the cause is not abandoned if the patient fails to awaken after the initial injection.

4. *Set about establishing the cause of the coma.* The first step is to decide if the coma is caused by structural brain damage (e.g., brain hemorrhage, infarct, tumor), drug intoxication, or metabolic disorder. Once this general distinction has been made, a more specific etiology can be sought in order to initiate treatment. It is helpful to invest a few minutes in watching the patient. Look for eversion of a paretic lower extremity or spontaneous movement of one side only, both signs suggesting a structural brain lesion. Watch the respiratory pattern and observe for posturing movements.

There are a few cardinal features that distinguish coma of structural or metabolic cause, and these need emphasis because of their diagnostic value.

1. Lateralizing motor signs (e.g., hemiplegia) are strong evidence for a structural cause for the coma. On the other hand, a rare patient with metabolic encephalopathy may show signs of corticospinal tract involvement and hemiparesis. In addition, a patient with old hemiparesis may also present in coma for a different cause.

2. Papilledema does not occur in metabolic encephalopathy. The only exception is the acute hypoparathyroid state which may follow thyroidectomy. Encephalopathy in the form of seizures may occur in these patients.

3. Absent pupillary reflexes almost always mean structural brain disease. Exceptions include glutethimide (Doriden) intoxication, in which the pupils are moderately dilated but fixed to light, and atropine poisoning, in which they are fully dilated and fixed to light. *— brainstem function*

4. Absent oculocephalic (doll's eyes) reflexes or response to caloric vestibular stimulation (ice water in the external auditory canal) argue strongly for structural cause of coma. Rarely, these signs, which depend on the integrity of the brainstem, may be lost in the presence of deep coma caused by metabolic encephalopathy or intoxication with phenytoin or phenobarbital. Eye movements must be carefully examined, for they provide a great deal of information about lesion localization. The oculocephalic reflexes are obtained by turning the patient's head briskly from side to side. The reflexes are intact if the eyes move conjugately in the opposite direction, completely filling the canthi. If this can be seen, there is no reason to do caloric testing, but the fact is that evaluation of the doll's head maneuver may be different in a comatose patient who is intubated and hard to examine. Caloric testing is performed after being certain that the tympanic membranes are intact, after which ice water is syringed in one ear at a time, observing the effect on eye movement. The normal response is that the eyes deviate conjugately to the side of the stimulation and nystagmus with the fast component to the opposite side (COWS—cold opposite, warm same) develops. The fast corrective phase of *eye deviation =* the nystagmus may be lost in deep coma for any reason, but absence of the *Brainstem* conjugate movement denotes a structural lesion affecting the vestibulo-ocular *pathway intact* pathways. Other valuable localizing information may appear. Failure of ad- *suggesting relatively intact Brainstem*

duction of the contralateral eye denotes internuclear ophthalmoplegia (interruption of the medial longitudinal fasciculus), and failure of abduction of the homolateral eye denotes 6th nerve palsy.

5. Tremor, myoclonus, and asterixis are common accompaniments of metabolic encephalopathy in the stages of declining consciousness. They disappear when the patient becomes comatose.

6. The electroencephalogram (EEG) is *always* abnormal in metabolic encephalopathy but can be normal in coma resulting from intrinsic structural brainstem disease. The type of EEG abnormality is sometimes helpful in distinguishing the cause of coma. For example, in barbiturate intoxication, fast-wave ($>$ 14/sec) activity is frequent; this never occurs in other types of metabolic encephalopathy. Rarely, status epilepticus exists in the absence of clinical seizure activity, and the patient appears only to be comatose; here the EEG may show the true electrical status, which certainly offers a special clue for management.

7. Respiratory irregularity is almost invariably a sign of structural brain disease: the greater the irregularity, the more caudal the lesion in the brainstem. Patients in coma from metabolic encephalopathy often show the respiratory characteristics that are secondary to the primary disease process, e.g., the Kussmaul respiration (deep hyperventilation) characteristic of diabetic coma or any metabolic acidosis, or the hypoventilatory pattern of chronic lung disease and severe carbon dioxide retention. Respiratory patterns may become irregular late in the course of a severe metabolic encephalopathy; this augurs ill for the patient. Although a great deal has been written about the various abnormal types of respiratory patterns which occur in lesions at various vertical levels of the neural axis, I have found them to be the least reliable of the clinical signs for distinguishing metabolic coma from that caused by a structural lesion. The examples given above which occur in metabolic disorders are the most useful. *Cheyne-Stokes* respiration is thought to signify loss of cortical control of respiratory rate and rhythm, so that the respiratory center is influenced almost exclusively by $PaCO_2$. *Central neurogenic hyperventilation* closely simulates metabolic acidosis and may actually cause respiratory alkalosis. When it can be documented, one can be reasonably sure that the patient has an extensive lesion in the upper pons, although such lesions may also occur without provoking respiratory abnormalities.

Causes of Metabolic Coma

The common causes of unconsciousness from lesions in the cerebral hemisphere have already been discussed briefly. It is re-emphasized that mass lesions of the cerebral hemispheres produce coma by virtue of their secondary pressure effect on the diencephalon or brainstem. The most frequent causes of metabolic coma are as follows.

Hypoglycemia

Because of its frequency in young diabetics with brittle control, hypoglycemia should always be considered first. Once the patient is unconscious, there are no distinguishing clinical features, although needle marks from insulin injection are an obvious clue. As previously mentioned, all patients with unknown cause of coma, suspected to be metabolic, should receive 50 g glucose intravenously immediately after blood has been drawn for glucose determination. The molecular mechanism whereby hypoglycemia produces encephalopathy and coma is only partially understood. Glucose is the most important substrate utilized by the brain for the generation of energy; indeed the normal brain utilizes about 80 mg glucose per minute, equivalent to about 70% of the total resting fasting glucose output by the liver. Many studies have demonstrated that the respiratory quotient (R.Q.) of the brain approximates 1.0, confirming the dependence of the brain on a steady glucose supply. As blood glucose falls, there are concomitant alterations in EEG activity (slow high-voltage waves), neurologic function, and cerebral metabolic rate, although cerebral blood flow remains normal. A fall in blood glucose to levels sufficient to produce coma is still not associated with decreased tissue ATP. The brain utilizes its endogenous substrates (glycogen, glucose, and amino acids) to generate sufficient energy to maintain the integrity of the cell membrane, although the patient may be comatose. Survival on endogenous substrate can last no more that 60 to 90 min, after which the ATP falls sharply and tissue autolysis begins. This is the point at which irreversible tissue injury occurs and the patient either dies or has permanent neurologic sequelae if he survives.

Hypoxia

Most patients who have suffered severe brain hypoxia have a clear antecedent history of cardiac arrest, respiratory failure, aspiration, suffocation, or carbon monoxide poisoning. In the last instance, the patients usually show a characteristic cherry-colored flush. The most frequent cause of accidental carbon monoxide poisoning is the use of gasoline heaters in inadequately ventilated rooms. Such patients must be removed from exposure immediately, of course, and treated by administration of 100% oxygen. Patients who have suffered temporary cardiac arrest are almost invariably acidotic, for which immediate treatment is required. Because severe hypoxia causes brain swelling, dexamethasone (24 mg i.v. in 24 hr) is often used to minimize this effect. It goes without saying that any respiratory cause of hypoxia requires immediate therapy. In the patient who has severe pulmonary fibrosis and emphysema, the hypoxia is accompanied by hypercarbia because of accumulation of carbon dioxide in the alveoli. These patients require mechanical respiratory assistance to reduce the hypercarbia while oxygen is administered, for their respiratory centers have become insensitive to carbon dioxide and are driven by hypoxia. Administration of oxygen without mechanical respiratory assistance may cause apnea and death.

Physiologically there is a considerable difference between the effects of pure hypoxia and global cerebral ischemia (cardiac arrest), which is probably the most frequent cause of nontraumatic brain death seen in the United States. The hypoxic brain is deprived of oxygen, without which it cannot function effectively for more than a few seconds. The normal brain utilizes about 60 ml oxygen per minute, about 20% of the resting oxygen consumption of the body. The brain's oxygen store is no more than 10 ml, adequate for only 10 to 12 sec before consciousness is lost. This sets into motion a complex series of biochemical events, including increased glycolysis, resulting in increased tissue lactate and a rapid drop in ATP. Irreversible changes, first noted in the mitochondrial cell membrane, appear within 5 to 6 min. In cardiac arrest the problem is more complex because there is cessation of cerebral blood flow and failure of delivery of all substrates to the brain. Changes in blood viscosity and capillary swelling may inhibit recirculation into the ischemic areas even if cardiac function is restored. Neurologic residuals, focal and diffuse, are common.

Diabetic Coma

The diagnosis of diabetic coma is sufficiently familiar to require little elaboration here. The blood picture is that of metabolic acidosis, with decreased arterial pH, HCO_3^- below 15 mEq/liter, decreased $PaCO_2$ (< 30 torr), and normal PaO_2. Blood and urine ketones are elevated, and blood glucose is almost invariably strikingly increased. The patient is stuporous or comatose but rarely shows asterixis, convulsions, or paralysis. Respirations are deep and rapid (Kussmaul). In the management of diabetic coma, serum K^+ must be carefully watched to avoid dilutional hypokalemia. A sudden fall in blood sugar should also be avoided because of the accompanying decrease in serum osmolality, which may, in turn, cause an excessively rapid shift of water into the dehydrated brain cells resulting in brain edema.

It is interesting to note that the reason for the coma in diabetic acidosis is not known. Cerebral oxygen and glucose consumption are substantially reduced, but there is an uncoupling of the usual flow-metabolism relationship and cerebral blood flow is normal. The depression of consciousness appears to be proportional to the severity of the systemic metabolic acidosis and ketosis; perhaps ketone ions pass across the blood-brain barrier and somehow interfere with cellular function.

Hepatic Encephalopathy

The usual precipitating causes for hepatic encephalopathy are gastrointestinal bleeding, severe infections, paracentesis, or the use of ammonia-producing drugs, e.g., chlorothiazides. A history of progressive liver failure or portocaval shunting is usually present, as are signs of liver disease. Although coma may occur precipitately, it usually is preceded by several days of restlessness, agitation, and delirium, with associated tremor, occasional myoclonus, and asterixis. Examination shows hyperventilation with resultant respiratory alkalosis, bilateral rigidity, decorticate and decerebrate posturing, bilateral extensor plantar signs, and not infrequently some evidence of focal or lateralizing neurologic signs. The last may be confusing and may incorrectly suggest structural brain disease. Convulsive seizures occasionally occur. Laboratory data do not always denote severe liver disease, and blood ammonia is not invariably elevated. The EEG shows bilateral slow-wave activity, but it is not diagnostic.

Coma in severe hepatic insufficiency is thought to be due to an adverse effect of ammonia on brain oxidative metabolism. Increased brain tissue ammonia increases the rate of α-ketoglutarate diversion to glutamate. The increased ammonia also favors increased conversion of glutamate to glutamine, a reaction which is energy-requiring, thus depleting available ATP. It has also been proposed that there is increased gamma aminobutyric acid (GABA) production from the glutamate, and that the GABA acts as an inhibitory neurotransmitter, affecting cells in the reticular activating system. Hepatic encephalopathy can usually be successfully treated provided massive portocaval shunts do not exist. Treatment is by administration of (1) neomycin orally or by enema after the gastrointestinal tract has been cleared of blood and (2) lactulose, an inert sugar that acidifies the bowel contents. Nothing presently known about the biochemistry of hepatic encephalopathy explains the remarkable proliferation of Alzheimer's type II astrocytes which occurs in this condition.

Hypo-osmolar and Hyperosmolar States

Already discussed briefly in reference to their role in acute dementia, hypo- and hyperosmolar states may also result in obtundation, stupor or coma, myoclonus, seizures, and focal neurologic deficits. The diagnosis can only be suspected clinically; it must be established by laboratory examination. The mechanism of the severe neurologic disorder accompanying the hypo-osmolar state is thought to be edema of brain cells. In hypo-osmolar states serum sodium is low from either excess water intake, excessive loss of sodium in the urine as in certain kinds of kidney disease or following use of diuretics, or inappropriate antidiuretic hormone (ADH) secretion, which results in water retention and hemodilution. Inappropriate ADH secretion can occur during a wide variety of medical or neurologic illnesses, following surgery, or after head trauma. The patients demonstrate increased urine and diminished serum osmolality. Plasma and urine osmolality determinations are usually available in a hospital laboratory, but plasma osmolality can be calculated quickly from readily available laboratory data. The formula used is:

$$2(NA + K) + \frac{glucose}{18} + \frac{BUN}{2.8} = mOs/liter$$

The normal value is 290 ± 10 mOs. Treatment is by restriction of fluid intake, not by salt replacement.

Hyperglycemic hyperosmolar aketonic coma usually occurs in middle-aged to elderly diabetics whose insulin requirements have been small. The patient may present during or after one or repeated seizures and may show lateralizing focal neurologic signs along with deep coma. The diagnosis is made by the finding of strikingly elevated blood sugar (400 to 2,000 mg%) and no ketonuria. Treatment is by rehydration and insulin. Failure to recognize this problem often results in the patient's death from severe brain dehydration.

Other Causes

The other causes of metabolic coma are less common. They include uremic encephalopathy, which infrequently causes deep coma, endocrine disturbances (e.g., myxedema or Addison's disease), other electrolyte disorders (including hypercalcemia from any cause), and rarely Wernicke's encephalopathy. In most instances, the diagnosis is not difficult to establish once it is considered.

Drug-Induced Coma

Statistically, the most important cause of coma is that caused by poisons or intoxicants, and particularly barbiturates or sedatives taken for suicidal purposes. This latter group comprises the greatest incidence of coma of undetermined cause and prompt appropriate action almost invariably saves the patient, whereas delay in initiating treatment because of failure to identify the problem may end in tragedy. Because historical data may not help in identifying the cause, all patients must be treated as if they are salvageable, as outlined earlier. The axioms of maintaining respiration and blood pressure and preventing pulmonary complications are particularly applicable in phenobarbital overdose, for these patients may be profoundly comatose, areflexic, and apneic, yet recover with no evident cerebral damage if their vital functions are patiently maintained. They may be unconscious for several days even after spontaneous respirations and reflexes return, and eventually they may recover completely.

It must be emphasized that there is no certain way to determine by examination alone that the coma results from a depressant drug. If an EEG is readily available, it may provide practical help, for the EEG pattern in barbiturate poisoning is that of fast-wave activity, quite different from structural or metabolic causes of coma. Many hospital laboratories have facilities for determining blood levels of barbiturates and other common depressant suicidal agents, e.g., phenothiazines, meprobamate, or glutethimide. An elevated blood level of such a drug usually, but not invariably, establishes the diagnosis and at least allows the physician to concentrate on the care of the patient, rather than looking further for cause of the coma; however, knowing the exact agent does not, in fact, alter the therapy for an overdose, which still consists of the principles previously outlined plus, in certain instances, careful diuresis and rarely hemodialysis.

Because severe depressant poisoning may result in brainstem signs (including decerebration, bilateral extensor plantars, respiratory depression, and loss of the oculocephalic reflexes and caloric responses), the major distinguishing feature is pupillary reactivity and symmetry. Patients comatose from poisoning always retain some reactivity to bright light, whereas unequal pupils, unreactive pupils, and disconjugate eye movements during caloric stimulation point to a destructive lesion of the brainstem.

Miscellaneous Causes of Coma

There are a host of other causes of coma, the majority of which are identifiable by history or fairly obvious accompanying signs. Bacterial meningitis and acute head injury are those which might produce diagnostic difficulties if there were no history available. Patients with bacterial meningitis are febrile and show nuchal rigidity; spinal fluid examination indicates the typical pattern of increased pressure, turbid fluid, pleocytosis with polymorphonuclear neutrophils predominating, increased protein, and decreased glucose. Occasionally, in young children coma develops so quickly in the course of *Haemophilus influenzae* meningitis that the antecedent signs may have been overlooked save for irritability, anorexia, and fever.

Most patients with acute head injury show obvious evidence of it or are found in a situation that suggests the diagnosis, but occasionally no clue is immediately available. The neurologic picture of cerebral concussion is coma with preserved brainstem reflexes, reactive pupils, and flaccidity; in most instances, recovery begins shortly after the injury. In all unconscious patients with history, however, the examiner should look carefully for evidence of head trauma, e.g., scalp lacerations or abrasions, scalp edema, and of course signs of more severe injury—the presence of blood behind the tympanic membranes, ecchymoses and edema over the mastoid processes (Battle's sign), and spinal fluid in the nose.

A discussion of coma would not be complete without a special word about subdural hematoma, for it may produce a picture of progressive obtundation to coma with few or no lateralizing signs and with no history of trauma to incite suspicion of the cause. The diagnosis must always be suspected, particularly if there is any chance of even remote injury; and it should be particularly suspected in the quiet, mildly demented patient who becomes increasingly drowsy. There is no classic history or clinical picture for subdural hematoma. It should be considered in all unconscious patients, for prompt surgical treatment usually allows full recovery, whereas if it is unrecognized the result is tragic.

STATES RESEMBLING COMA

One becomes involved in semantic subtleties when attempting to distinguish *akinetic mutism* from coma because the differentiation involves a specific definition of consciousness. There are two syndromes which fit into this category and which should be distinguished from "true" coma. In one the patient lies quietly, without voluntary movements, opening his eyes occasionally to strong stimuli and occasionally showing signs of decerebration. There may be paralysis of extraocular movements. Occasionally he looks as if he is aware of the existence of the examiner, but this can never be determined. The patient is mute. The cause is an upper brainstem (high pons, low mesencephalon) lesion, usually vascular in origin. A variation is a similar posture but no paralysis of ocular movements. The patient may look about vacantly, but without evidence that he perceives or understands. He may or may not move extremities in response to stimuli. He is also mute. Here the responsible lesion is thought to be in the medial, orbital, and anterior surfaces of the frontal lobes or adjacent cingulate gyri.

The *locked-in syndrome* can be distinguished from the above by careful examination. The patient is totally immobile and unable to speak or swallow. He can respond to simple questions by opening and closing eyes, and can perceive his environment. Bilateral pyramidal tract signs are present. Decerebrate posturing may occur. The lesion is in the basis pontis, involving the corticobulbar and corticospinal pathways, and presumably sparing the reticular activating system.

SUGGESTED READINGS

Arieff AI, and Kleeman CR: Studies on mechanism of cerebral edema in diabetic coma. *J Clin Invest* 52:571, 1973.

Bates D, Caronna JJ, Cartlidge NEF, Knill-Jones RP, Levy DE, Shaw DA, and Plum F: A prospective study of nontraumatic coma: methods and results in 310 patients. *Ann Neurol* 2:211, 1977.

Brown R: The physiological basis of consciouness. *Brain* 81:426, 1958.

Cairns H: Disturbances of consciousness with lesions of the brainstem and diencephalon. *Brain* 75:109, 1952.

Cravioto H, Silberman J, and Feigin I: A clinical and pathological study of akinetic mutism. *Neurology (Minneap)* 10:10, 1960.

Dila CJ, and Pappins HM: Cerebral water and electrolytes. *Arch Neurol* 26:85, 1972.

Finney LA, and Walker AR: *Transtentorial Herniation.* Charles C Thomas, Springfield, Illinois, 1962.

Fisher CM: The neurological examination of the comatose patient. *Acta Neurol Scand* 45:5, 1969.

Forester CF: Coma in myxedema. *Arch Intern Med* 111:734, 1963.

Fulop M, Tannenbaum H, and Dreyer N: Ketotic hyperosmolar coma. *Lancet* 2:635, 1973.

Goldberg M: Hyponatremia and the inappropriate secretion of antidiuretic hormone. *Am J Med* 35:293, 1963.

Goodman JI: Review: insulin (hypoglycemic) reactions in diabetic patients. *Metabolism* 2:485, 1953.

Howell DA: Longitudinal brainstem compression with buckling. *Arch Neurol* 4:572, 1961.

Jennett B, and Plum F: Persistent vegetative state after brain damage. *Lancet* 1:734, 1974.

Jennett WB, and Stern WE: Tentorial herniation: the midbrain and the pupil; experimental studies in brain compression. *J Neurosurg* 17:598, 1960.

Kernohan JW, and Woltman HW: Incision of the crus due to contralateral brain tumor. *Arch Neurol Psychiatry* 21:274, 1929.

Kubik CS, and Adams RD: Occlusion of the basilar artery—a clinical and pathological study. *Brain* 69:73, 1946.

Leavitt S, and Tyler HR: Studies in asterixis. *Arch Neurol* 10:360, 1964.

Locke S, Merrill JP, and Tyler HR: Neurologic complications of acute uremia. *Arch Intern Med* 108:519, 1961.

Lubash GD, Ferrari MJ, Scherr L, and Rubin AL: Sedative overdosage and the role of hemodialysis. *Arch Intern Med* 110:884, 1962.

Nordgren RE, Markesbery WR, Fukuda K, and Reeves AG: Seven cases of cerebro-medullospinal disconnection: the "locked-in" syndrome. *Neurology (Minneap)* 21:1140, 1971.

Norris FH, and Fawcett J: A sign of intracranial mass with impeding uncal herniation. *Arch Neurol* 12:381, 1965.

Pazzaglia P, Frank G, Frank F, and Gaist G: Clinical course and prognosis of acute post-traumatic coma. *J Neurol Neurosurg Psychiatry* 38:149, 1975.

Plum F, and Brown HW: The effect on respiration of central nervous system disease. *Ann NY Acad Sci* 109:915, 1963.

Plum F, and Caronna JJ: Can one predict outcome of medical coma? In: *Outcome of Severe Damage to the Central Nervous System*. Elsevier-Excerpta Medica, Amsterdam, 1975.

Plum F, and Posner JB: *The Diagnosis of Stupor and Coma*. Davis, Philadelphia, 1966.

Richardson JC, Chambers RA, and Heywood PM: Encephalopathies of anoxia and hypo-glycemia. *Arch Neurol* 1:178, 1959.

Ziegler DK, Zosa A, and Zileli I: Hypertensive encephalopathy. *Arch Neurol* 12:472, 1965.

12

Syndromes of the Neck and Low Back

Conventional textbooks of neurology which are disease-oriented usually consider painful conditions of the neck and low back under a variety of headings. Patients, however, usually present themselves to their physicians with simple complaints of neck and arm pain or low back and leg pain, sometimes accompanied by weakness, numbness, or dysesthesia. These particular complaints and the conditions which cause them appear to be increasing in frequency, perhaps as a consequence of automobile and industrial accidents as well as increased awareness, and hence reporting, by physicians. The disorders involved are the cause of considerable disability and comprise an important broad entity for discussion, particularly so because the neurologist, neurosurgeon, and orthopedic surgeon are often called on for advice in diagnosis and management. Like most seemingly confusing clinical disorders, painful lesions of the neck and low back are less mystifying if the physician approaches their diagnosis and management in an orderly, anatomically oriented manner.

NECK

General Conditions

The cervical vertebrae, the ligaments which bind them together, and the powerful strap muscles connecting the head to the trunk undergo a great deal of stress even during normal activity (e.g., flexion, extension, and rotation). This is augmented by any circumstance that causes excessive flexion or extension, as may occur in sudden acceleration or deceleration.

A review of the anatomy of the cervical spine is helpful in understanding the mechanisms of the various disorders that produce cervical symptomatology. There are only seven cervical vertebrae, although there are eight cervical spinal cord segments and sets of nerve roots. The cervical nerve roots exit through the neural foramina immediately above the corresponding vertebra, in contrast to the dorsal, lumbar, and sacral nerve roots, which always exit below the corresponding vertebra. For example, C-3 exits between C_2 and C_3, whereas D-5 exits between D_5 and D_6. The importance of this when localizing the vertebral level of a nerve root lesion is obvious.

The cervical vertebrae have small transversely elliptical bodies, so that when viewed from the anterior aspect, the upper concave surface of each overlaps the lower convex surface of the vertebra immediately above. This area of overlapping produces a false joint (joint of Luschka), false because there is no actual synovial articular surface. The constant flexion, extension, and rotation of the cervical spine causes these two opposing areas of the adjacent vertebrae to move on one another, and thus bony overgrowth and spurs are common. The "joints" of Luschka lie immediately adjacent (anterior) to the intervertebral neural foramina, through which the nerve roots pass. Immediately posterior to the neural foramina are the articular facets of the vertebra, the true joints that form the actual fulcrum of movement between the vertebrae. These joints are also subject to constant stress and commonly undergo mild subluxation caused by degeneration of the disc space or by excessive flexion or extension movements, producing bony hypertrophy and spurring. This further compromises the neural foramina, which are thus encroached on anteriorly and posteriorly, thereby producing radicular (nerve root) symptoms and signs. Actual disc protrusion is relatively uncommon in the cervical region compared to the lumbar, and most instances of cervical nerve root compression are caused by spondylitic (hypertrophic) changes.

The intraspinous ligamentous structures also probably play an important role in the pathogenesis of cervical symptomatology, particularly the syndrome of *cervical spondylosis*, in which there is evidence of spinal cord compression. This comes about when the cervical disc spaces narrow, due either to disc degeneration or acute trauma, causing a buckling and hypertrophy of the posterior longitudinal ligaments, which run vertically along the posterior surfaces of the vertebral bodies. This is not infrequently accompanied by hypertrophy and buckling of the ligamenta flava, which lie on the anterior surfaces of the vertebral arches. Even though the spinal cord normally occupies only a small part (less than 60%) of the total volume of the cervical spinal canal, it is tightly tethered by the nerve roots, vascular attachments, and dentate ligaments, so that localized ligamentous hypertrophy can narrow the spinal canal sufficiently to (1) produce continuous cord compression or (2) increase the chances of trauma to the anterior surface of the cord during vigorous neck flexion or extension.

There are, of course, many conditions that cause neck and upper extremity pain. Most important is the recognition that pain in the upper extremities may have its origin in the cervical spine, specifically the cervical nerve roots, and that the *location* of the upper extremity pain often is the key to which nerve root is involved. Several points should be remembered. Not all radicular pain is lancinating, radiating, electric-like, or burning in quality. *Any type of localizable upper extremity pain may have its origin in the cervical nerve roots.* The nerve roots are a far more frequent source of neurologic disturbances, including pain, in the upper extremities than is the brachial plexus. When the latter is involved, the neurologic involvement is usually diffuse. Evidence of *multiple* nerve root involvement unilaterally is the key to suspecting a more distal or plexus lesion, but cervical spondylosis can also be a diffuse process, and involvement of several nerve roots at the time of examination is not rare.

Cervical Spondylosis

The mechanism for cervical spondylosis, a common neurologic disorder of the middle-aged, has already been discussed. It is the result of nerve root and occasionally spinal cord compression by bony and ligamentous overgrowth. There is frequently a history of recurrent neck and shoulder pain and stiffness. The patient may never have any symptom other than pain, which may be localized in any part of an upper extremity or which may be typically radicular, with radiation along the distribution of a specific nerve root. The radicular pain may be localized entirely in the extremity with no associated neck pain. The pain may be accompanied by other signs of nerve root compression (e.g., muscle weakness, atrophy, hypalgesia, or hyperesthesia) and a diminished to absent deep tendon reflex. The latter may be the only sign on physical examination which confirms that the pain is due to radicular compression. Although nerve root entrapment is much more common, cervical spondylosis may also cause compression of the spinal cord as described above, evidenced by spastic weakness in the lower extremities. High cervical radiculopathy is infrequently encountered in cervical spondylosis, so involvement of a nerve root above C-4 should arouse suspicion of a different type of pathology, specifically tumor.

C-5 nerve root lesions may cause weakness and atrophy of the deltoid, biceps, supinator, and brachioradialis muscles, loss of the biceps reflex, and a sensory abnormality as outlined in the dermatome chart (Fig. 1.5). C-6 nerve root lesions involve the biceps, brachioradialis, supinator, and triceps. Lesions of C-7 and C-8 nerve roots cause sensory symptoms in the fingers. The sensory pattern of a C-8 lesion closely resembles that seen in ulnar nerve pathology. The motor defect in a C-7 nerve root lesion is weakness of the flexors of the wrist and extensors and flexors of the fingers; whereas in C-8 and D-1 lesions, the outstanding feature is "claw" hand in which there is atrophy of the intrinsic hand muscles.

When the spondylitic process causes spinal cord compression, upper motor neuron signs appear in the lower extremities. These consist of weakness, spasticity, and increased deep tendon reflexes. One must be particularly aware that cervical spondylosis can develop painlessly and sensory abnormalities may be minimal; hence the combination of atrophy of the hand muscles and upper motor neuron signs in the lower extremities must *always* be considered cervical cord compression until proved otherwise. In the past this was not uncommonly confused with amyotrophic lateral sclerosis for which there is no treatment, and the patient was dismissed as incurably ill.

The management of the patient with cervical spondylosis depends, of course, on the severity of the symptoms and signs. The first step is to establish the diagnosis, and the most important differentials to be excluded are spinal cord tumor or acute herniated cervical disc. Because cord tumor usually causes a nonrelenting progressive course, the history often is sufficient to establish that this is not the diagnosis. Acutely herniated cervical disc usually appears suddenly after unusual exertion or neck movement, whereas the symptoms of spondylosis are more indolent and are intermittent. X-ray films of the cervical spine may not differentiate among these possibilities. *Because substantial spondylitic changes are frequently observed by x-ray in asymptomatic individuals, their presence does not exclude other pathology.* X-ray films of the cervical vertebral should include anterior-posterior, lateral, and oblique views. The last are essential to visualize the neural foramina and to evaluate the extent of osteophyte encroachment on the foramina. The lateral views should be taken in the flexed, neutral, and extended positions to look for vertebral dislocations or displacement. Careful examination of the lateral x-rays often permits determination of whether the spinal cord is compressed; this is done by measuring the distance between the most posterior projection of the spondylitic spurs located on the posterior surface of the vertebrae and the roof of the laminar arch. A vertical distance of less than 11 mm is evidence of probable cord compression (Figs. 12.1–12.4).

Electromyography (EMG) is helpful in establishing if a nerve root is injured and, if so, which one it is. If a nerve root lesion is present, carefully performed EMG should reveal denervation potentials in some of the muscles innervated by that root. It is difficult to make the diagnosis of radiculopathy in the absence of this EMG abnormality.

Myelography is reserved for those patients in whom the diagnosis is in doubt, in those where there is a good possibility that a tumor may be present, or in those for whom surgery is contemplated because of intolerable pain or progressing neurologic signs. Metrizamide is now used by most centers as the contrast of choice in myelography because it is water-soluble, does not have to be removed afterward, and the needle can be removed immediately after injecting the dye, permitting the patient to be manipulated more easily. Combination of metrizamide myelography and computerized axial tomography (CAT) scanning of the cervical spine allows excellent definition of the spinal cord.

Management of cervical spondylosis depends on the exact nature of the pathology and the patient's clinical course. If the problem is pain alone, every effort should be made to treat the patient conservatively. This usually means:

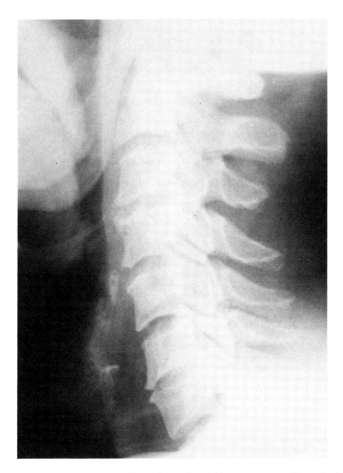

FIG. 12.1. Lateral x-ray in neutral position of a patient with upper extremity radicular pain and weakness and spasticity of lower extremities. This is a case of localized spondylytic disease. These films barely reveal the responsible lesion, which is severe posterior spurring between C-6 and C-7.

1. Adequate analgesia, avoiding narcotics if possible.

2. Soft cervical collar worn as much as possible but particularly at night. The collar probably helps by inhibiting neck movement, thereby reducing the possibility of further irritation of an injured partially entrapped nerve root.

3. Cervical traction. This is a controversial modality, but there is no doubt that a small number of patients benefit from it. Eight to 10 pounds of traction applied through a properly positioned halter with the patient in the supine position is usually adequate. Most patients do not tolerate more than 30 min of traction at a time.

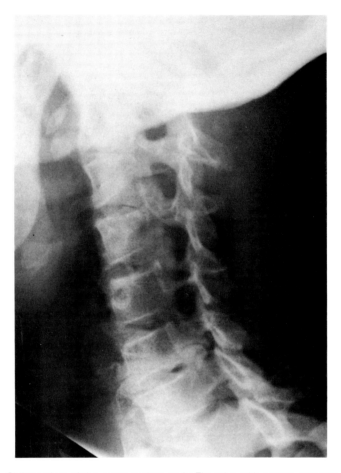

FIG. 12.2. Oblique view of the same patient as in Fig. 12.1 with severe osteophytic spurring encroaching on the neural foramen between C-6 and C-7. The other foramina appear reasonably normal. This invasion of the neural foramen is responsible for the patient's radicular pain into the left arm.

4. "Anti-inflammatory drugs." These include indomethacin, ibuprofen (Motrin), and steroids. There are no good studies from which to evaluate their effectiveness, and the response which occurs may be coincidental.

Surgery should be reserved for patients with intolerable and persistent radicular pain, those with progressing weakness of the muscles innervated by the entrapped nerve root, or patients with clinical evidence of worsening spinal cord compression and radiologic confirmation that the spinal cord lesion is caused by the cervical spondylosis. The value of surgical treatment of spinal cord compression caused by cervical spondylosis is, at best, limited. The longer the duration of the spinal cord compression, the less likely is there

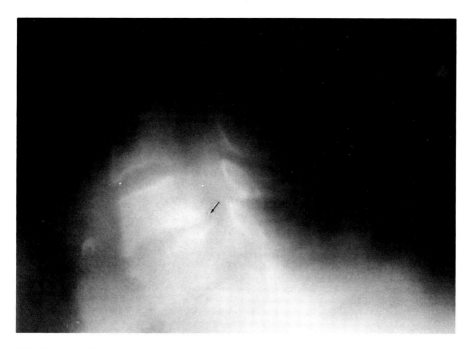

FIG. 12.3. Lateral tomography reveals the huge posterior eburnation between C-6 and C-7, barely visible on the plain films. This bony spur is compressing the spinal cord.

to be significant improvement in the spinal cord signs following surgery. A major objective of the surgery is to prevent progression of the spastic weakness of the lower extremities, even though the patient may not improve significantly from the preoperative state. On the other hand, surgery is quite helpful in providing relief from the pain and muscle weakness caused by a trapped cervical nerve root.

The operative procedure most widely used is the anterior discectomy. The surgeon removes the eburnated disc material from the anterior approach and usually fuses the two contiguous vertebral bodies by means of a bone plug taken from the patient's iliac crest. A foraminotomy is also done to decompress the involved nerve root. Laminectomy for cervical spondylosis is performed much less frequently than in prior years, and there are many neurosurgeons and orthopedic surgeons who regard it as an ineffective procedure.

It is speculated that the corticospinal signs in cervical spondylosis are due to repeated contusions of the cord by the protruding cervical bars, eventually damaging the arterial supply to the anterior two-thirds of the cord. The resultant infarction of a small segment of the cord is a permanent lesion, and it is for that reason that surgery may not be followed by recovery but only by stabilization of clinical signs. Fortunately, the great majority of patients with

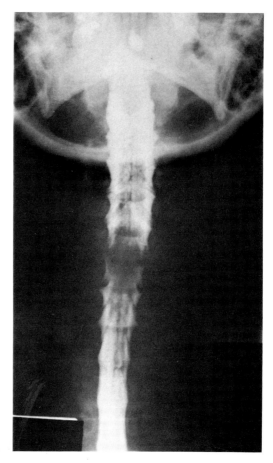

A

FIG. 12.4A and **B.** Pantopaque myelography on the same patient as in Fig. 12.3 confirms the presence of the localized bony spur between C-6 and C-7. The lateral view shows the indentation made on the dye column by the spur. Note that the spinal cord itself is not encroached on with the neck in the extended position. In the AP view the bar defect in the dye column is easily seen. *(Cont.)*

symptomatic cervical spondylosis causing nerve root signs have a benign course, with remission of symptoms and signs during conservative management; therefore a decision to operate should never be a precipitate one.

Cervical Whiplash

Cervical whiplash is a term in such common usage that it is heard in the repertory of television comedians. It refers to the neck (and other) symptoms

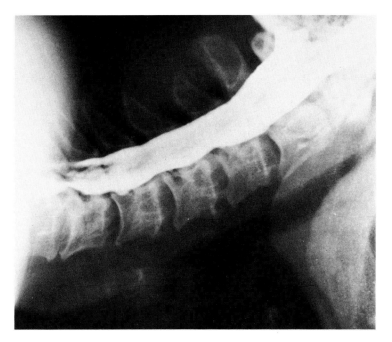

FIG. 12.4B.

that result from automobile accidents, particularly when a standing car has been struck from behind, but it is also used occasionally to describe the effects of industrial accidents in which the neck may be injured. True cervical whiplash injury is a sudden acceleration-deceleration injury in which the body is thrust forward suddenly, causing the head and neck to be strongly extended, following which the head and neck snap forward on the trunk. The cervical musculature is thus stretched and injured. In rare instances there may even be accompanying injury to the brainstem. Less infrequently, cervical radiculopathy may appear. Such patients should be treated conservatively with rest, analgesics, and sedation. Cervical spine films must always be obtained to be certain that no fracture or dislocation is present. The chronic management of these patients is not uncommonly complicated by the legal aspects of the problem. It has been my experience that, barring cervical fracture or dislocation, well-motivated patients recover fairly rapidly, although some neck stiffness or soreness may persist for several weeks or, less commonly, months, whereas compensable injuries of similar intensity in which a law suit is involved have a much more chronic course. This is not intended in a pejorative sense—it is a distillation of my own experience with this medicosocial problem.

Thoracic Outlet Syndrome

True thoracic outlet syndromes are extremely rare, and the diagnosis should be reserved for patients whose clinical picture meets specific criteria. The brachial plexus and subclavian artery and vein course between the anterior and medial scalene muscles. An extension of the lateral process of the 7th cervical vertebra, called a cervical rib, may disturb the anatomic relationships described above and cause compression or displacement of a part of the neurovascular bundle, just as the subclavian artery may be partially compressed at several points in its course out of the thorax, over the first rib, between the scalene muscles, beneath the clavicle, and finally under the pectoralis minor. Cervical ribs occur in 0.5% of the population, but fewer than 10% of these individuals have any symptoms.

Symptoms and signs include the following: (1) pain and dysesthesia in the shoulder, arm, and hand, most frequently in the distribution of the ulnar nerve; and (2) signs of compression of the subclavian artery, including unilateral Raynaud's phenomenon, ulcerated cyanotic fingers, edema of the hand, and pallor of the arm and hand on elevation of the arm. Adson's maneuver (turning the head toward the affected arm and the supinating arm) causes obliteration of the radial pulse, *but this test may be positive in normal individuals*. Nerve conduction velocity from the supraclavicular region to the arm is decreased, indicating brachial plexus involvement, *but the conduction velocity may also be decreased in asymptomatic individuals*. Angiography should establish the presence of subclavian artery compression. Operation (either resection of a portion of the first rib or sectioning of the anterior scalene muscle, should be reserved for those individuals who meet all the criteria described above. Direct crushing injury to the clavicle or supraclavicular region may precipitate this syndrome, but there is no convincing proof that it is caused by whiplash or jostling injuries.

Obviously there are many causes for neck pain in addition to cervical spondylosis or trauma. Extramedullary cervical tumors (e.g., neurofibroma) may cause classic cervical radiculopathy in the distribution of the involved nerve root. Tension headaches are not infrequently tension neck aches, the muscles of the neck bearing the full brunt of the spasm which causes discomfort. Cervicomedullary junction lesions (e.g., Arnold-Chiari syndrome or meningioma of the posterior rim of the foramen magnum) rarely present as pain problems, and the accompanying neurologic signs usually point to the diagnosis. Primary disease of the bones or joints of the cervical vertebrae [e.g., metastatic disease of the bone or cervical ankylosing spondylitis (rheumatoid arthritis)] causes cervical pain, usually of a relentless, nonradiating type that is accentuated by head or neck movement. X-ray examination of the cervical spine frequently allows the correct diagnosis to be made.

LOW BACK PAIN SYNDROMES

Diagnostic considerations in patients with low back and leg pain must include invasive or compressive lesions of the lumbosacral plexus, carcinoma of the prostate with spread into the adjacent sacrum, occlusive disease of the lower abdominal aorta or iliac arteries, Paget's disease, and sacral nerve root cysts. The historical features and physical findings of each of these are usually sufficiently distinctive to be suggestive. Persistent low back pain with scattered neurologic deficits (e.g., disparate local areas of muscle atrophy or high lumbar sensory loss) suggests a lumbosacral plexus lesion, and a retroperitoneal mass must be carefully sought. Severe local sacral or hip pain associated with rapidly developing urinary obstructive symptoms points to prostatic carcinoma. The correct diagnosis in most of these conditions can be confirmed by appropriate x-ray examination and blood chemistries.

By far the most important statistically is the *lumbar disc syndrome*, which to most physicians means herniated lumbar or lumbosacral disc but which should also include a group of disorders of the lumbosacral spine that results in symptomatology often indistinguishable from that of herniated disc and the presence of which must be recognized to avoid missing significant pathology. These include lumbar spondylosis, stenosis, or congenital narrowing of the spinal canal as well as congenital defects of the pars articularis of the lumbar vertebrae (spondylolysis and spondylolisthesis). Because the last diagnosis is often made simply by appropriate x-ray examination and is rarely responsible for a true lumbar disc syndrome, it is not considered further here.

The modern history of the lumbar disc syndrome began with Mixter and Barr in 1934, who identified the rupture of the intervertebral disc as a cause of nerve root and spinal cord compression. The role of disc herniation as a cause of low back radicular syndromes was emphasized to the exclusion of other causes until recently, when several investigators pointed out the importance of lumbar spondylosis and spinal stenosis in the genesis of what has become known as the lumbar disc syndrome.

As in the case of the cervical spine, a review of the important anatomic details of the lumbar vertebrae and disc spaces is in order. A functional unit of the spinal column consists of two vertebral bodies, the disc between them, the two posterior articular joints, and the ligamentous structures that bind the two vertebrae together. The soft tissue components of these units are innervated by the sinuvertebral nerve, which innervates the dura, the blood vessels, posterior longitudinal ligament, and the annulus fibrosus, whereas the posterior rami (branches of the posterior nerve roots) innervate the skin and muscles of the lumbar region, the intervertebral joints, and ligamenta flava. Acute tearing of the annulus fibrosus (as in acute disc herniation) stimulates the sinuvertebral nerve and causes a deep back pain associated with muscle spasm owing to the richness of the neural supply. This is quite different from the pain of nerve root compression, which usually extends into the buttock or posterior aspect of the leg.

The relationship of the lumbar nerve roots to the vertebral bodies elucidates the mechanism of symptoms in the lumbar disc syndrome. The roots leave the anterior dura opposite one vertebral body above their foramina of exit and, in their passage, cross the ventrolateral aspect of the disc below the vertebral body opposite which they emerged; thus the nerve root compressed by a disc or spondylitic spur always has its origin in the *spinal cord segment immediately superior to the disc space.*

The pathologic processes involved in the lumbar disc syndrome are complex and interdependent. The disc itself is adapted to withstand tremendous stress. The nucleus is composed of a protein-polysaccharide complex in which fibrils of collagen are embedded. It combines with the elastic annulus fibrosus, which is, in turn, covered by anterior and posterior longitudinal ligaments. The nucleus pulposus has no visible blood supply in the adult, and continuous stress results in degenerative changes associated with increased collagen content and the appearance of fenestrations in the annulus.

The degenerative process in the nucleus and annulus may result in narrowing or collapse of the disc space. This, in turn, causes a partial subluxation of the posterior articular joints and buckling and hypertrophy of the posterior longitudinal ligaments and ligamenta flava, so the spinal canal is encroached on from its anterior, posterior, and lateral aspects, and the neural foramen is compromised, producing lumbar spondylosis. It can be readily appreciated that the effect of all these changes would be exaggerated in a congenitally small spinal canal and the likelihood of cauda equina compression increased.

An alternate and sometimes concomitant pathologic sequence is actual protrusion of the disc material through the annulus, where it may point laterally, dorsally, or in the neural foramen. Lateral protrusion most likely occurs because that is where the fibers are thinnest, and the posterior longitudinal ligament is progressively stripped off the vertebral bodies, allowing the mass to migrate in any direction. Obviously the symptoms and signs depend on the direction of the protrusion, the size of the spinal canal, and the presence of spondylitic changes. It is easy to see how more than one nerve root may be involved and why certain positional changes may produce symptoms (Figs. 12.5 and 12.6).

Thus the characteristics of symptomatology in the lumbar disc syndrome depend on the pathology, which is far more complex and varied than was first suspected by Mixter and Barr. Back and radicular pain as well as signs of compression of one or more nerve roots may occur in the absence of actual extrusion of disc material; the most common pathology is a combination of two or more of the three conditions of herniated nucleus pulposus, spondylosis, and stenosis of the spinal cord.

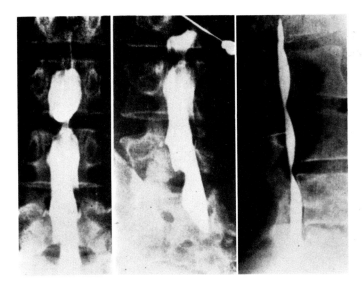

FIG. 12.5. Examples of myelographic pathology in the lumbar disc syndrome. The top film is a lateral view in a case of spinal stenosis, showing a small spinal canal. The other two films show an example of spondylosis between L2 and L3 and L4 and L5, as well as a herniated nucleus pulposus between L5 and S1 on the left.

A rare clinical manifestation of stenosis and spondylosis is intermittent claudication of the cauda equina, caused partly by postural effects (compression of cauda equina by ligamenta flava) and partly by nerve root ischemia. These patients often have a highly characteristic complaint—their legs feel as if they are encased in concrete or are extremely heavy or numb after relatively modest physical activity. The abnormal sensation subsides with rest, and even careful neurologic examination may fail to detect any abnormality. Eventually signs of urinary sphincter disturbance develop in these patients, usually in the form of urinary retention and overflow incontinence. The patient suspected of having this syndrome should be examined immediately after vigorous physical activity, for at that time neurologic abnormalities (e.g., muscle weakness or decreased deep tendon reflexes) may appear. In addition, urinary residual should be checked by catheterizing the patient immediately after voiding, for such residual may be substantial even in the absence of significant urinary symptoms.

The stenotic spinal canal may be impossible to identify by routine x-ray, although foraminal osteophytes and spondylitic spurs can often be seen. Lumbar puncture may be difficult and painful in patients with a stenotic canal because of the closely packed cauda equina, and the crowding may produce an unusual myelographic picture, which can be mistaken for extra-arachnoid dye injection.

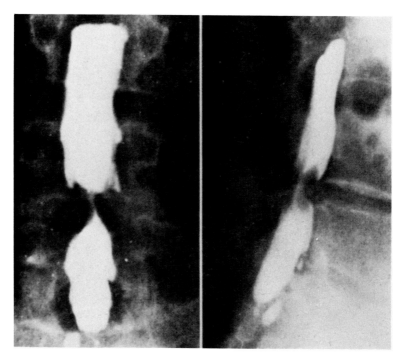

FIG. 12.6. Lumbar spondylosis. Note defects in Pantopaque anteriorly and posteriorly at the L4–5 interspace.

Evaluation of a patient with a low-back pain syndrome should include as much help as possible from clinical testing, electromyography (which may demonstrate *multiple* nerve root involvement), and of course from myelography. The principle is the same as in the cervical spine. Myelography is deferred until the patient's symptoms or signs, or both, require surgical intervention. Because the majority of instances of acute and subacute lumbar disc syndrome improve spontaneously, and because many patients have recurrent complaints after surgery, conservative (nonsurgical) management is indicated whenever possible. This consists of a trial of bed rest, sedation, pelvic traction, and even a brief trial of steroids. Improvement of symptoms, particularly pain, has been reported from the use of oral steroids in large doses (100 to 120 mg prednisone) for 1 week. The usual precautions associated with such therapy must be observed.

Concepts of surgical management of the lumbar disc syndrome have altered strikingly during the past decade. There is still general agreement that patients with abrupt onset of radicular pain, often after lifting a heavy object or twisting suddenly, associated with other signs of nerve root compression (e.g., muscle weakness and diminished deep tendon reflex) are likely to have a ruptured annulus fibrosus and herniated disc material. Persistence of motor signs or intractable pain are reasonable indications for laminectomy and disc removal. The management of the chronic low-back problem due either to proved lumbar spondylosis or injury or a recurrence after a prior laminectomy is much more controversial. There is good evidence to support caution and conservatism in the management of these patients. Repeated surgical procedures rarely provide relief and often complicate and worsen the situation. The stabilization of the lumbosacral spine following laminectomy by the insertion of bone struts is now infrequently used because subsequent overgrowth of the bony grafts often contributed to the narrowing of the lumbosacral canal. A patient with chronic lumbar disc syndrome who has progressive neurologic deficits (muscle weakness and atrophy, sphincter disturbances, sensory deficits, appropriate EMG abnormalities) must be strongly considered a surgical candidate, but pain alone should only rarely be considered a requirement for surgery. Every modality and approach for pain relief should be attempted in these patients before surgery is even considered.

SUGGESTED READINGS

Abdullah AF, Ditto EW, Byrd EB, and Williams R: Extreme-lateral lumbar disc herniations: clinical syndrome and special problems of diagnosis. *J Neurosurg* 41:229, 1974.

Alexander E: Significance of the small lumbar spinal canal: cauda equina compression syndromes due to spondylosis. Part 5. Achondroplasia. *J Neurosurg* 31:513, 1969.

Brain L, and Wilsonson M (eds): *Cervical Spondylosis and Other Disorders of the Cervical Spine*. Saunders, Philadelphia, 1967.

Brish A, Lerner MA, and Braham J: Intermittent claudication from compression of cauda equina by a narrowed spinal canal. *J Neurosurg* 21:207, 1964.

Clark K: Significance of the small lumbar spinal canal: cauda equina compression syndromes due to spondylosis. Part 2. Clinical and surgical significance. *J Neurosurg* 31:495, 1969.

Cloward RB: *Ruptured Lumbar Intervertebral Discs* (Signature Series). Codman and Shurtleff, Randolph, Mass.

Cyrias JH: *Cervical Spondylosis*. Appleton-Century-Crofts, New York, 1971.

Ehni G: Significance of the small lumbar spinal canal: cauda equina compression syndromes due to spondylosis. Part 1. Introduction. *J Neurosurg* 31:490, 1969.

Ehni G: Significance of the small lumbar spinal canal: cauda equina compression syndromes due to spondylosis. Part 4. Acute compression artifically-induced during operation. *J Neurosurg* 31:507, 1969.

Epstein JA: Diagnosis and treatment of painful neurological disorders caused by spondylosis of the lumbar spine. *J Neurosurg* 17:991, 1960.

Goff CW, Alden JO, and Aldes JH: *Traumatic Cervical Syndrome and Whiplash*. Lippincott, Philadelphia, 1964.

Gutterman P, and Shenkin HA: Syndromes associated with protrusion of upper lumbar intervertebral discs: results of surgery. *J Neurosurg* 38:499, 1973.

Harris RI, and Macnab I: Structural changes in the lumbar intervertebral discs: their relationship to low back pain and sciatica. *J Bone Joint Surg [Br]* 36B:304, 1954.

Jacobson RE, Gargano FP, and Rosomoff HL: Transverse axial tomography of the spine. Part I. Axial anatomy of the normal lumbar spine. *J Neurosurg* 42:406, 1975.

Jacobson RE, Gargano FP, and Rosomoff HL: Transverse axial tomography of the spine. Part II. The stenotic spinal canal. *J Neurosurg* 42:412, 1975.

Jones RAC, and Thomson JLG: The narrow lumbar canal: a clinical and radiological review. *J Bone Joint Surg [Am]* 50B:595, 1968.

Mixter WJ, and Barr JS: Rupture of the intervertebral disc with involvement of the spinal canal. *N Engl J Med* 211:210, 1934.

Onofrio BM: Injection of chymopapain into intervertebral discs: preliminary report on 72 patients with symptoms of disc disease. *J Neurosurg* 42:384, 1975.

Paine KWE, and Haung PWH: Lumbar disc syndrome. *J Neurosurg* 37:75, 1972.

Russell ML, Gordon DA, Ogryzlo MA, and McPhedran RS: The cauda equina syndrome of ankylosing spondylitis. *Ann Intern Med* 78:551, 1973.

Smith BH: *Cervical Spondylosis and Its Neurological Complications.* Charles C Thomas, Springfield, Illinois, 1968.

Spurling GR: *Lesions of the Cervical Intervertebral Disc.* Charles C Thomas, Springfield, Illinois, 1956.

Sussman BJ: Inadequacies and hazards of chymopapain injections as treatment for intervertebral disc disease. *J Neurosurg* 42:389, 1975.

Watts C, Hutchison G, Stern J, and Clark K: Comparison of intervertebral disc disease treatment by chymopapain injection and open surgery. *J Neurosurg* 42:397, 1975.

Watts C, Knighton R, and Roulhac G: Chymopapain treatment of intervertebral disc disease. *J Neurosurg* 42:374, 1975.

Wilson CB: Significance of the small lumbar spinal canal: cauda equina compression syndromes due to spondylosis. *J Neurosurg* 31:499, 1969.

Yamada H, Ohya M, Okada T, and Shiozawa Z: Intermittent cauda equina compression due to narrow spinal canal. *J Neurosurg* 37:83, 1972.

13

Neuromuscular Disorders

Although it is usually easy to distinguish weakness caused by lesions of the central nervous system—either brain or spinal cord—from that caused by disorders of the peripheral nerve or muscle, it is by no means a simple matter to decide clinically whether a disease originates in the anterior horn cell, nerve root, plexus, peripheral nerve, myoneural junction, or muscle. Peripheral neuropathy may occur without weakness if only sensory neurons or fibers are diseased. The combination of weakness, decreased tone, diminished tendon jerks, and diminution of sensation over the peripheral portions of the extremities establishes the location of the lesion as being in the peripheral nerve, although it does not identify whether the disease process is in the cell body, axon, or myelin sheath of the peripheral nerve. Classic nerve root lesions produce pain, muscle weakness, sensory loss, and reflex changes in the known distribution of that root, so localization is usually obvious. Muscle weakness without sensory abnormality may be either neural or muscular in origin. Muscle atrophy may occur in both instances, but profound muscle weakness without significant atrophy is suggestive of myopathy. Myopathy is said to cause proximal muscle weakness predominantly, and peripheral neuropathy to cause distal muscle weakness, but this is not always so. Weakness of neck extension is characteristic of myasthenia gravis, whereas weakness of neck flexion almost invariably connotes myopathy. Deep tendon reflexes are always diminished or lost in neural lesions causing severe weakness, whereas they are usually preserved in myopathy, even that associated with severe weakness. Muscle fasciculations are also a strong clinical indicator of neural disease.

Despite these many clues, it is still often necessary for the clinician to resort to various laboratory examinations, some of which require special training and experience, and even then final diagnosis may be difficult. Elevations of serum aldolase and creatine phosphokinase (CPK) are fairly reliable indications that the patient's weakness is myopathic in origin, but muscle necrosis from any cause (e.g., injury or even an intramuscular injection) may allow these enzymes to leak out of the damaged muscle cell and enter the blood, thereby confusing the diagnosis. Furthermore, myopathic disease, as confirmed by the clinical picture and muscle biopsy, may exist in the face of normal or only mildly elevated serum enzymes. In many instances the degree of elevation of muscle enzymes parallels the severity of the disease process, and this examination can therefore be used as a barometer of the effectiveness of treatment; unfortunately, this is not invariably the case. Creatine phosphokinase is also highly concentrated in brain and myocardium and may therefore be elevated in patients with myocardial or cerebral infarction. The different biochemical properties of CPK from the various tissues allow them to be distinguished in the laboratory.

Electromyography (EMG) and nerve conduction velocity studies are important adjuncts when attempting to distinguish the site of a lesion causing muscle weakness. Electrodiagnosis requires considerable skill and experience and must always be correlated with the clinical findings. Recording is made from concentric needle electrodes which are placed into the muscles to be studied. Although the needle diameter is small, the procedure is nevertheless uncomfortable for many patients. The major objective of the EMG is to detect evidence of denervation of muscle fibers, thereby establishing the existence of disease of the motor nerves, either in the cell nucleus, axon, or myelin sheath. Denervation is usually detected by increased insertional activity and by the presence of fibrillation or fasciculation potentials, but fibrillation potentials may be present in myopathic disorders due to destruction of the intramuscular nerve endings by the disease process. Low-amplitude, voluntary motor unit potentials of brief duration occur in myopathies—either inflammatory, degenerative, or metabolic—because of reduced numbers of fibers in the motor unit. On audio examination they produce a characteristic whining, crackling sound.

Characteristic responses to nerve stimulation are seen in the muscles of patients with myoneural junction abnormalities. Whereas muscle action potentials retain the same amplitude in normal muscle following repeated electrical stimuli of the innervating nerve at frequencies up to 30 to 40 per second, they decrease progressively following repetitive nerve stimulation at rates of 5 to 15 per second in many patients with myasthenia gravis. In the myasthenic syndrome (Eaton-Lambert syndrome) repetitive nerve stimulation causes the voltage of an initial low-amplitude muscle action potential to increase progressively until a normal range is achieved. Edrophonium (Tensilon) usually reverses the block seen in myasthenia gravis, and guanidine corrects the defect in the myasthenic syndrome. Figures 13.1 through 13.5 are illustrative of EMG abnormalities in specific typical disorders.

Motor and sensory conduction velocity studies augment the information obtained by EMG. The examination is performed by stimulating specific large peripheral nerves percutaneously and recording the summated muscle potential by skin leads placed over the belly of a muscle innervated by that nerve. The conduction time so recorded (in milliseconds) is the distal latency, which

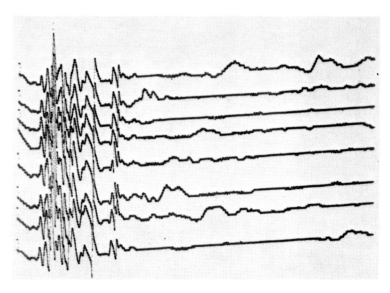

FIG. 13.1. Polyphasic motor unit potential of considerably increased duration indicative of reinnervation and characteristically seen in neuropathic disorders.

is comprised of the conduction time as well as nerve trunk, the conduction time of the impulse through the terminal branches of the nerve, the myoneural synapse, and the muscle itself. Motor nerve conduction velocity is calculated by subtracting the latency of a distal stimulation site from that of a site more proximal on the nerve trunk. This represents the maximal conduction velocity in the measured nerve segment between the two stimulating electrodes. Normal motor nerve conduction velocity in adults varies from 40 to 75 meters per second; it is much lower in infants. Decreased maximal conduction velocities are characteristic of peripheral neuropathies associated with segmental demyelinization, whereas neuropathies caused by or associated with axonal degeneration show normal conduction velocities, as do myopathic disorders.

Sensory nerve conduction velocities are obtained by measuring the maximal antidromic nerve impulse generated by distal stimulation. Reliable values

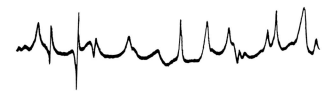

FIG. 13.2. Positive sharp waves and fibrillation potentials typically seen in denervated muscle but also seen in some myopathies.

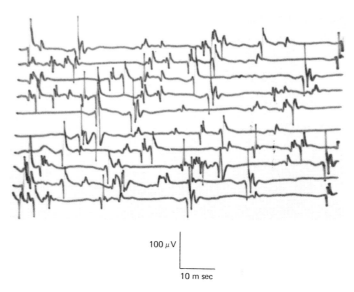

100 μV

10 m sec

FIG. 13.3. Numerous small, short-duration motor unit potentials on minimal contraction in a patient with Duchenne muscular dystrophy.

are often difficult to obtain because of technical problems in amplification and recording.

Muscle biopsy has become a valuable diagnostic tool in the differential diagnosis of neuropathic and myopathic disorders and in the differentiation among the causes or types of myopathy. It is particularly helpful in establishing the diagnosis of collagen vascular diseases and distinguishing metabolic and other presumably genetic muscle diseases. There are three distinct elements to a successful muscle biopsy: (1) surgical excision of the sample; (2) tissue handling (staining techniques, etc.); and (3) interpretation of the histology. All three elements must be of high quality for the examination to be of value, and the biopsy must be interpreted in the context of the clinical picture.

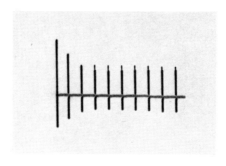

FIG. 13.4. Myasthenia gravis. Decremental response of the compound muscle action potential to 2/sec supramaximal stimulation.

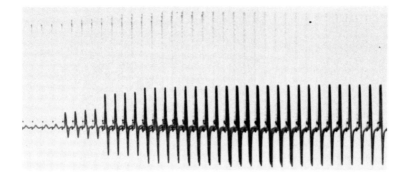

FIG. 13.5. Lambert-Eaton syndrome. Progressive increase in amplitude of the compound muscle action potential in response to 40/sec supramaximal stimulation.

The biopsy should be taken from an affected but not destroyed muscle which has had no recent needle punctures. The piece of muscle 1.0 to 2.5 cm in length is prevented from contracting by tying it in stretched position on a stick or keeping it in a special clamp. Details of the fixation process are beyond the scope of this presentation, but the examining laboratory should have the capacity to perform routine histologic stains, histochemical stains, and fixation and staining for electron microscopy. Finally, the finished slide should be interpreted only by an individual with specific training in the above techniques

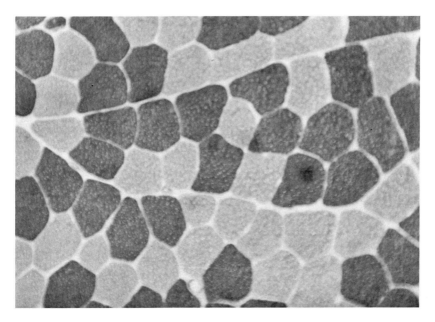

FIG. 13.6. Use of muscle biopsy in diagnosis. This is an alkaline preincubated ATPase stain demonstrating the normal pattern of type I (light) and type II (dark) myofibers.

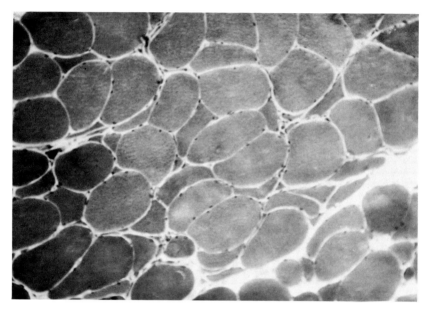

FIG. 13.7. Muscle biopsy. Modified trichrome stain (here in black and white) of a partially denervated muscle. Note the atrophic angular fibers as compared to the normal full globular ones.

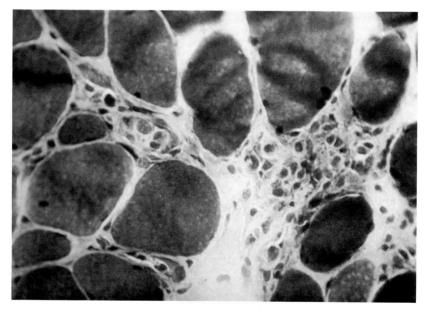

FIG. 13.8. Muscle biopsy. Modified trichrome stain of polymyositis. Note clusters of inflammatory cells and phagocytosis of muscle fibers.

and in examining such tissue. It is apparent that muscle biopsy is a highly specialized procedure and should not be attempted unless all the criteria indicated above can be met. Examples of the use of muscle biopsy in the diagnosis of neuromuscular diseases are shown in Figs. 13.6 through 13.10.

NEUROPATHIES

There are several ways to classify the neuropathies so the clinician can approach the differential diagnosis of the patient's problem in a practical manner. One approach is to classify them according to presumed etiology, recognizing that the pathogenesis may not be understood. Another is to classify them according to pathology. Neuropathy may be caused by: (1) Disease of the cell bodies of peripheral nerves, as the nucleus and the perinuclear cytoplasm produce the protein of the axis cylinder of a nerve fiber; this exoplasm moves peripherally in the axon to replace catabolized protoplasmic systems. (2) Disorder of the myelin sheath of the peripheral nerve; this may be primary as a result of disease of the Schwann cells or secondary to the axonal degeneration as in (1). Because an etiologic agent produces a consistent type of pathology and because the EMG and nerve conduction velocity studies may be different in the two pathologic types, it may be clinically helpful to think of neuropathies as being caused either by segmental

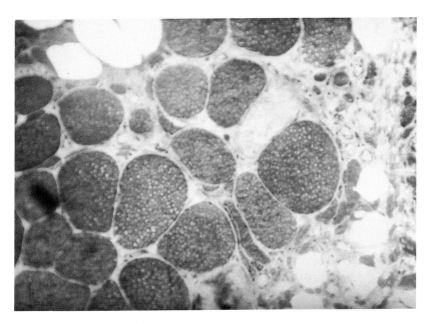

FIG. 13.9. Muscle biopsy. Modified trichrome stain of Duchenne dystrophy. This shows myofiber degeneration, endomysial connective tissue proliferation, fatty metamorphosis, and myofiber hypertrophy.

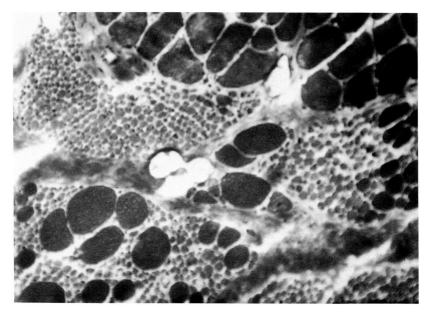

FIG. 13.10. Muscle biopsy. Infantile spinomuscular atrophy (Werdnig-Hoffman disease). Note the groups of markedly atrophic myofibers as well as individual and groups of hypertrophic myofibers.

demyelinization of the peripheral nerve or by disease of the neuron itself. Other useful parameters for classifying and identifying neuropathies include the predominant symptoms or signs (sensory, motor, mixed) of the disorder and the distribution of the neuropathy (polyneuritis, mononeuritis, mononeuritis multiplex).

The characteristic symptoms and signs of neuropathy include *muscle weakness or atrophy, diminished to absent deep tendon reflexes, pain, and sensory abnormalities*. The last may include all sensory modalities or only one or two, leaving others relatively intact. This is particularly true if the site of origin of the neuropathy is in the dorsal root ganglion. *Paresthesias* (numbness, tingling, burning sensations) are common in neuropathies, and *hyperpathia* (increased sensitivity and pain to touch) is also frequent. The pattern of sensory loss in polyneuropathy is most severe distally (in feet or hands) in the area covered by stockings or gloves. This pattern of sensory change immediately excludes nerve root localization and is extremely helpful when making a diagnosis. Of course, sensory loss also establishes that the primary pathology cannot be in the muscle even though severe weakness may be present. Some neuropathies are predominantly motor, others sensory, others mixed, but *the diagnosis of neuropathy must be questioned unless the tendon reflexes are diminished or absent*. Muscle fasciculations (twitching) may occur in peripheral neuropathy, but their presence should always alert the examiner to think of the anterior horn cells in the spinal cord as the source of pathology and therefore consider the diagnosis of amyotrophic lateral sclerosis. Autonomic disturbances are common in many types of neuropathies. These include altered sweating, loss of hair over the affected area, and skin discoloration and atrophy.

As previously discussed, electromyography and nerve conduction velocity studies are particularly helpful for confirming the diagnosis of neuropathy because they should indicate whether the muscle weakness originates from the anterior horn cell, peripheral nerve, myoneural junction, or muscle. As mentioned, impaired conduction velocity suggests segmental demyelinization of the peripheral nerve and therefore aids in establishing etiology. Local nerve pathology, as in an entrapment neuropathy, is often characterized by a specifically localizable conduction defect (viz., carpal tunnel syndrome).

The diagnosis of neuropathy can usually be made readily from the history and physical examination, but sometimes the findings are confusing; the clinician must then revert to the principles enunciated in Chapter 1 to distinguish between lesions of the peripheral nerve and those of muscle, the myoneural junction, or the spinal cord. Intramedullary spinal cord lesions (e.g., syringomyelia or spinal cord ependymomas) may also simulate peripheral neuropathy, and compressive lesions of the cauda equina may present special problems in differential diagnosis. Peripheral neuropathy may also coexist with central nervous system (CNS) disease, thereby further complicating the diagnosis.

Having determined that the patient's problem is a neuropathy, the clinician's next responsibility is to look for the etiology, which determines management. This involves careful evaluation of the patient's entire medical status, social and occupational history, exposure to toxins, and genetic disorders. Laboratory evaluation is aimed at assessing these factors.

The following classification of neuropathies is based on presumed etiology, and the order of listing is generally proportional to the incidence of these types of neuropathy as they are seen in the usual clincial practice. This list is not intended to be encyclopedic, and there could be some argument about the proper etiology for some of the neuropathies. The various mononeuropathies associated with acute trauma are not discussed. The symptoms and signs are similar in all neuropathies and were discussed earlier, so they are not described in each instance here unless they are sufficiently distinctive to be pertinent.

Nutritional Neuropathies

Mild forms of nutritional neuropathy are commonly seen in the United States; far more severe deficiency neuropathies are frequent occurrences in those parts of the world where malnutrition is the rule. The common feature is a deficiency of one or more of the B vitamins; no other vitamin deficiency is known to cause neuropathy. The vitamin deficiency is caused by poor nutrition, whether from dietary faddism, alcoholism, severe recurrent vomiting, malabsorption states, or simple starvation, as has occurred in prisoner-of-war camps.

Nutritional neuropathy is usually motor and sensory, but the patients complain early of paresthesias and numbness in feet and hands, so early evaluation may indicate only sensory abnormalities. The neuropathy of chronic alcoholism is often associated with other evidence of alcoholism, e.g., tremor, hallucinosis, dementia, or signs of liver disease.

Although thiamine deficiency is most frequent, other states of B vitamin deficiency are occasionally seen, including pellagra, which classically results in neuropathy, diarrhea, dermatitis, and dementia. Vitamin B_{12} deficiency (pernicious anemia) is caused by lack of the gastric intrinsic factor necessary for absorption of B_{12} by the small bowel. Such patients may show distal paresthesias in hands and feet in addition to the more typical subacute combined degeneration of the spinal cord. Vitamin B_6 (pyridoxine) deficiency has been associated with prolonged isoniazid therapy for tuberculosis. Isoniazid increases pyridoxine excretion, the result of which may be a severe polyneuropathy, which can be prevented simply by prophylactic administration of pyridoxine.

Malabsorption states (sprue, Whipple's disease, regional ileitis) can be accompanied by severe nutritional neuropathy, which can be prevented or managed by taking vitamin B.

Diabetic Neuropathies

Neuropathy is an extremely common complication of diabetes mellitus. Its cause has been debated for years, some experts considering that it is a metabolic abnormality of the nerves secondary to the diabetes, and others that it is caused by occlusive disease of the vasa nervorum. The most common diabetic neuropathy is the predominantly sensory neuropathy of the lower extremities seen in elderly individuals with mild diabetes. In many instances the neuropathy, which may significantly impair ambulation, presents prior to the recognition of the diabetes, which must always be the primary suspect in unexplained neuropathy of the elderly. In young diabetics the peripheral neuropathy may be so severe as to be totally incapacitating, with mixed polyneuropathy and autonomic nervous system involvement manifested by orthostatic hypotension, loss of sexual libido, urinary retention, and nocturnal diarrhea. Peripheral sensory loss may be so severe that the patient acquires arthropathy (Charcot's joints) in the lower extremities or in the lumbosacral region.

Diabetic amyotrophy is characterized by gradual onset of diffuse leg pain, proximal weakness and wasting in the lower extremities, and loss of patellar reflexes. No sensory abnormalities are observed. Cerebrospinal fluid (CSF) protein is often elevated, and some authors have reported accompanying evidence of spinal cord pathology. The neurologic findings are frequently asymmetrical.

The anatomic site of the lesion producing this unusual neurologic complication of diabetes is unknown; some believe the primary pathology to be in the spinal cord, others in the motor roots, and others in the lumbar plexus. It is particularly interesting in that it is the only form of diabetic neuropathy that consistently responds to strict diabetic control.

A variety of mononeuropathies have been described as complications of diabetes, perhaps the best known being the cranial nerve palsies and specifically those of the 3rd and 6th nerves. The patients are in the second half of life. They present with painless 3rd or 6th nerve palsies. Pupillary function is always spared, an important point in differentiating a "diabetic" 3rd nerve palsy from compression of the 3rd nerve by carotid aneurysm. The pathology is not certainly understood but is thought to be caused by nerve infarction from small vessel occlusion. In any event, the syndrome is always self-limited, with spontaneous recovery occurring within a few weeks to months. There is some doubt that these extraocular palsies have any specific relationship to diabetes, as they are also seen in patients with normal glucose tolerance.

Although hard evidence is lacking, there is some reason to believe that good diabetic control is helpful in the management of the various diabetic neuropathies. There is no evidence that vitamin therapy is of value.

Postinfectious or Autoimmune Neuropathies

Using a classification of "postinfectious or autoimmune" neuropathies is probably presumptuous because the actual mechanisms responsible for the neuropathies grouped in this section are not identified. They are considered together on the basis of the current thinking that some sort of auto-immunologic mechanism is responsible for them. By far the most important and frequent of these disorders is the *Guillain-Barré* syndrome (called by some Landry-Guillain-Barré, by others Guillain-Barré-Strohl). An eponym is appropriate, as the clinical criteria have become quite flexible and the etiology is unknown. Current belief has it that the illness is caused by invasion and destruction of the myelin sheaths and eventually the axons of peripheral nerves by lymphocytes which have been transformed by an immunologic response. In more than 50% of cases there is a history of minor infection (e.g., coryza, tracheobronchitis, or gastroenteritis) followed after some days by paresthesias and progressive weakness of the lower extremities. Classically the involvement is mainly motor, but sensory abnormalities are also frequently seen. Typically also, the weakness is ascending, progressive, and associated with diminished or absent deep tendon reflexes. Sphincter involvement is infrequent but can occur. Facial diparesis or diplegia is common.

Other cranial nerve involvement is infrequent, but the bulbar musculature is involved often enough that the treating physician must always be prepared to provide an artificial airway. The primary threats to life are the involvement of the bulbar muscles and respiratory paralysis, *so these patients must be managed where airway and respiratory assistance can be provided until it is certain that the progression of the paralysis has stopped.*

Elevated CSF protein in the absence of pleocytosis (cell count less than 5/mm³) is characteristic, but the protein may be only minimally elevated early in the sickness and the cell count occasionally increased. The protein level is usually highest about the third week of the illness; there is no correlation between clinical severity and degree of protein elevation. CSF glucose is normal.

The course of the illness is variable. In the mildest forms there is flaccid weakness of the lower limbs and relatively little involvement of the upper extremities; improvement begins within 2 or 3 weeks.

The more severe forms involve all four limbs, respiratory muscles, and bulbar muscles. These patients must be watched very carefully, for it is indeed a tragedy for an individual with a self-limited illness to die of respiratory paralysis or aspiration pneumonitis. Regression in the severe cases may not begin for several weeks to months, and complete recovery may require more than a year. Permanent sequelae are rare if the patient receives vigorous physical and rehabilitative therapy.

A small percentage of patients with Guillain-Barré syndrome have a course of relapse, with symptoms and signs returning and regressing over a period of many months.

The differential diagnosis includes any type of progressive (primarily motor) neuropathy. Poliomyelitis, rarely seen now, is characterized by a great deal of pain, fever, rapid progression, absence of sensory abnormalities, and asymmetry of motor involvement. The CSF shows pleocytosis. Acute intermittent porphyria, hypokalemia, and familial periodic paralysis must all be considered. Diphtheritic paralysis is extremely rare in the United States, but botulism may simulate one form of Guillain-Barré syndrome, i.e., that characterized by ophthalmoplegia (with pupillary involvement), ataxia, and areflexia.

Management of these patients must emphasize the need for providing respiratory and airway assistance before it is too late. These should never be done after the fact but, rather, anticipated and prepared for. The value of corticosteroid therapy is open to question; and as is well known, steroid administration is not free from hazard. For these reasons it has been our practice not to use steroids unless the patient's course is relentlessly progressive, in which circumstance we consider that a trial on large doses (prednisone up to 120 mg/day) is in order. If the patient shows no improvement after 7 days of steroid therapy, the drug is discontinued; if his condition is improved, the steroid dosage is gradually reduced.

Other autoimmune causes for neuropathy are rare. A few have been re-ported following administration of typhoid-paratyphoid vaccine or as a part of the syndrome of serum sickness, and the latter is occasionally said to cause brachial plexus neuritis. In our experience, the syndrome of brachial plexus neuritis characterized by painful paresis of shoulder girdle muscles is not preceded by a history of serum or vaccine injection.

Compression and Entrapment Neuropathies

Compression and entrapment probably have a common pathogenesis in that the nerve fibers are injured or the blood supply to the nerve is obstructed by pressure. In the first instance the problem is acute and the compressing agent externally applied, whereas in the latter the neural compression occurs by mechanical irritation from an impinging anatomic neighbor. Compression neuropathies are not uncommon. They usually occur in individuals who are comatose, anesthetized, or drunk, so the discomfort of the compression is not noted and the extremity is immobile for a considerable period. Occupational compression neuropathies are uncommon, although much discussed in the literature, whereas "Saturday night palsy" of the drunk who falls asleep with his arm over a park bench and compresses the radial nerve against his humerus, or any similar phenomenon, is not uncommon. Ulnar nerve palsies following prolonged use of arm boards during intravenous administration are well known. Fortunately, compression neuropathies usually recover spon-taneously, although in severe instances this may require several months.

Entrapment neuropathies are also fairly common, particularly the carpal tunnel syndrome of median nerve compression and meralgia paresthetica caused by entrapment of the lateral femoral cutaneous nerve as it pierces the ilioinguinal ligament or the fascia lata. Ulnar nerve entrapment at the olecranon process has been reported many years after an old ulnar fracture or may appear without a history of prior trauma. In the last example, the anatomic problem is not so much actual entrapment as chronic stretching and repeated trauma of the nerve.

The carpal tunnel syndrome serves as a model for this type of neuropathy. It is caused by compression of the median nerve at the wrist by the transverse carpal ligament and is probably the most common cause of acroparesthesia (numbness and burning) in the fingers on one hand. This symptom was formerly attributed for the most part to the cervical outlet or scalenus anticus syndrome, but in our experience this is extremely rare, the carpal tunnel being far more common. The symptoms are those of acroparesthesia, often occur-ring mainly at night, and the aching may extend high up the forearm. In more advanced cases, one sees atrophy of the proximal portion of the thenar eminence associated with weakness of opposition of the thumb. Demonstra-ble sensory loss in the thumb and first two fingers is rare, although the patient complains that they feel numb. When the flexor surface of the wrist is struck

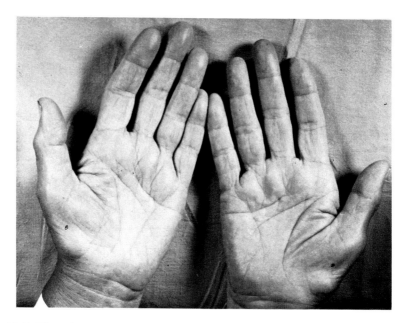

FIG. 13.11. Bilateral carpal tunnel syndrome. Note wasting of proximal portion of thenar eminence (opponens muscles) bilaterally resulting in weakness of opposition of thumb and little finger.

with a reflex hammer, the patient states that an unpleasant burning or electric sensation extends into the thumb and first two fingers. Nerve conduction studies reveal partial or complete block at the level of the transverse carpal ligament (Fig. 13.11).

This syndrome may occur in healthy individuals but should alert the physician to look for a cause, e.g., old fracture of one of the carpal bones, rheumatoid arthritis, myxedema, gout, or acromegaly. It may also occur during pregnancy. Treatment depends on severity. Local injection into the carpal tunnel with a small quantity of lidocaine (Xylocaine) and steroid often causes remission of symptoms. Some patients obtain relief from wearing a plastic splint designed to dorsiflex the wrist, particularly at night. Relief from discomfort may be rapidly forthcoming. If there is a progression of motor signs, the transverse carpal ligament must be sectioned, although perfect results cannot be anticipated in every instance.

Meralgia paresthetica, a syndrome characterized by burning discomfort and numbness on the lateral surface of the thigh, is occasionally confused with a lumbar disc syndrome, and the patient is subjected to an unnecessary myelogram. It may occur from constriction by tight undergarments. Some believe it follows weight loss and the consequent unpadding of the lateral superficial femoral cutaneous nerve. In most instances a cause cannot be found. Treatment should be with analgesics or a brief trial of carbamazepine.

Ulnar nerve entrapment is first treated by splinting the elbow in a slightly flexed position. This produces remission in a significant number of patients, making nerve transposition unnecessary.

Toxic Neuropathies

One must always think of and attempt to exclude a toxic etiology in any peripheral neuropathy of undetermined etiology. The work-up should therefore explicitly include blood and urinary lead and arsenic determinations and arsenic levels in hair. Although many potential toxic agents have been reported to cause neuropathy, by far the most frequent in the United States is lead, with arsenic second in importance. Lead and arsenic produce their toxic effects by binding the sulfhydryl radicals of enzymes, thereby rendering them inactive, so that almost any organ system can be involved. CNS signs are prominent in acute and chronic intoxications from both. Lead may produce a polyneuropathy but is known for the characteristic involvement of the radial nerves with bilateral wrist drop and little or no sensory involvement. Arsenic ingestion may result in a severe polyneuropathy, particularly in the lower extremities, with painful paresthesias and motor, sensory, and autonomic involvement.

Probably the main source of lead poisoning in the United States is *pica*, the chewing of paint and putty peelings from window sills and other sources by small children. This causes a severe, often fatal encephalopathy. The main sources in adults are bootleg whisky (lead-lined pipes in stills) and burning salvaged lead-containing battery casements for fuel, although isolated cases have been reported from a variety of sources. Arsenic is used in insecticides, the largest series being reported in North Carolina (tobacco), and is still a favorite drug in quiet homicide. In acute arsenic poisoning, gastrointestinal symptoms (e.g., abdominal pain, nausea, vomiting, and diarrhea) are common; but in slow, chronic arsenic poisoning these signs may be absent and the neuropathy the only clinical evidence. White transverse lines on the fingernails (Mee's lines) (Fig. 13.12) are helpful in the diagnosis of arsenic poisoning and actually denote the time of most intense exposure to arsenic. In chronic arsenic poisoning the fingernails, toenails, and hair (usually pubic) are examined for arsenic levels, for urinary excretion of arsenic will likely be normal.

Lead neuropathy is treated by Versene and arsenic neuropathy by BAL. In the case of arsenic neuropathy, however, once peripheral neuropathy has developed, it is doubtful if treatment other than rehabilitative efforts is useful.

For historic interest, mercury should be mentioned, not only because of the famous allusion by Lewis Carroll to the "Mad Hatter" but also because it figured powerfully in a crisis of modern ecology, i.e., the notorious Japanese Minamata Bay affair in which the mercury-containing effluent of a large chemical plant emptied into this body of water. The fish and shellfish concentrated the mercury and were ingested by humans; the mercury was then

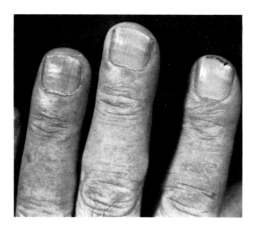

FIG. 13.12. Mee's lines. Pale transverse lines on fingernails denote time of arsenic poisoning.

released by the digestive processes, with resultant intoxication characterized by CNS and peripheral nervous system involvement.

Collagen Vascular Neuropathies

Collagen vascular diseases are probably inappropriately named for collagen may be only minimally involved. They have in common diffuse involvement of the connective tissue and small arteries in the pathologic process. Traditionally, these include rheumatoid arthritis (by far the most common), systemic lupus erythematosus, polymyositis and dermatomyositis, polyarteritis nodosa, and systemic sclerosis (scleroderma). This group of diseases is discussed again later in the chapter when muscle diseases are considered. In fact, peripheral neuropathy is an uncommon complication in collagen-vascular diseases. When it occurs it is most likely secondary to local or widespread small artery occlusion with peripheral nerve ischemia. Occasionally, mononeuropathies are reported in lupus erythematosus, and neuropathies secondary to joint inflammation and swelling are seen in conjunction with rheumatoid arthritis. The systemic features of each of these illnesses are usually paramount and call attention to the diagnosis. Treatment of the neuropathy, as well as the primary disorder, involves the use of adrenal cortical steroids.

Metabolic and Genetic Neuropathies

In a sense, all neuropathies, like all diseases, are "metabolic" in origin. In the clinical sense metabolic disorders usually mean abnormalities secondary to organ dysfunction (liver or kidney), electrolyte abnormalities, or acute infection. In this context, the only peripheral neuropathy that merits mention is the sensory neuropathy occasionally seen in severe uremia; prolonged dialysis may also be complicated by neuropathy.

The genetic neuropathies are more frequent and in some instances are part of a generalized disorder relating to an enzymatic defect. The more common of these are mentioned briefly. For more detailed information the reader is referred to a text on inherited diseases, a neurology text, or both.

Peroneal muscular atrophy (Charcot-Marie-Tooth syndrome) is an autosomal dominant disorder with great variation in the extent of clinical involvement. It may be so mild that the patient's only sign is high arches; or in the same family it may be severe, with high arches, varus deformity of the feet, hammer toes, atrophy of peroneal and anterior tibial muscle groups, diminished to absent deep tendon reflexes, minimal sensory abnormalities, enlargement of the peripheral nerves, and, late in the course, atrophy of the hand muscles. *Slow course, leg braces needed,*

Hypertrophic interstitial neuropathy (Déjèrline-Scotta's disease) is characterized by symmetrical motor and sensory neuropathy with palpable enlargement of the nerves, associated cerebellar and pupillary abnormalities, kyphoscoliosis, sporadic or familial history, and onset during infancy or early childhood.

Hereditary sensory neuropathy manifests with painless mutilating foot ulcers during childhood. Although all sensory modalities may be affected, pain and temperature loss are most prominent.

Heredopathia atactica polyneuritiformis (Refsum's syndrome) is a lipid-storage disease seemingly caused by deficiency of phytanic acid alpha-hydroxylase. It is characterized clinically by chronic remitting polyneuropathies, cerebellar signs, retinitis pigmentosa, nerve deafness, ichthyosis, and cardiomyopathy. Elevation of CSF protein is characteristic.

Primary amyloidosis may affect the peripheral nerves (*amyloid neuropathy*) as well as other organs. The neuropathy is mainly sensory, along with involvement of the peripheral autonomic nervous system. Pain and orthostatic hypotension are the main symptoms. Diagnosis is made by gingival or rectal biopsy.

Acute intermittent or tardive *porphyrias* may constitute baffling diagnostic problems and should be considered in any setting of peripheral neuropathy, particularly in association with gastrointestinal or psychiatric symptoms. The classic syndrome is mainly an ascending motor neuropathy that may involve the trunk and bulbar muscles, thus resembling Guillain-Barré syndrome. The neurologic picture is usually accompanied by severe abdominal pain, obstipation, psychotic behavior, and rarely seizures. An attack may be precipitated by barbiturates, sulfonamides, alcohol, and other drugs. The diagnosis is made by finding elevated porphyrobilinogen and δ-aminolevulinic acid in the serum and urine. Treatment is by high carbohydrate diet.

Riley-Day syndrome is a rare autosomal recessive disorder which occurs almost entirely in Ashkenazi jews. It is characterized by peripheral motor and sensory neuropathy, gastrointestinal and respiratory disorders, insensitivity to pain, and evidence of disease of the autonomic nervous system, viz., anhidrosis, orthostatic hypotension, and absence of tears.

Miscellaneous enzymatic disorders should always be considered in the diagnosis of unexplained progressive neuropathy, particularly in children; all show signs of multiple organ system involvement. The following particularly require noting: (1) *Metachromatic leukodystrophy neuropathy* due to deficiency of the enzyme aryl sulfatase. Look for metachromatic granules in the urine or in rectal or peripheral nerve biopsies. The patients manifest changes in speech and mental status, nystagmus, ataxia, tremor, and peripheral neuropathy. (2) *Bassen-Kornzweig syndrome*, with absent beta-lipoproteins in blood. Look for acanthocytosis and decreased total serum lipids and cholesterol. (3) *Angiokeratosis diffusum (Fabry's disease)* is caused by abnormal lipid storage of ceramide dihexoside and trihexoside. Angiokeratosis is scattered over the buttocks and legs, and there is a sensory neuropathy.

Infectious Neuropathies

Herpes zoster (shingles) is thought to be due to a spontaneous reactivation of an ancient varicella infection which remains latent in the sensory ganglia following chickenpox. It occurs mainly in middle-aged to elderly individuals and is characterized by a burning or aching pain in the distribution of a nerve root, followed by a typical vesicular rash in the same distribution. Involvement of motor fibers and ensuing palsies also occur ("geniculate" herpes, Ramsay-Hunt syndrome), and sensory deficits and severe pain may persist in the distribution of the involved nerve root after the acute infection has subsided. It is this postherpetic neuralgia which may be debilitating and extremely difficult to manage successfully. Carbamazepine is the initial treatment of choice. The association of shingles with malignancy has been noted. It occurs in 10 to 25% of patients with lymphoma, in particular those who received radiotherapy or had splenectomy.

Diphtheritic neuropathy is said to occur in 2 to 20% of patients in various epidemics. The most characteristic lesion is palatal paralysis, but any cranial nerve may be involved and combined motor and sensory polyneuropathy may also occur.

Botulism follows ingestion of tainted canned food and is characterized by paralysis of the muscles of accommodation of the iris, ophthalmoplegia, dryness of mucous membranes, dysphagia, dysarthria, weakness of extremities, hyporeflexia, and constipation. Treatment is by administration of the antitoxin and guanidine, a drug which enhances acetylcholine release into the synaptic cleft at the myoneural junction.

Leprosy is said to be the commonest cause of neuropathy worldwide and is thought still to be endemic in southern Florida and the southwestern United

States. It is a form of mononeuritis multiplex, producing local anesthesia and hypopigmentation. It is treated with chaulmoogra oil and sulfones.

Sarcoidosis is not known to be infectious and is usually classified as a chronic granulomatous disease. It has a predilection for Blacks; it involves the cranial nerves mainly, particularly the facial nerves, but may also cause a peripheral mononeuritis multiplex. Although steroid therapy is advocated, its efficacy is still debated.

Neoplastic Neuropathies

"Neoplastic neuropathies" is a generic term used to classify the polyneuritis (motor and sensory) that may occur with carcinoma, particularly of the lung. Hidden carcinoma is always looked for in a patient with neuropathy of undetermined cause. Severe neuropathy may occur in the course of any of the syndromes characterized by hypergammaglobulinemia (immune or immunoglobulin), specifically multiple myeloma and macroglobulinemia. The cause of the neuropathy is not known.

Ischemic Neuropathies

The ischemic neuropathies refer specifically to the neuropathies which may occur in occlusive peripheral vascular disease. The major clinical problem is pain or paresthesia in the distal part of an extremity. Evidence of occlusive peripheral vascular disease is usually obvious. True symmetrical polyneuropathy does not occur and, if present in a patient with peripheral vascular disease, is attributable to some other cause. The burning distal pain characteristic of ischemic neuropathy is sometimes made worse by activity or may be relieved by keeping the foot dependent.

MOTOR NEURON DISEASES

The group of disorders referred to as motor neuron diseases are "neuropathic" only in the sense that the lesion is predominantly in the motor neurons of the CNS (brain and spinal cord). Moreover, to the extent that they all produce muscular weakness and atrophy, they must be considered in the differential diagnosis of neuromuscular diseases. The one common feature in all of these disorders is that there are no associated sensory abnormalities.

Amyotrophic Lateral Sclerosis

Amyotrophic lateral sclerosis is a sporadic, noninherited disorder that occurs usually during middle age and twice as frequently in men; it has a mean survival time of 4+ years. It is characterized by progressive muscle weakness, atrophy, fasciculations, and, at some time in the illness, evidence of corticospinal tract involvement (hyperactive deep tendon reflexes, positive Babinski signs), and no sensory or sphincter dysfunction. Bulbar involvement is common, causing dysphagia and dysarthria, along with a paralyzed, atrophic tongue. The CSF is normal. The EMG shows diffuse denervation, fibrillations, and fasciculations, as well as giant action potentials, and is so characteristic that the diagnosis can be safely made by it. It is important not to confuse this illness with cervical spondylosis, which causes atrophy and weakness in the upper extremities and weakness and spasticity in the lower, because the latter entity is surgically treatable, whereas there is no known therapy for amyotrophic lateral sclerosis.

Two related entities are *infantile muscular atrophy* (Werdnig-Hoffmann disease) and *juvenile muscular atrophy* (Kugelberg-Welander syndrome). The former is a major cause of floppiness in infants. It is an inherited disease characterized by progressive motor weakness beginning almost at birth, muscle atrophy, loss of deep tendon reflexes, hypotonia, and (usually) death from aspiration by the age of 2 years. The EMG shows fasciculations in all muscle groups. Juvenile muscular atrophy begins from early childhood and continues to early adult life. It is characterized by proximal muscle weakness in the extremities and particularly in the legs, so the patient has difficulty arising from a chair or climbing stairs. The patients appear to have muscular dystrophy, but muscle fasciculation is evident, the EMG shows evidence of denervation, and muscle biopsy shows neurogenic patterns. The signs are usually slowly progressive. Like the other two similar disorders, there is no known treatment.

MYONEURAL JUNCTION DISORDERS

Myasthenia Gravis

There is a reduction in the number of functional acetylcholine receptor sites in myasthenia gravis, as revealed by studies utilizing radioactively labeled α-bungarotoxin. Moreover, circulating antibodies detected in the serum of almost all patients with myasthenia gravis cross-react with receptor proteins. These two findings are compelling evidence that the conduction defect in myasthenia is postsynaptic and is caused by an antibody. These proofs have been strengthened by the observations that experimental myasthenia can be induced in rabbits by injecting purified acetylcholine to produce an antibody, and that injections of immunoglobulins from patients with myasthenia causes a myasthenic picture in mice. These exciting observations confirmed what had been long suspected—that myasthenia gravis is an autoimmune disease. The increased evidence of association of thyrotoxicosis, rheumatoid arthritis, lupus erythematosus, and polymyositis, in addition to the known association of myasthenia and thymic tumor or hyperplasia, have long suggested an immunologic basis for the disease.

Myasthenia gravis is difficult to define, although it is readily recognized once the diagnosis is considered. It is a syndrome of muscle weakness and excessive fatigability, spontaneously varying in intensity, involving cranial nerves particularly, and improved partially by drugs which inhibit the action of acetylcholinesterase. Deep tendon reflexes are normal. There are no sensory abnormalities. Extraocular muscles commonly cause diplopia and ptosis, and facial and bulbar weakness are frequently present. All age groups from infancy to old age are affected, the peak incidence occurring in the 20- to 30-year-old age group; it occurs three times as commonly in women as in men. Thymic tumors develop in about 15% of the patients, most frequently in elderly males.

The muscle weakness is most evident after activity and least apparent on awakening in the morning. There may be progressive difficulty in masticating solid foods and an inability to swallow. Jaw weakness may produce an open, drooling mouth, and weakness of the facial muscles may transform an intended smile into a grimace. The extraocular muscle pareses are such that they cannot be mistaken for lesions of individual extraocular nerves, and pupillary reflexes are normal. The extensor muscles of the neck are usually much weaker than the flexors, so the patient may have difficulty keeping his head erect. Extremity weakness without cranial nerve involvement is infrequent. Sphincter disturbances do not occur. The most threatening signs are those of bulbar and/or respiratory paralysis. The course is quite variable, and spontaneous remissions of varying duration occur in many patients.

Diagnosis

A high index of suspicion is the most important aspect of the diagnosis of myasthenia; confirmation of the diagnosis depends on consistent observable improvement following the administration of anticholinesterase drugs. Edrophonium (Tensilon), 2 mg, is given intravenously, and the patient is checked carefully for improvement in muscle strength versus any untoward response (increased weakness, nausea, diarrhea) after 30 to 45 sec. An additional 8 mg edrophonium is then given over a period of 1 min. The examiner looks for improvement in extraocular movements, speech, or muscle strength. The response is frequently dramatic; a ptotic eye may open widely or the patient's dysphagia disappear. The effect of edrophonium lasts only 5 to 6 min. Neostigmine (1 to 2 mg i.m.) may also be used; its effect is noticeable within 15 to 20 min and peak action is at 1 to 2 hr. As previously described, EMG demonstrates a rapid decline in the amplitude of muscle potentials during repetitive stimulation of the innervating nerve. This defect in neuromuscular transmission may be corrected by administration of anticholinesterase drugs.

Evaluation of the patient must include chest x-rays to look for thymic tumor. Although routine views may be sufficient, small tumors can be visualized only by tomography of the mediastinum.

The curare sensitivity test has been used in difficult, doubtful cases, but it may be hazardous and difficult to interpret. Antibodies to muscle receptor proteins occur in almost all myasthenics and are not found in other diseases or normals.

Treatment

The management of patients with myasthenia has been changed dramatically by the use of steroids; the trend has been to attempt to induce a remission by the use of steroids or thymectomy, rather than continued supportive care by anticholinesterase drugs. This is an important concept which is still being tested and debated. It is safe to say that universally acceptable standard therapy does not yet exist.

pyridostigmine + atropine

Anticholinesterase treatment

The drugs most commonly used in the United States are pyridostigmine (Mestinon) and neostigmine. Therapy is usually initiated with 60 mg pyridostigmine q.i.d. Atropine may be required to counteract nausea, abdominal cramping, or diarrhea. The quantity and frequency of the dose are then adjusted to the patient's requirements; the objective is to achieve the maximum benefit with the fewest complications. Patients who respond well to anticholinesterase treatment may be maintained on it indefinitely. When the toxic therapeutic margin of the drug narrows, other therapy can be considered. The patient must be aware that his dosage requirements will vary and adjustments will be necessary. In instances in which it is difficult to decide whether a patient requires additional anticholinesterase medication, 2 mg edrophonium may be given intravenously 1 hr after the oral dose of the patient's medication. If strength is improved by the injection, the dosage of the patient's medication can be increased.

Corticosteroid therapy

Corticosteroid therapy has been effective in inducing prolonged remissions in many patients. The safest approach is to administer small, increasing, alternate-day doses, beginning with 10 to 15 mg prednisone and increasing by 5 to 10 mg on alternate days to a level of 100 to 120 mg on alternate days. Anticholinesterase drugs should be discontinued if possible. If the patient's symptoms subside, the steroids are reduced gradually. If symptoms reappear, the dosage can be increased; if not, the patient should be weaned as far as possible. The ideal objective of chronic corticosteroid therapy is to induce a remission, and, in the judgment of many, it is highly effective.

Thymectomy

Thymectomy has been utilized in the treatment of myasthenia since 1939. Despite this long and extensive clinical experience, there has been no convincing controlled, prospective study, and there is considerable controversy about its use. Thymomas should probably be removed because they are potentially malignant, but removal of the thymoma may not improve the patient's myasthenia. Indeed thymectomy is not considered essential for anterior mediastinal masses by some authorities.

Thymectomy is not recommended for patients who are well controlled with anticholinesterase drugs or corticosteroid therapy. It is said to be most effective in young (< 50 years) patients with progressive myasthenia who are not well controlled by medication and who have had the disease less than 2 years. Medication failure is a definite indication for thymectomy in a patient with progressive myasthenia of any age if the surgical procedure is not contraindicated for some other medical reason. Although the mortality rate of thymectomy in experienced hands is less than 2%, the patient requires highly skilled pre- and postoperative care. It is now believed that successful thymectomy requires removal of all traces of the thymus, so extensive mediastinal exploration is required at surgery.

[handwritten: Cholinergic crisis – blockade of activation of muscarinic receptors (esp. GI)]

Myasthenic crisis

[handwritten: myasthenic crisis – block of cholinergic receptor (mostly muscles)]

Myasthenic crisis is a rapid worsening of the patient's weakness despite active therapy. Bulbar and respiratory paralysis are the most important ingredients of myasthenic crisis. Such worsening is sometimes induced by excessive administration of cholinergic drugs (cholinergic crisis), but the differential diagnosis between myasthenic and cholinergic crisis may be extremely difficult. The patient should be in an intensive care unit and the respiratory function controlled. Intubation or tracheostomy should be performed promptly if required and respirator assistance administered in an expert fashion using intermittent positive pressure breathing. Control of the respiratory problem allows the clinician to determine whether the crisis is myasthenic or cholinergic, a distinction not easily made. Unless edrophonium testing unequivocally demonstrates improvement in muscle strength, all cholinergic drugs are discontinued and the patient is maintained on a respirator for 72 hr before a trial of cholinergic drugs is cautiously reinstituted. Patients in true myasthenic crisis may remain refractory to cholinergic drugs for an indefinite period. Such patients should be given corticosteroids or ACTH. High-dose corticosteroid therapy (prednisone 80 to 100 mg daily) may intensify weakness at first but usually induces a remission within 10 to 12 days. Low-dose, alternate-day therapy usually takes longer. The method of therapy may be individualized, but the principle is the same: Patients in crisis caused by failure of cholinergic therapy should be treated by steroids, maintaining tracheal toilet and respiratory function. In a modern intensive care unit, death during myasthenic crisis should now be a rare event.[1]

Special Considerations in Myasthenia Gravis

Patients with myasthenia have some pharmacologic sensitivities. Quinine, succinylcholine, and morphine may increase weakness. All sedatives and narcotics, as well as quinidine and procainamide, should be administered with great caution. Aminoglycoside antibiotics, polymyxin, viomycin, and colistin may have a neuromuscular blocking effect. Ocular myasthenia may be difficult to control completely with cholinergic drugs, and massive doses rarely improve the situation. Eye patches or lid crutches are useful devices and certainly to be preferred to thymectomy; and a course of corticosteroid therapy is justified. The effect of pregnancy in a patient with myasthenia is unpredictable, but therapeutic abortion is not helpful if the patient's symptoms have been worsened by pregnancy. Labor is normal.

Myasthenic Syndrome (Eaton-Lambert Syndrome)

The myasthenic syndrome is a rare disturbance of neuromuscular transmission thought to be caused by a deficiency of acetylcholine release into the synaptic cleft. It is characterized by generalized muscle weakness, depressed-to-absent deep tendon reflexes, no cranial nerve pathology, and inconsistent or no response to acetylcholinesterase inhibitors. It occurs in patients with carcinoma (usually oat cell carcinoma of the lung), but the syndrome may appear before such a lesion has been demonstrated. Unlike myasthenia, the weakness improves with exercise, which can be demonstrated physiologically by EMG, in which repetitive nerve stimulation results in gradual increase in the amplitude of muscle action potentials. The syndrome should be suspected in an individual who complains of muscle weakness, even though none can be demonstrated on formal testing, if the deep tendon reflexes are absent. Removal of the tumor, if it can be found, may result in improvement in the syndrome. Guanidine HCl (30 to 40 mg/kg/day divided into three doses) is inconsistently beneficial.

DISEASES OF MUSCLE

The group of disorders to be discussed as diseases of muscle are characterized by weakness or disturbed speed of muscular contraction and relaxation with no evidence of neural disease or neuromuscular block. Although it is apparent that the clinical diagnosis of a myopathic disorder depends to a substantial degree on the exclusion of disease of other structures (the CNS or peripheral nervous system, myoneural junction, joint disease, etc.), there are nevertheless clinical and laboratory features, most of which

---

[1]See *Note Added in Proof,* p. 271.

have been defined during the past 25 years (EMG, muscle histochemistry), which allow the clinician to localize the causative pathology to the muscle. All myopathic disorders, no matter what the presumed etiology, have in common an extreme paucity of knowledge of the biologic mechanisms underlying the disorder in muscle function and the pathology as visualized in the light and electron microscopes. This is true despite the accumulation of a staggering array of knowledge of normal and pathologic anatomy and the biochemistry and physics of muscle contraction. There is, indeed, a remarkable apparent similarity of basic anatomy and physiology in all striated muscle; nevertheless various diseases consistently involve only certain groups of muscles and even specific types of muscle fibers, sparing others completely. It is this topographic distribution of pathology which, along with other clinical features, allows classification of the dystrophies, although there is no explanation for it as yet forthcoming. Certain anatomic features (e.g., the fact that extraocular muscles have an extremely high neural/fiber ratio, each motor unit being comprised of only 6 to 10 nerve fibers, as compared to extremity muscles in which each motor unit may contain 1,500 fibers) are tantalizing reasons for explaining certain clinical phenomena, viz., the frequent involvement of extraocular muscles in myasthenia gravis.

Having said this, it is evident to the reader that there is still no completely satisfactory classification or grouping of muscle disorders. *Enzymatic disorders* or deficiencies are probably responsible for the largest group of myopathies:

1. Muscular dystrophies
2. Glycogen storage diseases
3. Familial periodic paralyses
4. Familial myoglobinurias
5. Congenital myopathies
6. Mitochondrial myopathies

"Inflammation" of the muscle, its connective tissue, and its vascular supply either primary or secondary to a collagen vascular disease is classified as *polymyositis* or *dermatomyositis*. *Metabolic disorders* may cause muscle weakness, and *toxic agents and trauma* are responsible for disturbances of muscle function reflected in several clinical syndromes.

This classification is not intended to satisfy purists with special expertise in muscle disease but, rather, to assist the clinician in focusing on those disorders of muscle function which might be amenable to treatment.

Enzymatic Disorders

Muscular Dystrophies

The muscular dystrophies represent a group of genetically determined diseases of muscle characterized by progressive weakness, usually but not necessarily beginning during childhood. Because no treatment other than genetic counseling is currently available, the major practical benefit to be derived from classifying the dystrophies is to be able to offer prognostic data to the patient and family. The muscle pathology in the various dystrophies does not allow distinction among types, nor are the biochemical abnormalities type-specific.

Concepts as to the mechanisms responsible for muscular dystrophy are the subject of extensive basic science investigation. There is no direct evidence of an enzymatic abnormality, but it is strongly suggested by the fact that the dystrophies are genetically determined. McComas challenged the hypothesis that the dystrophies are caused by disease intrinsic to the muscle fiber by purporting to demonstrate that the number of functional motor units is diminished in all types of muscular dystrophy, suggesting that the disorder is neurogenic. Other investigators have not confirmed his findings. The major thrust of recent research has been to identify the biochemical abnormality common to the dystrophies. Much emphasis has been placed on the concept that the muscle membrane in dystrophy is sick and therefore unable to maintain a proper biochemical environment for the cell. In this regard studies on the membranes of erythrocytes, a somewhat easier model, have begun to have an interesting harvest which may well bear on this interesting and important problem.

The laboratory investigation of patients with muscular dystrophies does not distinguish among the types. They may all show similar EMG abnormalities and elevation of urinary creatine, serum creatine phosphokinase and aldolase. Muscle biopsies are not type-specific. They reveal variable degrees of loss of muscle fibers, degeneration of muscle fibers with phagocytosis, persistent muscle fibers haphazardly arranged and of various sizes, increased lipocytes, and fibrosis.

Duchenne muscular dystrophy begins during the first 3 to 6 years of life, occurs almost exclusively in males, shows a sex-linked recessive inheritance, and is the most rapidly progressive of all dystrophies. The weakness involves proximal muscle groups first and is accompanied by pseudohypertrophy. The appearance is typical: The patients stand with protruding abdomen, lordotic posture, and legs wide apart for better support. They waddle when they walk and climb up their own extremities to achieve a standing position from a sitting or lying posture (Gower's sign). These patients usually require a wheelchair by midadolescence and die, usually of respiratory failure, in their twenties.

Limb-girdle dystrophy is a group of dystrophies with slowly progressive shoulder and pelvic girdle weakness, and sporadic or with family history. Its onset is during late adolescence, and it has a gradual, unpredictable course.

Fascioscapulohumeral dystrophy is an autosomal dominant dystrophy, beginning at the end of the first decade of life. It is characterized by weakness and wasting of facial, scapular, and upper arm muscles. It may be compatible with a normal life span.

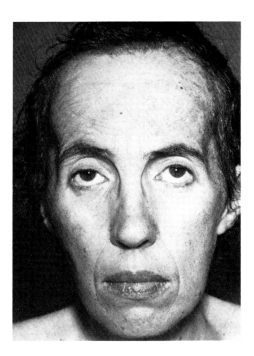

FIG. 13.13. Myotonic dystrophy. Note atrophy of temporalis muscles, frontal hair loss, and absence of facial expression resulting from weakness of facial muscles.

Myotonic muscular dystrophy is an autosomal dominant disorder associated with myotonia, cataracts, frontal baldness, and testicular atrophy. Mental deficiency is common. The facial muscles are involved earliest, and all other muscle groups are gradually involved. The patients have a characteristic appearance: facial diplegia, ptosis, high forehead, and wasted temporal muscles (Fig. 13.13). Myotonia can usually be demonstrated by percussing the thenar eminence or the tongue. The patients also complain of difficulty in releasing their grasp, particularly in cool weather. Pharyngeal and laryngeal weakness is common. Decreased pulmonary ventilation results in recurrent pulmonary infections. The electrocardiogram (ECG) often reveals a prolonged P-R interval and bradycardia.

Glycogen Storage Myopathies

Five types of glycogen storage disease involving muscle and associated with specific enzymatic defects have been described. These disorders have served as models in clarifying normal metabolic processes in muscle. Unfortunately, they are genetically heterogeneous, and there is considerable variation in symptomatology. Two of these merit mention.

McArdles disease (phosphorylase deficiency) is characterized by muscle cramping upon exercise, poor stamina, weakness, and muscle stiffness. It is a familial disorder, occasionally appearing sporadically. When the patient exercises the extremity, lactate in the venous effluent does not increase appropriately, denoting a metabolic defect in the glycolytic cycle. Muscle atrophy occurs in older patients.

There are several forms of *acid maltase deficiency* (Pompe's disease). In the infantile form glycogen accumulation in the muscle, heart, brain, and spinal cord is massive. In later developing forms the accumulation is confined to striated muscle, and the course resembles Duchenne dystrophy. Diagnosis can be made by muscle biopsy and with glycogen visualized by electron microscopy. Acid maltase activity is absent in cultured fibroblasts, liver, and muscle. Affected infants are floppy, weak, and show cardiomegaly and respiratory difficulty.

Familial Periodic Paralysis

Familial periodic paralysis comprises a group of at least four clinical and metabolic syndromes. The presumption that they are due to enzymic abnormality is just that; there is no proof. All are characterized by periodic disturbances in potassium metabolism and muscle weakness.

Hypokalemic periodic paralysis. The symptoms usually begin during adolescence; onset of weakness is during sleep, often after a heavy carbohydrate meal or strenuous activity. Weakness begins in the lower extremities and may eventually involve even the cranial nerves. The weakness may last a few hours or even several days. Serum potassium is reduced, and this is reflected in the electrocardiogram. The attack can be aborted by administration of 4 to 5 g potassium chloride, repeated as often as every 1 to 2 hr, with careful ECG monitoring. The attacks spontaneously lessen with advancing age.

Hyperthyroid periodic paralysis. This occurs mainly in Orientals and is characterized by recurrent attacks of hypokalemic paralysis associated with hyperthyroidism.

Adynamia episodica (hyperkalemic periodic paralysis). The attacks are brief (30 to 60 min), begin during early childhood, follow physical exercise, and are aborted by additional exercise. The serum potassium is usually elevated, and an attack may be precipitated by ingestion of potassium.

Paramyotonia congenita. This may be a variant of adynamia episodica, the major difference being the association of myotonia. Exposure to cold precipitates an attack in both groups of patients.

Familial Myoglobinuria

Familial myoglobinuria is a rare disorder and one of the least common causes of myoglobinuria. It is familial and may be associated with myopathy or dystrophy. The attack of myoglobinuria is precipitated by vigorous exercise or infection. The patients complain of muscle aching, swelling, tenderness, and weakness. Biopsy reveals degenerating and regenerating muscle fibers. These patients should avoid physical exertion because the myoglobin may cause permanent renal disease.

Congenital Myopathies

The term congenital myopathy is used to describe a rare group of disorders that are present during early childhood and for which no specific genetic pattern has emerged. There is no known enzymatic defect. Furthermore, the disorder may not become clinically evident until middle life. They were discovered after the development of specific histochemical techniques, and their features were defined by electron microscopy.

Central core disease is characterized by proximal muscle weakness, no atrophy, and slow progression. The central part of the muscle fibers show a dense hyaline change in the myofibrils.

Nemaline myopathy is similar to central core disease, but the muscles are hypoplastic. The nemaline bodies seem to arise from the Z lines.

Mitochondrial Myopathies

Mitochondrial myopathies include an amorphous group of myopathies in which the muscle fibers contain excessive numbers of large mitochondria containing abnormal inclusions. The clinical syndromes are diverse, consisting of weakness, fatigability, and cramps.

Progressive Ophthalmoplegia (Ophthalmoplegia Plus, Kearns-Sayre Syndrome)

Progressive ophthalmoplegia is a difficult entity to classify because it is difficult to differentiate myopathic from neuropathic changes in biopsies of affected extraocular muscles. There is a spectrum of clinical abnormalities, varying from progressive external ophthalmoplegia alone to ophthalmoplegia plus retinitis pigmentosa, varying degrees of heart block, short stature, small musculature, and elevated CSF protein. Onset of this disorder is during childhood, and the patients not uncommonly succumb to the consequences of the heart block, which may require implantation of a cardiac pacemaker. Some authorities classify the syndrome as a form of muscular dystrophy, but the typical pathology includes lipid inclusions in type I muscle fibers and abnormal mitochondria (by electron microscopy). The enzymatic abnormality (if such it is) responsible for this syndrome has not been discovered.

Inflammatory Diseases of Muscle

Muscle inflammation can be caused by a wide variety of infections and infestations, but these are actually quite unusual in clinical practice in the United States. Bacterial infection of the muscle can be caused by any pathogen. *Clostridial* muscle necrosis (gas gangrene) may be the best known, but tuberculous and leptospiral infections have also been described. *Viral* myopathies, in particular *Bornholm's disease* and *Coxsackie B virus*, are associated with aching, tender muscles, fever, and a septic course. Parasitic infestation of muscle, particularly *trichinosis*, may cause muscle pain, fever, periorbital swelling, and eosinophilia. *Echinococcus*, *toxoplasmosis*, and *schistosomiasis* may invade muscle and produce local and systemic symptoms.

The commonest and therefore most important of the inflammatory diseases of muscle are *polymyositis* and *dermatomyositis*. Authorities differ as to whether these represent different entities. Some believe that dermatomyositis is a fairly homogeneous syndrome, occurring often during childhood; in adults it is frequently associated with carcinoma. Polymyositis, on the other hand, appears to be a syndrome of multiple etiologies, viz., lupus erythematosus, polyarteritis, systemic sclerosis, rheumatoid arthritis, and carcinoma. Of these, only systemic sclerosis and carcinoma are associated with dermatomyositis.

The muscle pathology is similar in both disorders, consisting of necrotic muscle fibers and cellular infiltrate. Intimal hyperplasia and inflammation of small arteries is said to occur more commonly in dermatomyositis.

In dermatomyositis either the rash or muscle weakness may appear first. The classic skin lesion is a pinkish-violet (heliotrope) colored maculopapular rash over the cheeks, bridge of the nose, eyelids, forehead, and fingers. Widespread subcutaneous calcification may develop in time. The myopathy of dermatomyositis and polymyositis involves predominantly the proximal limb muscles and the flexors of the neck. Dysphagia is not uncommon and may be due to esophageal involvement. Muscle weakness varies from barely detectable to total paralysis. Deep tendon reflexes are preserved, although they may be reduced. Muscles are usually not tender.

Arthralgia and low-grade fever are common. As previously noted, systemic lupus erythematosus, scleroderma, polyarteritis, and rheumatoid disease are present in about 35 to 50% of cases of polymyositis. Carcinoma has been encountered in about 20% of patients, especially those with dermatomyositis, and the frequency of association increases after age 50, particularly in males.

The laboratory confirmation of polymyositis or dermatomyositis is made by the increase in serum CPK and aldolase, myopathic EMG, and muscle biopsy. The etiology of these illnesses is as yet unknown, although evidence is accumulating that altered immunologic mechanisms are responsible.

Treatment of polymyositis and dermatomyositis is far from satisfactory. A well-planned, controlled prospective study is needed to evaluate the effects of corticosteroid and other immunosuppressive therapy. There is no doubt that there is a high failure rate (> 30%), and the natural history of the disorders is known to be variable, with exacerbations and remissions. Nevertheless, treatment is usually by prednisone, 20 to 30 mg t.i.d., along with potassium supplement and antacids. Recovery is judged by improvement of strength and a reduction of serum enzymes and the erythrocyte sedimentation rate (ESR), following which the dose of steroids is reduced slowly to the smallest level consistent with maintaining clinical and laboratory improvement.

Patients who respond poorly to steroids may be treated with azathioprine in doses sufficient to suppress the blood leukocyte count to 3,500/mm³.

The prognosis of polymyositis and dermatomyositis depends to a considerable extent on the diseases with which it is associated or presumed to be caused by. All the collagen vascular diseases are serious and restrict life span: Rheumatoid disease is the least malignant; and myositis associated with carcinoma, despite the poorly understood relationship, implies a poor prognosis. In fact, few patients recover completely from polymyositis or dermatomyositis. Most are left with weakness of the shoulder girdle and hip muscles. A few die of cardiac, pulmonary, or renal complications. In short, despite the best therapy available, these are serious disorders, with the outlook for complete recovery poor.

Metabolic Myopathies

Endocrine Myopathies

Thyroid disease

Hyperthyroidism is probably associated with muscle weakness and evidence of myopathy by EMG in over 75% of cases, but the problem is usually mild. In some instances the weakness becomes disproportionately severe. These patients usually improve after treatment of the hyperthyroid state; propranolol, a beta-adrenergic blocking agent, may provide dramatic and rapid improvement. As previously mentioned, myasthenia gravis also accompanies thyrotoxicosis.

Myxedema is commonly associated with decreased speed of muscle contraction and relaxation as well as pseudomyotonia, which is an electrically silent local swelling of muscle following percussion. Rarely, a true myopathy develops in patients with myxedema, and this usually responds to treatment of the primary condition.

Thyroid eye disease or ocular myopathy occurs in the hypo- and hyperthyroid states; the clinical picture is that of diplopia caused by weakness of one or more extraocular muscles. The pathology seems to be an infiltrative and scarring lesion in the muscle so that surgical correction may be required. Treatment of the primary endocrine abnormality may not be helpful.

Adrenal disease

Muscle weakness is common in patients with Cushing's syndrome and responds to treatment of the primary disorder.

Parathyroid disease

The severe weakness which accompanies hyperparathyroidism is probably a manifestation of hypercalcemia, which may also occur consequent to other disorders (sarcoid, metastatic disease).

Pituitary disease

Severe muscle weakness with characteristic electrical signs of myopathy occurs in acromegaly.

The Myoglobinurias

When myoglobin appears in the urine, it is an indication of damaged muscle cell membranes. Probably the most common cause of myoglobinuria is trauma, specifically the crush syndrome, but other extrinsic causes include intoxications, electric shock, carbon monoxide poisoning, and heavy alcohol ingestion. Diabetic acidosis, hypothermia, barbiturate or heroin intoxication, and ingestion of amphotericin B and licorice have all been incriminated as rare causes of myoglobinuria. Unusually heavy exercise may cause myoglobinuria. Idiopathic paroxysmal myoglobinuria begins during childhood, probably has a genetic basis, is not related to trauma or exertion, and may cause death due to renal failure.

The clinical picture is similar, whatever the cause. The affected muscles are weak, tender, and may be swollen; they are usually those that have been subjected to the heaviest physical stress. These symptoms are accompanied by urinary pigmentation and elevation of serum enzymes. The identification of the urinary pigment as myoglobin and its differentiation from hemoglobin or porphyrins requires special laboratory techniques.

The major objective of therapy in myoglobinuria is to protect the kidneys, but there is no certain evidence that the usual measures, particularly the use of osmotic diuretics, which produce a dilute urine, are helpful. The myoglobinuria accompanying crush injuries is a reflection of severe muscle damage.

Drug-Induced Myopathies

The term myopathy is used loosely in the classification "drug-induced" myopathy because there is no typical pathology or electrical abnormality in most cases of weakness induced by drugs; however, one should be aware that certain drugs can cause rather severe and prolonged weakness. Probably the best-known drug-induced weakness is that caused by agents which produce hypokalemia, particularly diuretics. Thyroid hormone and steroid administration may result in progressive weakness. Serum potassium should be measured in any patient with relatively rapid onset of weakness. In most instances the cause is evident.

Alcoholics also acquire a severe myopathy which resembles polymyositis. The patients may complain of leg cramps on walking, trunk and proximal extremity weakness, and rarely myoglobinuria. The myopathy subsides along with decreased alcohol ingestion. Other drugs which induce weakness include vincristine, glycyrrhizate, and colchicine.

Cramps and Myotonia

Muscle cramps are common and have been experienced by almost all normal individuals. A cramp is a painful involuntary muscle spasm which is sometimes relieved by stretching the involved muscle. Cramps occur particularly after exercise, and they may be induced during exercise by sodium depletion. Other conditions associated with susceptibility to cramps include myxedema, uremia, partial denervation of a muscle, and a number of myopathies. The important point is that most muscle cramps are benign and should not be a source of anxiety. Nocturnal cramps experienced by elderly individuals can often be relieved by quinine 300 mg at bedtime.

Stiff-man syndrome is clearly more than a series of simple cramps but can logically be described here. It is a sporadic, rare disorder characterized by painful spasms and chronic muscular rigidity. It may become progressively more severe, resembling the opisthotonic spasms of tetanus late in the disease. The EMG shows constant motor unit activity indicative of muscle contraction while the patient is at rest. It is believed that this disorder is caused by some yet unexplained type of CNS hyperexcitability. Diazepam in doses of 25 to 50 mg daily is quite effective in managing most patients.

Myotonia is a rare, interesting phenomenon in which muscle contraction, either voluntary or mechanical, is followed by slowed relaxation. The abnormality responsible for the persistence of muscle action potentials probably resides in the muscle fibers. The biochemical basis for the phenomenon is still not understood; defects in lipid composition of muscle membranes or inability of membranes to bind calcium have been postulated.

The clinical features include muscle stiffness or difficulty in relaxing a contracted muscle as observed when the patient is unable to release a grasped object. Facial spasms after eye closure or spasms of the pharynx and tongue may be quite troublesome. Mechanical myotonia can be demonstrated by percussing the thenar eminence or any other available muscle. The contraction induced by the blow is followed by a slow return to the normal configuration.

Myotonia congenita is a genetically determined disorder characterized by myotonia, striking muscular hypertrophy, and normal strength. It is present from early childhood and, in extreme forms, may cause great difficulty in running or pursuing normal physical activity.

Diazocholesterol produces myotonia in humans and experimental animals. As previously described, myotonia is also a prominent feature of myotonic dystrophy. Pseudomyotonia, or what appears to be delayed muscle relaxation to voluntary or mechanical contraction but without appropriate EMG abnormalities, occurs in myxedema. All myotonia is worsened by exposure to cold.

Treatment with phenytoin or procainamide or steroids has been quite successful in most cases.

SUGGESTED READINGS

Peripheral Neuropathies

Etiology and Pathogenesis

Aetiology of Bell's palsy. *Br Med J* 4:2, 1971.

Appenzeller O, Kornfeld M, and MacGee J: Neuropathy in chronic renal disease: a microscopic, ultrastructural, and biochemical study of sural nerve biopsies. *Arch Neurol* 24:449, 1971.

Bleehan S et al: Mononeuritis multiplex in polyarteritis nodosa. *Q J Med* 32:193, 1963.

Brain R, and Henson RA: Neurological syndromes associated with carcinoma: the carcinomatous neuropathies. *Lancet* 2:971, 1958.

Brain WR, Wright AD, and Wilkinson M: Spontaneous compression of both median nerves in the carpal tunnel. *Lancet* 1:277, 1947.

Chawla LS, et al: Meralgia paraesthetica. *Acta Neurol Scand* 42:483, 1966.

Cracchiolo A, and Marmor L: Peripheral entrapment neuropathies. *JAMA* 204:431, 1968.

Croft PB, Urich H, and Wilkinson M: Peripheral neuropathy of sensorimotor type associated with malignant disease. *Brain* 90:31, 1967.

Dawson CW, et al: Charcot-Marie-Tooth disease. *JAMA* 188:659, 1964.

Denny-Brown D: Primary sensory neuropathy with muscular changes associated with carcinoma. *J Neurol Neurosurg Psychiatry* 11:73, 1948.

Denny-Brown D: Hereditary sensory radicular neuropathy. *J Neurol Neurosurg Psychiatry* 14:237, 1951.

Denny-Brown D: Clinical problems in neuromuscular physiology. *Am J Med* 15:368, 1953.

Dolman CL: The pathology and pathogenesis of diabetic neuropathy. *Bull NY Acad Med* 43:773, 1967.

Drachman DA: Ophthalmoplegia plus: the neurodegenerative disorders associated with progressive external ophthalmoplegia. *Arch Neurol* 18:654, 1968.

Dreyfus PM, Hakim S, and Adams RD: Diabetic ophthalmoplegia. *Arch Neurol Psychiatry* 77:337, 1957.

Eames RA, and Lange LS: Clinical and pathological study of ischaemic neuropathy. *J Neurol Neurosurg Psychiatry* 30:215, 1967.

Gamstorp I: Polyneuropathy in childhood. *Acta Paediatr Scand* 57:230, 1968.

Garland HT: Diabetic amyotrophy. *Br Med J* 2:1287, 1955.

Henson RA, Russell DS, and Wilkinson M: Carcinomatous neuropathy and myopathy: a clinical and pathological study. *Brain* 77:82, 1954.

Heyman A, et al: Peripheral neuropathy caused by arsenical intoxication. *N Engl J Med* 254:401, 1956.

Jones KK, and Walsh JR: Diabetic amyotrophy. *Postgrad Med* 37:342, 1965.

Kocen RS, and Thomas PK: Peripheral nerve involvement in Fabry's disease. *Arch Neurol* 22:81, 1970.

Koeppen AH, Messmore H, and Stehbens WE: Interstitial hypertrophic neuropathy. *Arch Neurol* 24:340, 1971.

Leading article: Tick paralysis. *Br Med J* 2:314, 1969.

Locke S, et al: Diabetic amyotrophy. *Am J Med* 34:775, 1963.

Martin MM: Diabetic neuropathy: a clinical study of 150 cases. *Brain* 76:594, 1953.

Meadows JC, Marsden CD, and Harriman DGF: Chronic spinal muscular atrophy in adults. I. The Kugelberg-Welander syndrome. *J Neurol Sci* 9:527, 1969.

Meadows JC, Marsden CD, and Harriman DGF: Chronic spinal muscular atrophy in adults. II. Other forms. *J Neurol Sci* 9:551, 1969.

Pleasure DE, Mishler KC, and Engel WK: Axonal transport of proteins in experimental neuropathies. *Science* 166:524, 1969.

Raff MC, Sangalang V, and Asbury AK: Ischemic mononeuropathy multiplex associated with diabetes mellitus. *Arch Neurol* 18:487, 1968.

Rundles RW: Diabetic neuropathy: general review with report of 125 cases. *Medicine (Baltimore)* 24:111, 1945.

Sullivan JF, Twitchell TE, Gherardi GJ, and Vanderlaan WP: Amyloid polyneuropathy. *Neurology (Minneap)* 5:847, 1955.

Swash M: Acute fatal carcinomatous neuromyopathy. *Arch Neurol* 30:324, 1974.

Thomas PK, and Lascelles RG: The pathology of diabetic neuropathy. *Q J Med* 35:489, 1966.

Victor M: Alcohol and nutritional diseases of the nervous system. *JAMA* 167:65, 1958.

Victor M, Banker BQ, and Adams RD: The neuropathy of multiple myeloma. *J Neurol Neurosurg Psychiatry* 21:73, 1958.

Walsh JC: Neuropathy associated with lymphoma. *J Neurol Neurosurg Psychiatry* 34:42, 1971.

Weber RB, Daroff RB, and Mackey E: Pathology of oculomotor nerve palsy in diabetics. *Neurology (Minneap)* 20:835, 1970.

Symptoms and Signs

Bartley O, Brolin I, Fagerberg S-E, and Wilhemsen L: Neurogenic disorders of the bladder in diabetes mellitus: a clinical roentgenological investigation. *Acta Med Scand* 180:187, 1966.

Thomashefsky AJ, Horwitz SJ, and Feingold MH: Acute autonomic neuropathy. *Neurology (Minneap)* 22:251, 1972.

Tsairis P, Dyck PJ, and Mulder DW: Natural history of brachial plexus neuropathy. *Arch Neurol* 27:109, 1972.

Turner JWA, et al: Neuralgic amyotrophy (paralytic brachial neuritis). *Lancet* 2:209, 1957.

Diagnosis

Brodal A, Böyesen S, and Frövig AG: Progressive neuropathic (peroneal) muscular atrophy (Charcot-Marie-Tooth disease): histological findings in muscle biopsy specimen in fourteen cases, with notes on clinical diagnosis and familial occurrence. *Arch Neurol Psychiatry* 70:1, 1953.

Lamontagne A, and Buchthal F: Electrophysiological studies in diabetic neuropathy. *J Neurol Neurosurg Psychiatry* 33:442, 1970.

Podivinsky F: Factors influencing the measurement of conduction velocity in the human peripheral nerve. *J Neurol Sci* 5:493, 1967.

Treatment

Ellenberg M: Treatment of diabetic neuropathy. *Mod Treatm* 4:44, 1967.

Killian JM, and Frowin GH: Carbamazepine in the treatment of neuralgia. *Arch Neurol* 19:129, 1968.

Myopathies

Etiology and Pathogenesis

Affi AK, Bergman RA, and Harvey JC: Steroid myopathy: clinical, histological and cytological observations. *Johns Hopkins Med J* 123:158, 1968.

Arundell FD, Wilkinson RD, and Haserick JR: Dermatomyositis and malignant neoplasms in adults. *Arch Dermatol* 82:772, 1960.

Astrom KE, Kugelberg E, and Muller R: Hypothyroid myopathy. *Arch Neurol* 5:472, 1961.

Bradley WG, Hudgson P, Gardner-Medwin D, and Walton JN: Myopathy associated with abnormal lipid metabolism in skeletal muscle. *Lancet* 1:495, 1969.

Byers RK, et al: Steroid myopathy. *Pediatrics* 29:26, 1962.

Campbell MJ, McComas AJ, and Petito F: Physiological changes in ageing muscles. *J Neurol Neurosurg Psychiatry* 36:174, 1973.

Denny-Brown D: Clinical problems in neuromuscular physiology. *Am J Med* 15:368, 1953.

Engel WK (ed): *Current Concepts of Myopathies*. Lippincott, Philadelphia, 1965.

Engel WK, McFarlin DE, Drews GA, and Wochner RD: Protein abnormalities in neuromuscular diseases. Part I. *JAMA* 195:754, 1966.

Faris AA, and Reyes MG: Reappraisal of alcoholic myopathy. *J Neurol Neurosurg Psychiatry* 34:86, 1971.

Floyd M, Ayyar DR, Barwick DD, Hudgson P, and Weightman D: Myopathy in chronic renal failure. *Q J Med* 63:509, 1974.

Frame B, Heize EG, Block MA, and Manson GA: Myopathy in primary hyperparathyroidism. *Ann Intern Med* 68:1022, 1968.

Gaan D: Chronic thyrotoxic myopathy with involvement of respiratory and bulbar muscles. *Br Med J* 3:415, 1967.

Gamstorp I: A study of transient muscular weakness. *Acta Neurol Scand* 38:3, 1962.

Lynch PG: Alcoholic myopathy. *J Neurol Sci* 9:449, 1969.

Mastaglia FL, Barwick DD, and Hall R: Myopathy in acromegaly. *Lancet* 2:907, 1970.

Myerson RM, and Lafair JS: Alcoholic muscle disease. *Med Clin North Am* 54:723, 1970.

Nickel SN, et al: Myxedema neuropathy and myopathy. *Neurology (Minneap)* 11:125, 1961.

Pearson CM: Polymyositis. *Annu Rev Med* 17:63, 1966.

Penn AS, Rowland LP, and Fraser DW: Drugs, coma, and myoglobinuria. *Arch Neurol* 26:336, 1972.

Ramsay ID: Muscle dysfunction in hyperthyroidism. *Lancet* 2:931, 1966.

Ramsay ID: Thyrotoxic muscle disease. *Postgrad Med J* 44:385, 1969.

Riddoch D, and Morgan-Hughes JA: Prognosis in adult polymyositis. *J Neurol Sci* 26:71, 1975.

Shy GM: Rare myopathies. *Med Clin North Am* 47:1525, 1963.

Walton JN, and Nattrass FJ: On the classification, natural history and treatment of the myopathies. *Brain* 77:169, 1954.

Zundel W, et al: The muscular dystrophies. *N Engl J Med* 273:537, 1965.

Diagnosis

Brooke MH, and Kaplan H: Muscle pathology in rheumatoid arthritis, polymyalgia, rheumatism and polymyositis: a histochemical study. *Arch Pathol* 94:101, 1972.

Munsat T, and Cancilla P: Polymyositis without inflammation. *Bull Los Angeles Neurol Soc* 39:113, 1974.

Rose AL, Walton JN, and Pearce GW: Polymyositis: an ultramicroscopic study of muscle biopsy material. *J Neurol Sci* 5:457, 1967.

Treatment

Engel AG: Treatment of metabolic and endocrine myopathies. *Mod Treatm* 3:313, 1966.

Mulder D: Steroid therapy in patients with polymyositis and dermatomyositis. *Ann Intern Med* 58:969, 1963.

Rose AL, and Walton JN: Polymyositis: a survey of 89 cases with particular reference to treatment and prognosis. *Brain* 89:747, 1966.

Vignos PJ Jr, Bowling GF, and Watkins MP: Polymyositis: effect of corticosteroids on final result. *Arch Intern Med* 114:263, 1964.

Dermatomyositis

Arundell FD, Wilkinson RD, and Haserick JR: Dermatomyositis and malignant neoplasms in adults. *Arch Dermatol* 82:772, 1960.

Banker B, and Victor M: Dermatomyositis (systemic angiopathy) in childhood. *Medicine (Baltimore)* 45:261, 1966.

Myasthenia Gravis

Etiology and Pathogenesis

Abdou NI, Lisak RP, Zweiman B, Abrahamsohn I, and Penn AS: The thymus in myasthenia gravis: evidence for altered cell populations. *N Engl J Med* 291:1271, 1974.

Engel WK, Festoff BW, Patten BM, Swerdlow ML, Newball HH, and Thompson MD: Myasthenia gravis. *Ann Intern Med* 81:225, 1974.

Fambrough DM, Drachman DB, and Satyamurti S: Neuromuscular junction in myasthenia gravis decreased acetylcholine receptors. *Science* 182:293, 1973.

Havard CWH: Progress in myasthenia gravis. *Br Med J* 3:437, 1973.

Ito Y, Miledi R, Vincent A, and Newson-Davis J: Acetylcholine receptors and end-plate electrophysiology in myasthenia gravis. *Brain* 101:345, 1978.

Namba T, Brown SB, and Grob D: Neonatal myasthenia gravis: report of two cases and review of the literature. *Pediatrics* 45:488, 1970.

Nastuk WL, and Plescia OJ: Current status of research on myasthenia gravis. *Ann NY Acad Sci* 135:664, 1966.

Osserman KE, and Whipple HE: Myasthenia gravis. *Ann NY Acad Sci* 135:1, 1966.

Richman DP, Patrick J, Arnason BGW: Cellular immunity in myasthenia gravis. *N Engl J Med* 294:694, 1976.

Satyamurti S, Drachman DB, and Slone G: Blockade of acetylcholine receptors: a model of myasthenia gravis. *Science* 187:955, 1975.

Thornell L-E, Sjöström M, Mattsson CH, and Heilbronn E: Morphological observations on motor end-plates in rabbits with experimental myasthenia. *J Neurol Sci* 29:389, 1976.

Toyka KV, Drachman DB, Griffin DE, et al: Myasthenia gravis: study of humoral immune mechanisms by passive transfer to mice. *N Engl J Med* 296:125, 1977.

Vetters JM, and Simpson JA: Comparison of thymic histology with response to thymectomy in myasthenia gravis. *J Neurol Neurosurg Psychiatry* 37:1139, 1974.

Diagnosis

Bennett AE, and Cash CPT: Myasthenia gravis; curare sensitivity: a new diagnostic test and approach to causation. *Arch Neurol Psychiatry* 49:537, 1943.

Borenstein S, and Desmedt JE: New diagnostic procedures in myasthenia gravis. *New Dev Electromyogr Clin Neurophysiol* 1:350, 1973.

Osserman KE, and Kaplan LI: Rapid diagnostic test for myasthenia gravis: increased muscle strength, without fasciculations, after intravenous administration of edrophonium (Tensilon) chloride. *JAMA* 150:265, 1952.

Osserman KE, Kaplan LI, and Besson G: Studies in myasthenia gravis: edrophonium chloride (Tensilon) test as a new approach to management. *Mt Sinai J Med NY* 20:165, 1953.

Treatment

Brunner NG, Namba T, and Grob D: Corticosteroids in management of severe generalized myasthenia gravis: effectiveness and comparison with corticotrophin therapy. *Neurology (Minneap)* 22:603, 1972.

Jankins RB: Treatment of myasthenia gravis with prednisone. *Lancet* 1:765, 1972.

Levasseur P, Noviant Y, Miranda AR, and Lebryan H: Thymectomy for myasthenia gravis: long-term results in 74 cases. *J Thorac Cardiovasc Surg* 64:1, 1972.

McQuillen MP, and Leone MG: A treatment carol: thymectomy revisited. *Neurology (Minneap)* 27:1103–1105, 1977.

Mertens HG, Balzereit F, and Leipert M: The treatment of severe myasthenia gravis with immunosuppressive agents. *Eur Neurol* 2:323, 1969.

Namba T, Brunner NG, Shapiro MS, and Grob D: Corticotropin therapy in myasthenia gravis: effects, indications, and limitations. *Neurology (Minneap)* 21:1008, 1971.

Osserman KE, and Genkins G: Studies in myasthenia gravis: short-term massive corticotropin therapy. *JAMA* 198:699, 1966.

Seybold ME, and Drachman DB: Gradually increasing doses of prednisone in myasthenia gravis. *N Engl J Med* 290:81, 1974.

Walker MB: Some discoveries on myasthenia gravis: the background. *Br Med J* 2:42, 1973.

Myasthenic Syndrome

Eaton LM, and Lambert EH: Electromyography and electric stimulation of nerves in diseases of motor unit: observations on myasthenic syndrome associated with malignant tumors. *JAMA* 161:1117, 1957.

McQuillen MP, and Johns RJ: The nature of the defect in the Eaton-Lambert syndrome. *Neurology (Minneap)* 17:527, 1967.

Guillain-Barré Syndrome

Abramsky O, et al: Cell-mediated immunity to neural antigens in idiopathic polyneuritis and myeloradiculitis. *Neurology (Minneap)* 25:1154, 1975.

Asbury AK, Arnason BG, and Adams RD: The inflammatory lesion in idiopathic polyneuritis: its role in pathogenesis. *Medicine (Baltimore)* 48:173, 1969.

Criteria for diagnosis of Guillain-Barré syndrome. *Ann Neurol* 3:565, 1978.

Fisher M: An unusual variant of acute idiopathic polyneuritis (syndrome of ophthalmoplegia, ataxia and areflexia). *N Engl J Med* 255:57, 1956.

Guillain-Barré syndrome: Ascending knowledge? *Lancet* July 29:243, 1978.

Haymaker WE, and Kernohan JW: The Landry-Guillain-Barré syndrome; clinicopathologic report of 50 fatal cases and critique of literature. *Medicine (Baltimore)* 28:59, 1959.

McFarland HR, and Heller GL: Guillain-Barré disease complex: a statement of diagnostic criteria and analysis of 100 cases. *Arch Neurol* 14:196, 1966.

Thomas PK, Lascelles RG, Hallpike JF, and Hewer RL: Recurrent and chronic relapsing Guillain-Barré polyneuritis. *Brain* 92:589, 1969.

Periodic Paralysis

DeGraeff J, and Lameijer LDF: Periodic paralysis. *Am J Med* 39:70, 1965.

Layzer RB, Lovelace RE, and Rowland LP: Hyperkalemic periodic paralysis. *Arch Neurol* 16:455, 1967.

Resnick JS, Dorman JD, and Engel WK: Thyrotoxic periodic paralysis. *Am J Med* 47:831, 1969.

Entrapment Neuropathies

Chawla LS, et al: Meralgia paresthetica. *Acta Neurol Scand* 42:483, 1966.

Cracchiolo A, and Marmor L: Peripheral entrapment neuropathies. *JAMA* 204:431, 1968.

Brain WR, Wright AD, and Wilkinson M: Spontaneous compression of both median nerves in the carpal tunnel. *Lancet* 1:277, 1947.

Ecter AD, and Woltman HW: Meralgia paraesthetica: a report of one hundred and fifty cases. *JAMA* 110:1650, 1958.

Edwards WG, Lincoln CR, Bassett FH III, and Goldner JL: The tarsal tunnel syndrome: diagnosis and treatment. *JAMA* 207:716, 1969.

Hamlin E, et al: Carpal-tunnel syndrome. *N Engl J Med* 276:849, 1967.

Purnell DC, et al: Carpal-tunnel syndrome associated with myxedema. *Arch Intern Med* 108:751, 1961.

Botulism

Scaer RC, Tooker J, and Cherington M: Effect of guanidine on the neuromuscular block of botulism. *Neurology (Minneap)* 19:1107, 1969.

Stiff-Man Syndrome

Gordon EE, Januszko DM, and Kaufman L: A critical survey of the stiff-man syndrome. *Am J Med* 42:582, 1967.

Myotonia

Magee KR: Paramyotonia congenita: association with cutaneous cold sensitivity and description of peculiar sustained postures after muscle contraction. *Arch Neurol* 14:590, 1966.

Malathion Poisoning

Namba T, Greenfield M, and Grob D: Malathion poisoning: a fatal case with cardiac manifestations. *Arch Environ Health* 21:533, 1970.

Myoglobinuria

Hinz CF, Drucker WR, and Larner J: Idiopathic myoglobinuria: metabolic and enzymatic studies in three patients. *Am J Med* 39:49, 1965.

Penn AS, Rowland LP, and Fraser DW: Drugs, coma, and myoglobinuria. *Arch Neurol* 26:336, 1972.

Rowland LP: Myoglobinuria. *Arch Neurol* 10:537, 1964.

Rowland LP, and Penn AS: Myoglobinuria. *Med Clin North Am* 56:1233, 1972.

Note Added in Proof (ref. p. 256):

Plasmapheresis has been shown to be of value in the treatment of patients with severe myasthenia gravis who have responded poorly to all forms of appropriate management and who require respiratory assistance. It is a procedure that requires a specially trained team in addition to the plasma exchange apparatus and is best performed in an intensive care setting. Several exchanges are usually necessary before significant improvement is seen. It is expensive and entails some risk and should be reserved for seriously ill patients. It can be given in conjunction with immunosuppressive drugs.

Recent reports have attributed some success to the use of plasma exchange in other diseases that have an immunologic basis, viz, polymyositis, Guillain-Barre syndrome, and multiple sclerosis. It is important to caution that, as of this writing, controlled series have not been reported and further evaluation of the modality is necessary.

14

Gait Disorders

Difficulty walking is a fairly frequent major complaint and reason for consulting a physician. A brief introduction to the evaluation of gait is given in Chapter 1; and the subject is discussed at greater length here because of its importance. Elderly patients in particular have difficulty walking, and unfortunately many find it hard to verbalize their symptoms properly. They may complain of weakness, frequent falling, unsteadiness, stiffness of the legs, or difficulty starting or stopping; or they simply say that they find it increasingly difficult to get about and for that reason are confined to home and to a chair.

Fortunately, it is possible to analyze gait disorders sufficiently accurately that the etiology of the problem can usually be identified; it requires only careful history-taking and examination. The objective of the evaluation is to establish the mechanism of the gait abnormality (i.e., which part of the nervous system is involved) and then to relate the anatomic defect to a causative agent if possible. It is important to obtain as much historical data as possible, so a careful system review is essential. A patient who complains of weakness and stiffness of his legs, causing him to fall, and who also has had urinary incontinence must be suspected of having a spinal cord lesion. Dementia accompanying gait disorder usually denotes a cortical location of pathology. Unsteadiness of gait in association with slurring of speech suggests cerebellar abnormality, and weakness in climbing stairs or getting up from a chair in conjunction with complaints of easy fatigue of the proximal muscle groups of the upper extremities should suggest a myopathic disorder. The complaint of upper extremity tremor in conjunction with trouble walking suggests parkinsonism. Diabetes, poor nutrition, or exposure to heavy metals may cause the gait abnormalities of peripheral neuropathy. A history of recurrent vestibular symptoms or administration of ototoxic antibiotics may clarify the cause of unsteady gait or poor equilibrium.

Inadequate space not infrequently prevents a proper evaluation of the patient's gait; there must be enough room to permit him to walk back and forth freely. Attention is paid to the smoothness of the gait, associative movements of the upper extremities, and whether the feet are in normal position relative to each other or are spread apart to provide a wide base. The patient is asked to walk on his toes and heels to observe for weakness of dorsiflexion or plantar flexion of the feet, and to walk in tandem to look for subtle signs of ataxia. He is asked to start and stop suddenly and to turn quickly to determine if there is rigidity, hypokinesia, festination, or propulsion. The patient should be watched as he stands up from a chair and initiates walking and as he approaches an obstruction or threshold.

In general, gait disorders are caused by disorders of the motor systems, the sensory systems, or poorly localizable cortical structures, the last causing a gait abnormality sometimes referred to as apraxia. The following section lists some of the characteristics of the gait disturbances that occur from lesions in specific anatomic locations or systems.

MOTOR DISORDERS CAUSING GAIT ABNORMALITIES

Central Nervous System Lesions

Corticospinal Lesions

The characteristics of gait disorders caused by lesions of the corticospinal pathways, either in the brain or spinal cord, are spasticity and weakness. The gait of a *hemiplegic patient* is well known. There is weakness of hip flexors and dorsiflexors of the foot, so the patient swings (circumabducts) the entire lower extremity through an arc, scraping the foot along the ground, as he leans on and toward the sound leg. The weak upper extremity is usually less useful than the weak leg; is kept flexed at the elbow, wrist, and fingers and is held close to the chest. There may be variations of this picture, depending on the severity of the brain lesion. The commonest cause is cerebral infarction, but brain tumor, head trauma, cerebral hemorrhage, or infantile hemiplegia are other causes.

A *paraparetic gait* is almost always the result of a *spinal cord* lesion, although parasagittal meningioma is a rare etiology. The nature of the spinal cord lesion can often be inferred from accompanying signs or by history. There may be only spasticity of both lower extremities with little or no demonstrable weakness. The patient usually slowly slides his feet along the ground in such a way that the advancing extremity may partially cross over the other, resulting in a scissoring action. There is obvious spasticity of the legs, which are usually strongly extended. Severe spasticity may be accompanied by clonus at the ankles and knees when the patient places his foot on the floor, increasing the difficulty in walking.

Extrapyramidal Disease: Parkinsonism

The abnormality of gait is an integral and distinctive feature of parkinsonism. The patient is usually stooped and walks rigidly with short, shuffling steps. There is decreased to absent arm swing, and the upper part of the body moves ahead of the legs. There is difficulty initiating movement and stopping or turning smoothly, the last being accomplished by short mechanical movements. On ocasion the patient's steps become shorter and more rapid (festination), and he may fall (propulsion and retropulsion). Thresholds may produce sticking of the feet to the floor, the patient becoming immobile.

Huntington's chorea may cause a bizarre dancing, almost ataxic, gait occasioned by the choreiform movements of the legs and associated with facial grimacing and chorea of the upper extremities.

Dystonia is most commonly the result of excessive dopaminergic drugs but also may appear spontaneously during childhood as dystonia musculorum deformans. The earliest sign may be an involuntary forced inversion or plantar flexion of one foot resulting in an awkward limp. Early in the disease the dystonic movement may disappear when the patient is sitting or lying, raising the question of a psychogenic disorder.

Cerebellar Disorders

The gait abnormality of diffuse cerebellar or spinocerebellar lesions consists of staggering from side to side, walking with feet wider apart than normal, and variation in the size of steps. The patient is unable to walk in tandem and to stand steadily with feet together. The gait disorder is usually accompanied by ataxia of the extremities when not walking, manifested by incoordination in heel-to-shin testing and, if the upper extremities are involved, in finger-to-nose and finger-to-finger testing.

The most frequent causes of cerebellar ataxia are tumor, multiple sclerosis, heredofamilial cerebellar degeneration, drug overdose, or alcoholism. Tumors which involve the midline cerebellar structures (vermis), e.g., medulloblastoma, produce profound ataxia when walking as well as truncal ataxia when the patient is sitting. These patients may have no extremity incoordination on testing. Alcoholic cerebellar degeneration involves primarily the anterior lobe of the cerebellum, the anatomic area concerned with lower extremity coordination, and the gait ataxia is therefore not accompanied by unsteadiness of the hands or arms. Cerebellar ataxia caused by overdose of drugs (anticonvulsants) or acute alcohol ingestion is accompanied by slurred speech, nystagmus, and usually drowsiness.

Peripheral Nerve or Muscle Disorders

Lesions of the lower motor neuron cause muscle weakness and atrophy no matter whether the pathology is in the anterior horn cell or peripheral nerve. There is no characteristic gait abnormality, unless it is the steppage gait of foot drop.

Myopathy of any cause usually involves the proximal muscles more than the distal ones, so the patient has difficulty arising from a chair or walking upstairs. Patients with muscular dystrophy, particularly in Duchenne's variety in children, walk with a waddling, swaying motion associated with accentuated lordosis, all due to weakness of the paraspinal, gluteal, and proximal leg muscles.

GAIT ABNORMALITIES CAUSED BY DISTURBANCES OF SENSATION

Impairment of joint position sensibility causes ataxia characterized by unsteadiness, slightly widened base, foot stamping when walking, and worsening in the dark. The lesion may be in large fibers of the peripheral nerves, dorsal roots, or posterior columns of the spinal cord. The disturbance of position sensibility is readily confirmed by examination. Etiologies include peripheral neuropathy, tabes dorsalis, vitamin B_{12} deficiency, or spinal cord compression by tumor.

CORTICAL LESIONS

Difficulty walking is, as previously mentioned, a not infrequent and usually difficult to diagnose symptom in elderly people. Examination reveals that the ataxia is not caused by muscle weakness, loss of sensation, or rigidity. The severity of the disorder varies from mild uncertainty and hesitancy when walking to total inability to walk unassisted. The characteristic abnormality is that the patient seems to lean backward on assuming the standing posture and seems to have forgotten how to initiate and carry out the movements of walking. The term gait apraxia is often used, although it can be argued that the term apraxia is inappropriate for this circumstance. In conjunction with dementia, psychomotor retardation, and urinary incontinence, the diagnosis of normal-pressure hydrocephalus must be considered (see Chapter 3). The lesions responsible for gait apraxia are thought to be in the frontal lobe and bilateral, but there is no characteristic pathology. The management of these patients is usually a difficult and frustrating experience for the patient, family, and physician.

VESTIBULAR LESIONS

Rarely, lesions of the vestibular nuclei or the vestibular end-organs (as by vestibulotoxic drugs) may result in a gait abnormality which is difficult to evaluate adquately. The patients complain of a persistent sensation of disequilibrium; and sudden movements of the head or trunk or being jostled in a crowd may accentuate the unsteadiness. Gait examination reveals only slight unsteadiness with no clear cerebellar abnormalities.

Rarely, patients are observed to have gait abnormalities that do not conform to any of the patterns described and which are bizarre, inconsistent, and associated with other features in the history or physical examination which suggest conversion reaction or hysteria. Such a diagnosis should never be made on the basis of exclusion alone.

15

Intracranial and Spinal Tumors

It is difficult to adapt a discussion of tumors to the purposes for which this book was intended, for the temptation is to attempt to be complete and to point the discussion toward a classification. Such biologic classifications are available to the interested reader in many publications, some of which are listed in the *Suggested Reading* section of this chapter. The intent of this presentation is, rather, to focus the attention of the clinician on a few useful concepts about this problem in order to assist him in the evaluation of patients suspected of tumor or to suggest in which instances the level of suspicion must be high.

INTRACRANIAL TUMORS

Although frequently suspected because they are also feared by patients, intracranial tumors are relatively uncommon, comprising only a small percentage of the usual busy neurologic practice. Statistics vary depending on the institution; however, a reasonable figure is that intracranial tumors comprise about 0.5% of hospital admissions and are found in a little more than 1% of all autopsies. It is estimated that about 8,500 patients die from primary brain tumors annually in the United States, but a much larger number have intracranial metastases from cancers in other parts of the body at the time of death. No age group is immune, for brain tumors are found from childhood through old age, but certain types of tumor seem to be characteristic of the two extremes of life.

For purposes of this discussion there are five general types of intracranial tumor that should be described briefly, as the clinical presentations, rapidity of course, methods of treatment, and prognosis vary in each. *Gliomas* are neoplastic proliferations of the glial cells of the brain, usually the *astrocytes* but rarely the *oligodendroglia*. They comprise the commonest type of primary intracranial tumor. Cushing originally classified as gliomas such special types of tumor as *ependymomas*, *pinealomas*, and *medulloblastomas* —although the cell types of these three are quite different and their true cell of

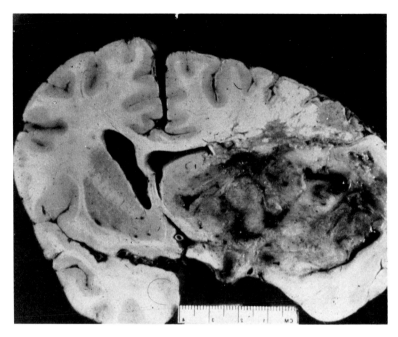

FIG. 15.1. Glioblastoma of left cerebral hemisphere. Note extensive areas of necrosis and hemorrhage and the swelling of the hemisphere, causing compression of the left lateral ventricle and a massive shift of the midline structures to the right.

origin is debated by pathologists. The astrocytomas are of varying grades of malignancy, ranging from extremely slow-growing and relatively confined (grade I) to rapidly growing, invasive, and anaplastic in appearance (grade III or IV), sometimes called *glioblastoma multiforme* (Fig. 15.1). All of these tumors share the characteristic of arising from intraparenchymal brain cells and therefore of being invasive in (and part of) the brain. This of course immediately denotes that they are malignant in the sense of their location, for their extirpation requires that part of the brain also be removed.

This characteristic distinguishes them from the other major groups of intracranial tumors, which are separate from, even if not outside, the brain parenchyma. *Meningiomas* are, as the name implies, tumors derived from the meninges, specifically from arachnoidal cells, and they affect the brain or cranial nerves by compression. In overall frequency they are second to gliomas among primary brain tumors. Meningiomas are thought of as "benign" intracranial tumors because they are generally not invasive into brain parenchyma, but it should be pointed out that the location of these tumors in regions difficult to reach surgically, particularly those in the middle and posterior fossae, results in their causing considerable morbidity and mortality, even in those identified and surgically attacked. Meningiomas are slow-growing and may be present many years before producing symptoms or being recognized. Occasionally, relatively asymptomatic meningiomas are not operated on in elderly individuals in the belief that the patient's anticipated life span may be briefer than the time required for the tumor to cause serious deficits (Fig. 15.2).

Pituitary tumors are discussed in Chapter 16. As the name denotes, these tumors arise from various cells in the pituitary itself and basically produce two kinds of symptoms and signs, endocrine and visual, the latter resulting when the tumor has grown out of the pituitary fossa and compressed the optic nerves or chiasm. *Craniopharyngiomas* are not of pituitary origin, although they are usually considered together with pituitary tumors because they also cause visual and special endocrine disturbances. These tumors arise from squamous epithelial rests which lie in the parts tuberalis of the pituitary and then expand superiorly, ultimately compressing the floor of the 3rd ventricle and causing symptoms of hypothalamic dysfunction. The craniopharyngioma is a much more difficult therapeutic problem than the pituitary adenoma.

Tumors which arise from the *sheaths of cranial nerves* are not uncommon, by far the most frequent being that from the sheath of the 8th nerve, called *schwannoma* because its histologic arrangement is characterized by parallel rows of Schwann cell nuclei. Such tumors may occur rarely on other cranial

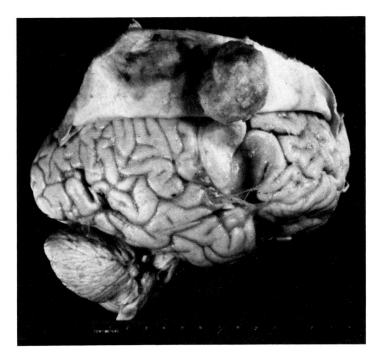

FIG. 15.2. Meningioma of right posterior frontal cerebral convexity. Note that the tumor is easily lifted out of its bed, is attached to the dura, and leaves a deep indentation in the surface of the brain. This tumor caused focal left-sided and generalized seizures.

nerves, particularly the 5th. The special clinical characteristics of this tumor are discussed in the chapter on dizziness (Chapter 6), for this is often the earliest presenting sign of this tumor, which also causes deafness, facial paralysis and numbness, and cerebellar signs (e.g., ataxia and nystagmus). The importance of early recognition of these tumors cannot be over-emphasized because they can be surgically excised in a large percentage of cases.

Metastatic brain tumors are also extraparenchymal, in a strict sense, for although the metastatic deposit may lie within the brain tissue it is still separate and distinct, often separated by a clear margin or a structure like a capsule; moreover, in many cases it can be totally excised without much damage to adjacent brain tissue. The problem is that cerebral metastases are often multiple, under which circumstances surgical therapy is usually not feasible, and other metastatic lesions may also be lodged in other organs. Another special characteristic of metastatic brain tumors is that signs caused

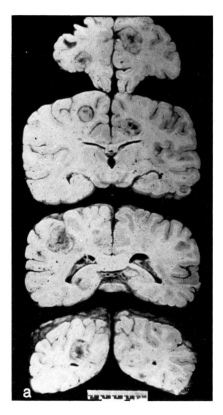
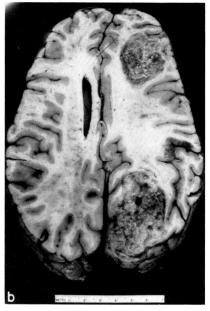

FIG. 15.3. Two brains showing multiple metastatic deposits. **a:** Numerous lesions in every section. The primary was a carcinoma of the breast. **b:** Two large right hemisphere metastases from bronchogenic carcinoma. Both lesions are accompanied by some edema.

by them often respond well to treatment with steroids and occasionally to radiation therapy (Figs. 15.3 and 15.4).

There are several other varieties of intracranial tumor, less common than those mentioned above, where diagnosis and management are usually more complex and specialized. Although all tumors cause signs dependent on the tumor's location and biologic characteristics, a few of the less common types of tumor should at least be mentioned because of the very special nature of their symptomatology. *Intraventricular tumors*, in particular *colloid cysts of the 3rd ventricle*, cause signs of acute or subacute ventricular obstruction (headache, vomiting, loss of consciousness) which may be relieved by changing the position of the head. Other intraventricular tumors, e.g., *papillomas of the choroid plexus*, cause hydrocephalus by increased cerebrospinal fluid (CSF) production. *Hemangioblastomas* are unique in that they occur almost exclusively in the cerebellar hemispheres and are commonly associated with retinal angiomatosis and polycythemia.

Although they are rare, mention should be made of tumors of the pineal region because they produce an interesting and fairly consistent group of signs. Pineal region tumors may be true *pinealomas* or a variety of *teratomas* and *gliomas*. The location of pineal tumors results in compression of the tectum of the midbrain, the classical signs of which are paralysis of conjugate movements of the eyes vertically (*Parinaud's syndrome*) along with the other features of the *Sylvian aqueduct syndrome*, i.e., convergence nystagmus,

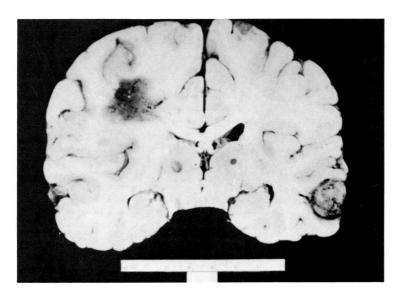

FIG. 15.4. Metastatic malignant melanoma. Note multiple deposits of melanin-containing tumor with a hemorrhagic focus adjacent to one. Hemorrhage is commonly seen in metastatic melanoma.

nystagmus retractorius, pathologic lid retraction, and impaired or absent pupillary responses to light and accommodation. As the tumors grow, aqueductal obstruction occurs and signs of increased intracranial pressure (headache, vomiting, papilledema) appear (Fig. 15.5). In children, precocious puberty may also be associated with pineal region tumors, and it has been suggested that this syndrome is due to pineal gland destruction, thereby removing normal pineal inhibition of gonadal development. The diagnosis of these tumors is usually not difficult clinically and their extent can be well identified by computerized axial tomography (CAT) scan, angiography, and/or air study. Surgical removal is difficult as these are usually intraparenchymal masses. Signs of increased intracranial pressure may be relieved temporarily by a shunting procedure, but the best definitive treatment may be a combination of surgery, radiation, and chemotherapy, depending on the cell type of the tumor.

Nasopharyngeal carcinomas, which invade the base of the skull and involve cranial nerves, are not uncommon. These cancers arise from the mucosa of the nasopharynx, usually near the Eustachian tube, often causing a sensation of ear stuffiness. Cranial nerve involvement is frequent, particularly one or more branches of the 5th nerve, causing facial pain and eventually numbness. Diagnosis is made by biopsy of the nasopharynx. Skull x-rays may reveal erosion of a portion of the skull base and a nasopharyngeal mass.

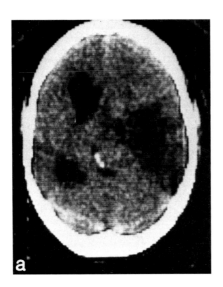 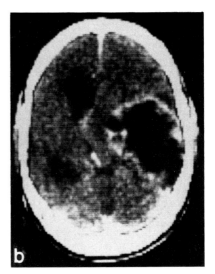

FIG. 15.5. Glioma of right frontal-parietal regions. **a:** A large irregular area of decreased density is seen in the right posterior frontal and parietal regions of the cerebrum. The lateral ventricles (frontal horns) are severely displaced to the left, as is the pineal gland and the suprapineal cistern. **b:** Following contrast there is a rim of increased density around the area of decreased density. This may mark the outer borders of the tumors. There is evidence of spread of the glioma across the midline.

Chordomas are derived from notochordal vestiges and are usually located on the clivus or the sacrum. Although rare, chordoma should be suspected in instances of progressive cranial nerve or cauda equina palsies. As it enlarges, it may destroy the clivus and present into the posterior pharynx. Diagnosis can be made by skull x-rays, tomography of the clivus, CAT scan, and, if necessary, angiography or pneumoencephalography. Treatment is by surgery and irradiation.

Glomus jugulare tumors arise from nonchromaffin paraganglioma cells which are in abundance in the dome of the jugular bulb. The tumor is a highly vascular one which grows into the skull. It first causes cranial nerve palsies and may eventually compress the brainstem and temporal lobe. Because the majority of these tumors arise near the jugular foramen, they cause unilateral 9th and 10th nerve palsies, but also may involve the 7th, 8th, 11th, and 12th nerves, as well as the cerebellum. The tumor may encase the carotid artery, causing Horner's syndrome, and may bulge against the tympanic membrane. Diagnosis is made by x-ray, CAT scans, angiography, and, if possible, biopsy of the tumor through the middle ear. Treatment is by conservative surgical dissection; radiation therapy is of disputed value.

The clinical manifestations of tumor cover the gamut of neurology, of course, and vary with location and type. Any part of the brain and any group of cranial nerves may be involved, and the signs usually reflect the site of involvement. There may be no exact correlation between severity of symptoms and size of the tumor; indeed, huge hemisphere tumors may exist with minimal symptomatology. The severity of neurologic deficit is often a function of the rapidity of growth and location of the tumor rather than of its size. Headache is an overrated tumor symptom. When an intracranial tumor produces headache, it is ordinarily far advanced and the diagnosis is fairly evident by examination. The usual mechanism of headache production is ventricular obstruction and increased intracranial pressure, and this occurs earliest in posterior fossa tumors and is often, but not invariably, accompanied by papilledema. Certain types of headache are said to be suspect. An individual, essentially free of headache in the past, who develops headaches of progressive severity and frequency certainly must be suspected of having a brain tumor. Some believe that headaches which awaken patients in the early morning or during the night also suggest tumor, but this is not a reliable sign since many type of vascular headaches occur during these hours. Severe headaches of abrupt onset unimproved by the leaning forward posture, accompanied by vomiting and occasionally syncope, suggest intermittent ventricular block by tumor. Posterior fossa tumors may cause rather severe occipital or upper cervical headaches when the cerebellar tonsils begin to herniate through the foramen magnum, compressing branches of cranial nerve 11 or the root of C2. In brief, headache, unless accompanied by other signs of increased intracranial pressure, is not reliable as a sign of brain tumor.

Tumors of the cerebral hemisphere not infrequently cause *epileptic seizures* even though no abnormalities can be observed in the neurologic examination. For this reason the onset of seizures in an adolescent or adult must always be investigated to the point that the physician can exclude tumor as the cause. In the past, this represented a considerable problem because such an investigation might involve invasive procedures (e.g., angiography or pneumoencephalography), which physician and patient were reluctant to undertake. The CAT scan eliminates that concern and should be part of the work-up of every patient with seizures. This technique detects tumors in a significant percentage of instances in which no abnormal neurologic signs are present.

Mental symptoms are also associated with brain tumors in the minds of many patients. In fact, only a few types of tumor cause such symptoms because of their special location. Of course, mental symptoms and signs may be a part of the clinical picture in any advanced tumor with increased intracranial pressure, but these do not usually present diagnostic difficulties. Dementia characterized by personality change, slovenliness, poor judgment, antisocial behavior, and a progressive state of withdrawal is characteristic of frontal lobe tumors, and in particular of subfrontal meningiomas (Fig. 15.6). This represents, then, a curable form of dementia. Progressive dementia may occur with any midline tumor and often accompanies gliomas of the corpus callosum, even in the absence of other neurologic deficits. Temporal lobe tumors, particularly those encroaching on the medial surface of the temporal lobes, may cause seizure activity that manifests in abnormal behavior, which may be construed as a disturbance of the mental state.

Cerebral hemisphere tumors may also cause hemiparesis, aphasia, parietal lobe syndromes, visual field deficits, and disorders of higher function, e.g., apraxias and agnosia. These signs assist in the localization of the tumor. The course of the illness is usually slowly progressive, but it may also be saltatory and, on rare occasions, may develop so rapidly it stimulates a cerebral vascular accident. Rapid onset and progression of signs may denote a hemorrhage into a tumor (bronchogenic carcinoma, choriocarcinoma, melanoma) or a sudden increase in contiguous brain edema.

Cerebral hemisphere tumors may produce nonlocalizing signs because of the associated progressive increase in intracranial pressure. Papilledema always means increased intracranial pressure, but it may also be absent in the presence of increased intracranial pressure (particularly in children) and in the presence of congenital obliteration of the optic nerve sheaths. Sixth nerve palsies not uncommonly occur in patients with increased intracranial pressure, presumably because of stretching of, or traction on, the long intracranial portions of these nerves. Expanding hemisphere tumors also cause herniation of brain from one compartment to another. Subfalcial herniation of the ungulate gyrus is common in the presence of large hemisphere masses; there is no specific clinical syndrome associated with this. Transtentorial herniation of the medial portion of the temporal lobe may occur fairly abruptly and results

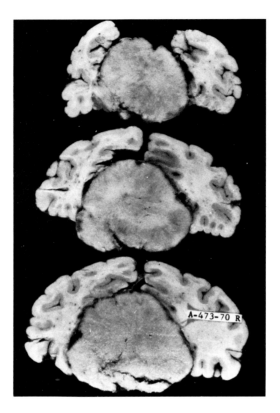

FIG. 15.6. Subfrontal meningioma. This orange-sized tumor caused progressive dementia and finally resulted in coma. The size of the tumor suggests that it is probably several years old, but symptoms had been present for less than a year. The distinct separation of the tumor mass from the brain parenchyma, which is compressed, can be readily seen.

in homolateral 3rd nerve palsy, stupor or coma, and a variety of other brainstem signs as described in Chapter 11.

The types of tumor and therefore their signs vary with the age of the patient. Cerebral hemisphere tumors are uncommon in children, whereas posterior fossa tumors, particularly *cerebellar astrocytomas*, *medulloblastomas*, and *brainstem gliomas*, are more frequent; *craniopharyngiomas* and *optic nerve gliomas* are also more common in children and adolescents. The *medulloblastoma* usually grows from the roof of the 4th ventricle, causing an ataxia of a special kind. These children have great difficulty walking but may have no appendicular ataxia on examination. Infiltrating gliomas may enlarge the brainstem (medulla and pons) substantially before causing symptoms and signs, usually of cranial nerve and gaze palsies, along with long tract signs. Craniopharyngiomas were previously mentioned. *Optic gliomas* often occur in children with signs of neurofibromatosis and cause progressive monocular blindness. The enlarging optic nerve erodes and expands the optic foramen, causing the sella turcica to take on a fairly typical J shape radiologically. They occasionally cause proptosis. It is now believed that surgery does not improve the prognosis of these patients.

The _cerebellar astrocytoma_ is probably the commonest brain tumor in children and is of particular importance because in many instances it can be completely cured surgically. The clinical history and physical findings are typical of any posterior fossa lesion, although unilateral cerebellar signs may signal the localization of the lesion to one cerebellar hemisphere. Many of these tumors are cystic, and removal of the mural nodule may be sufficient to provide a cure or relief from symptoms for many years.

In middle and old age there is an increased frequency of high-grade cerebral gliomas and metastatic brain tumors, which not infrequently produce neurologic symptoms or signs even before a primary lesion is suspected (Fig. 15.4). Bronchogenic carcinoma, for example, may present first because of cerebral metastases, the primary lesion being discovered only after the patient has consulted a physician for the neurologic problem. The commonest cerebral metastatic lesions are from cancers of the lung, breast, gastrointestinal tract, kidney, and skin (melanoma). The management of patients with cerebral metastases is complicated by the frequency with which multiple cerebral metastatic deposits occur, the existence of metastatic disease in other organs, and occasionally difficulty in establishing the origin of the primary. The pace of development of neurologic signs is rapid, and the neurologic deficit is often disproportionately severe in comparison to the size of the tumor. These characteristics are likely caused by the prominent edema which surrounds each of the metastatic nodules. The CAT scan has immeasurably decreased the difficulty of evaluating these patients and, specifically, of determining if there are multiple cerebral lesions. Management of these patients depends on the nature of the patient's neurologic deficit, the type of tumor, and the number and location of metastases. As a rule, surgical intervention is contraindicated if more than one cerebral lesion is present.

The neurologic deficits from cerebral metastatic disease are usually rapidly improved by the use of dexamethasone in doses of 24 to 96 mg daily, reducing the dosage as the patient improves. The biologic effect of steroids is not completely understood, although it now seems evident that there is not only relief of edema in tissue adjacent to the tumor but also an effect on the growth rate of the tumor itself. This applies to some rapidly growing gliomas as well, although the effects are far less consistent than in metastases.

In reference to cerebral metastases, mention should be made of the unusual and frequently puzzling symptomatology produced by _meningeal carcinomatosis_, widespread meningeal (arachnoid) invasion by carcinoma. This is an extremely serious problem, the average survival time after diagnosis being about 6 weeks. The time between the onset of neurologic symptoms and diagnosis averages about 2 months. The most frequent symptoms are headache, leg pains, backache, ataxia, dysesthesias of extremities, seizures, and diplopia. The progress is relentless, and multiple cranial nerve lesions and dementia eventually appear. Since a primary site of cancer is not initially suspected in about half the cases, the diagnosis is difficult. Examination of the CSF is probably the most helpful approach; the fluid shows increased protein and decreased glucose, and malignant cells can often be found by careful examination of dried smears from samples of centrifuged fluid. Treatment is by irradiation and intrathecal chemotherapy, although the prospect of substantial improvement is poor.

Brain Tumors Which Impair Vision

Impairment of vision is an important and sometimes poorly interpreted sign of tumors in the general region of the sella turcica and the junction of the orbit with the intracranial cavity. The most important of these, because of frequency of incidence and curability, are the pituitary tumors, which are also discussed briefly in Chapter 16. There are three basic types of pituitary adenoma, characterized by cell type; and each type produces a different endocrine abnormality. The commonest is a mixture of chromophobe and eosinophilic cells, occurring predominantly in young adults and usually destroying much of the functioning pituitary. These are large tumors that not only enlarge the sella but often rupture through the diaphragma sellae to compress the optic chiasm, optic nerves, or the base of the brain. The cardinal signs of this type of pituitary adenoma are visual disturbances, headache, and signs of hypopituitarism, e.g., altered menses, changes in sexual function, and signs of hypothyroidism and hypoadrenalism. The eosinophilic adenoma, much less common, causes overproduction of growth hormone, resulting in either giantism or acromegaly depending on whether the disorder begins before or after epiphyseal closure. The eosinophilic adenoma also produces headache and visual disturbances indistinguishable from those caused by the mixed cell or chromophobe adenoma. The basophilic adenomas of the pituitary are the least common and infrequently extend out of the sella turcica to cause visual symptoms. These tumors occur in conjunction with the clinical state of Cushing's syndrome, which is the result of excessive secretion of adrenal cortical hormone.

The extrasellar expansion of the pituitary adenoma results in compression of the optic chiasm and optic nerves. These structures are trapped between the anterior cerebral and anterior communicating arteries superiorly and the adenoma inferiorly. The visual abnormality, of course, depends on which part of the visual apparatus is involved, but bitemporal hemianopsia or monocular blindness with a temporal cut in the field of the other eye are common. The funduscopic examination reveals optic atrophy on the side of the compressed optic nerve. Extraocular palsies are not infrequent, particularly of those muscles innervated by the oculomotor nerve, which may be involved if the tumor extends into the wall of the cavernous sinus. As the tumor expands into the intracranial cavity, other structures are involved, producing appropriate symptomatology, e.g., temporal lobe seizures, anosmia, or signs of hypothalamic involvement.

Craniopharyngiomas may also compress the optic chiasm, but compression is often from the superior or posterior aspect, as these tumors may arise from the floor of the 3rd ventricle.

Meningiomas that grow from any of the structures at the junction of the orbit and intracranial cavity also cause monocular blindness and field defects. The sites of origin of these tumors may be the tuberculum sellae or any area adjacent to the optic foramen. They are slow-growing tumors which may not cause a significant amount of pain and therefore result only in progressive monocular blindness and optic atrophy. Unlike the pituitary adenomas, these tumors may not enlarge the sella turcica and may cause only subtle thickening of the bony structures underlying their attachment. *It is for that reason that progressive monocular blindness and optic atrophy must be considered to be caused by tumor even if the plain x-rays of the skull are normal.*

The diagnosis of pituitary tumor or of a tumor affecting the visual apparatus is usually suspected because of the patient's symptoms and signs. Plain x-rays of the skull may reveal the diagnosis by demonstrating a ballooned sella turcica with a double floor and thinning of the posterior clinoids and dorsum sellae in the case of a pituitary tumor (Fig. 15.7), sclerosis of a portion of the lesser wing of the sphenoid bone due to a meningioma, or speckled calcification in the suprasellar region in a craniopharyngioma. Polytomography of the sella turcica is extremely helpful in outlining the dimensions of a pituitary tumor and particularly its inferior extent. A CAT scan may reveal the tumor, and coronal sections may demonstrate the extent of its extrasellar extension (Figs. 15.8 and 15.9). Angiography is still utilized to make certain that the tumor is not an aneurysm and to further delineate its effect on the adjacent carotid and anterior cerebral arteries.

In the context of enlarged sella turcica observed in skull x-rays, the *empty sella syndrome* should be mentioned because the x-ray appearance may simulate tumor. It results from a defect in the diaphragma sellae that permits access of the arachnoid into the sella. The pulsations of the CSF gradually enlarge the sella and compress the pituitary. This syndrome may also appear after any destructive lesion of the pituitary, either infarction or surgical trauma.

Pituitary apoplexy is the term applied to the dramatic clinical state that ensues when a pituitary adenoma becomes infarcted or hemorrhagic. There is acute or subacute (over a period of hours) onset of severe, worsening headache, obtundation, extraocular palsies, visual loss, and circulatory collapse— all due to the sudden enlargement of the tumor mass along with the destruction of functioning pituitary tissue. If the existence of the tumor has not been recognized prior to the apoplectic event, the diagnosis may be difficult,

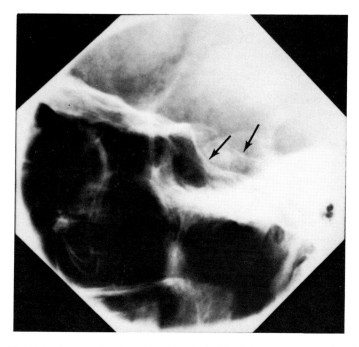

FIG. 15.7. Plain lateral x-rays of sella turcica in patient with pituitary tumor. Note that the sella is ballooned, the dorsum is eroded, and there is a double floor (*arrows*), denoting asymmetry of tumor growth.

although the constellation of signs clearly points to the location of the lesion, and the skull film almost invariably reveals signs of tumor. The management of these patients is by administration of ACTH or adrenal cortical steroids to combat the acute adrenal insufficiency, and by early surgical decompression of the tumor mass.

Although the treatment of pituitary adenomas has been a subject of considerable controversy over the relative merits of surgical extirpation and radiation therapy, the refinement of the transsphenoidal surgical approach by the use of an operating microscope has clearly weighted the argument in favor of surgery. There is fairly universal agreement that tumors which threaten visual acuity must be treated surgically if possible. Radiation therapy alone might be considered in a patient with unequivocal endocrine signs of a pituitary tumor and no visual signs, but there is never any assurance that irradiation will be effective in any given case because the tumor may be cystic. Certainly, radiation therapy alone should never be used unless the clinician can distinguish with absolute certainty that the tumor to be treated is a pituitary adenoma and not a craniopharyngioma or meningioma.

The diagnosis of brain tumor has been literally revolutionized by computerized tomography of the brain. It is important to recall that certain tumors

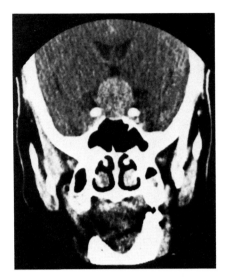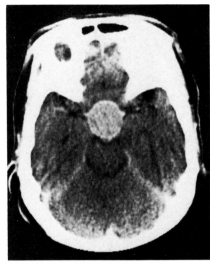

FIGS. 15.8, 15.9. Axial and coronal views by CAT scan with contrast of large pituitary tumor which has extended superiorly out of the sella turcica to the floor of the 3rd ventricle, producing compression of the optic chiasm.

may achieve great size without producing a neurologic deficit that can be detected by the most careful neurologic examination. The patient may have presented with a single seizure or several episodes of early morning headache and vomiting, and the clinician finds no neurologic abnormality. In the past such patients were studied first by innocuous, noninvasive techniques, e.g., roentgenology of the skull, electroencephalography (EEG), and isotope brain scanning. If these did not reveal any abnormality, then the clinician was forced to decide whether to proceed with an invasive procedure such as angiography and, in some instances, pneumoencephalography. Since these procedures have a small morbidity rate and can be uncomfortable, the decision to perform them in a patient without a neurologic deficit on examination was sometimes an agonizing one. The CAT scan eliminates this dilemma because it is a highly accurate and noninvasive procedure. The risk is only that of the intravenous injection of the iodide dye, and that is minor indeed. The dividends are enormous, for the CAT scan reveals the size of the tumor and its effect on cerebral structures (e.g., ventricular displacement), and often tells a great deal about the histologic type. Multiple metastatic lesions may be visualized, offering great assistance in deciding if surgery should be performed and, if so, what type of surgical procedure is indicated. It is, of course, invaluable for following patients postsurgically by allowing evaluation of remaining tumor, brain edema, or postsurgical bleeding. Figures 15.10 through 15.18 illustrate the effectiveness of the CAT scan in brain tumor diagnosis.

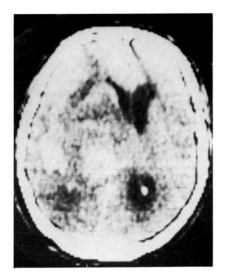
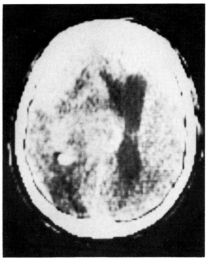

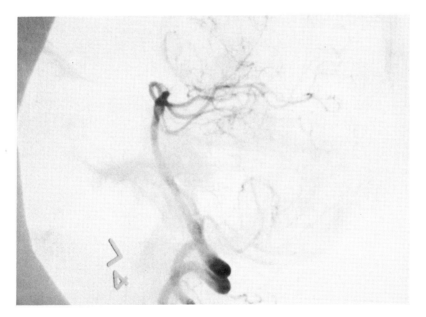

FIGS. 15.10, 15.11, 15.12. CAT and angiographic correlation of massive left hemisphere glioblastoma, which has extended across the midline in the corpus callosum. The CAT scan is shown with contrast, and the intense enhancement of the tumor can be seen. The left lateral ventricle is pushed across the midline under the falx. The vascular nature of the tumor can be seen in the vertebral angiogram, which shows a blush outlining part of the tumor, which is receiving much of its vascular supply from the posterior cerebral artery.

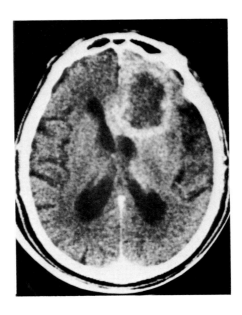

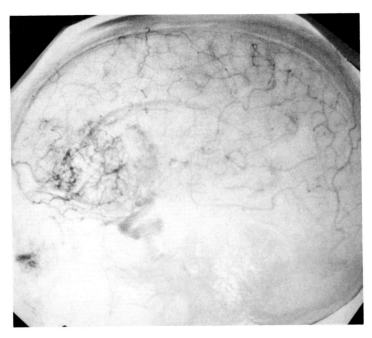

FIGS. 15.13, 15.14. Right frontal glioblastoma. Note enhancement of the peripheral margins of the tumor, which has crossed the midline in the corpus callosum and obliterated the right frontal pole of the lateral ventricle. The angiogram confirms the intensely vascular nature of the mass in the late arterial phase. Early filling veins are also evident.

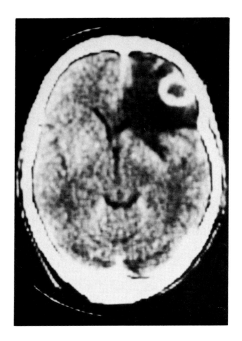

FIG. 15.15. Large right frontal metastases from bronchogenic carcinoma. The ring enhancement and large contiguous area of edema (decreased density) are typical of metastatic disease but may also be produced by abscess and less commonly by gliomas.

A detailed discussion of the treatment of brain tumors is obviously beyond the scope of this book, as it must always be individualized to conform to the needs of the patient and the capabilities of the treating institution. Mention must be made, however, of two therapeutic advances that have greatly influenced the results of intracranial surgery in general: the operating microscope and the use of steroids. The former has permitted the neurosurgeon to handle tissues more delicately and delineate the boundaries of lesions, blood supply, etc. so much better that operative results have improved substantially. The use of steroids preoperatively has also improved surgical results by reducing the incidence of postoperative shock as well as the brain edema that frequently accompanies the tumor and that which ordinarily follows surgical manipulation of the brain. The reduction of tumor-induced edema facilitates the operation mechanically. In addition, there is considerable evidence that steroids have some as yet unexplained action on the biologic characteristics of certain brain tumors, in particular metastatic lesions and certain gliomas, which inhibits the growth rate of the tumor. Finally, neuroanesthesia advances have also contributed greatly to the improvement of neurosurgical

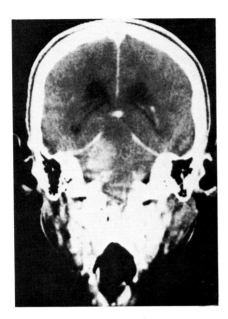 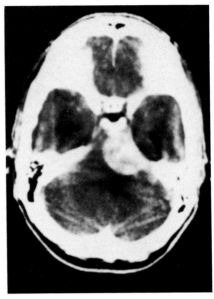

FIGS. 15.16, 15.17. CAT scan, with contrast, showing meningioma attached to the inferior surface of the tentorium and presenting as a cerebellopontine angle tumor. The tumor could be accurately localized by CAT scan and distinguished by its tentorial attachment from a schwannoma of the 8th nerve. Axial and coronal views are shown.

procedures, for the patients may now be kept in a more physiologic state for the lengthy operative periods required of the careful dissection performed under the operating microscope, and the brain volume can be manipulated by regulating the patient's arterial carbon dioxide tension.

The guiding principle in the treatment of brain tumors should be the preservation of the best possible quality of life for the patient. There can be no argument about the indication for surgical removal of an accessible symptomatic meningioma. On the other hand, there is little likelihood of a cure and considerable risk of causing increased neurologic deficit if the patient has a deep (thalamic or basal ganglionic or corpus callosal) glioma and particularly if the tumor is in the dominant hemisphere. A major problem is that diagnosis of histologic type cannot be made with certainty without a biopsy even though the CAT scan and angiography offer powerful clues to the biology of the tumor. Clearly it would be tragic to treat a brain abscess or tuberculoma by radiation therapy.

The problem is compounded in the instance of metastatic brain disease. In the presence of a known primary cancer and evidence of more than one intracranial metastasis, surgery is not indicated except in the most unusual circumstances. Such patients should be treated with steroids, radiation, and, if appropriate, chemotherapy. A single metastatic nodule to the brain should

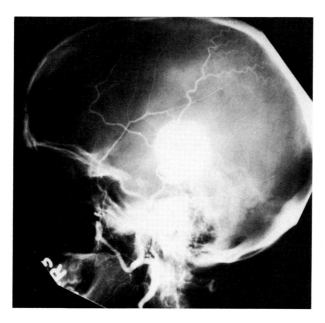

FIG. 15.18. Meningioma low on convexity of brain. Note the intense blushing after selective injection of the *external* carotid artery with renografin. This clearly establishes the diagnosis of meningioma.

probably be removed, particularly if the primary is not known, because of the small but definite possibility that one is dealing with a renal cell carcinoma or choricocarcinoma, either of which may present with a single metastasis. Finally, of course, the metastatic nodule removed from the brain may greatly assist in locating the primary lesion and in directing appropriate therapy.

Some degree of professional agreement has been achieved during the past 5 years with respect to the management of malignant (grades III and IV) astrocytoma and glioblastoma multiforme, primarily as a result of the publications of the Brain Tumor Study Group sponsored by the National Cancer Institute. On the basis of duration of survival, the ideal therapy would be surgical resection of as much tumor as is possible without worsening the neurologic deficit, followed by radiation therapy to a total of 5,500 to 6,000 rads, three-fourths of which is whole brain irradiation and one-fourth of which is directed to the hemisphere containing the tumor, followed or accompanied by chemotherapy. The addition of radiation therapy to tumor resection increases mean survival twofold, and the addition of chemotherapy allows more patients to live longer than 18 months. The chemotherapeutic agents presently available are not outstandingly effective and do produce some complications. The nitrosoureas appear to be the most effective, particularly BCNU (dose = 80 mg/meter²/day intravenously for 3 days, repeated every 6 to 8 weeks) or CCNU (dose = 130 mg/meter² orally every 6 to 8 weeks).

Steroid dosage should be reduced as promptly as possible after surgery or following initiation of radiation therapy to avoid the complications of prolonged steroid usage.

The data supporting the above regimen are persuasive. Although there remain arguments about the necessity for surgical resection, there are no disagreements about the value of radiation therapy. It is unfortunate that the therapeutic dosage is so close to the brain toxic effect of radiation, and radiation necrosis has become a well-defined clinical and pathologic syndrome. Much of the delayed radiation effect on the central nervous system (CNS) appears to be the result of a progressive obliterative vasculopathy which causes tissue necrosis. There is no known effective treatment for radiation necrosis of the brain or spinal cord.

Although the extant chemotherapeutic agents are far from perfect, it is encouraging to realize that substantial progress has been made in the search for effective drugs, with a reasonable hope for more effective, less toxic agents in the future.

SPINAL TUMORS

Tumors of the spinal canal, either within or causing compression of the spinal cord or cauda equina, are much rarer than intracranial tumors. Fortunately, the majority of such tumors are benign in the sense that they originate outside the cord and produce symptomatology by compressing it, and can therefore be excised without damaging the cord. Even some spinal cord gliomas (e.g., astrocytomas and ependymomas) can be removed without significantly damaging the cord further. In this sense, therefore, spinal tumors offer a more favorable prognosis than intracranial tumors.

The most important of the primary tumors from the point of frequency are neurofibromas, meningiomas, and gliomas. Of the gliomas, ependymomas are the commonest. Metastases to the spinal canal or compression of the cord by lymphoma or multiple myeloma are not uncommon during middle age and beyond.

The clinical signs of spinal tumors depend, of course, on the location and type of tumor. It is frequently taught that extramedullary tumors cause radicular pain at the level of the lesion, and that this pain is accentuated when the patient lies down so he is forced to sit up at night in order to sleep. It is further taught that intramedullary tumors infrequently cause pain, but if they do the pain is deep and boring. It is not wise to rely on this distinction as many patients with spinal cord compression may become paraplegic without ever having a significant amount of localizing pain.

Other features that may distinguish extramedullary from intramedullary tumors are:

1. Extramedullary tumors cause spasticity, weakness of lower extremities, hyperreflexia, and positive Babinski signs early, whereas these signs occur late in patients with intramedullary tumors.

2. The sensory level caused by extramedullary tumors is often several segments below the level of the lesion because of the lamination which occurs in the lateral spinothalamic tracts, whereas the sensory abnormalities caused by intramedullary tumors are at the level of the lesion and may be dissociated, as they are in syringomyelia, and there may be sparing of the sacral dermatomes because of the aforementioned lamination.

3. Sphincter disturbances occur much earlier in intramedullary lesions.

Extramedullary tumors comprise about 90 to 95% of all spinal tumors. Because the majority are surgically treatable, early diagnosis is essential, before irreversible cord damage has occurred.

Syndromes Associated with Spinal Cord Tumors at Various Locations

Tumors of the Cervical-Medullary Junction

Tumors at the cervical-medullary junction are usually meningiomas, often growing from the posterior rim of the foramen magnum, but high dumbbell-type neurofibromas may also occur at this level. Motor involvement may be confusing, for the patient may show paraparesis, quadriparesis, hemiparesis, or monoparesis depending on the major site of compression. These patients may also have nystagmus; rarely, compression of the most caudal portion of the descending root of the 5th nerve may result in hypalgesia over part (usually the upper) or the whole half of the face. Fibers of the 11th cranial nerve may also be involved, resulting in weakness or atrophy of the trapezius and/or sternocleidomastoid muscles. Unsteady gait may result from involvement of the posterior columns or spinocerebellar pathways. Pain in the shoulder, neck, or occiput may be precipitated by head movement. Sensory abnormalities may also be confusing because levels of pain and temperature loss are less common than in lower lesions, and compression of the posterior columns may produce impairment of proprioception in the hands and arms, causing confusion with peripheral neuropathy. Respiratory failure always is a threat. Down-beating nystagmus may occur from lesions of the cervicomedullary junction. Arnold-Chiari syndrome may be confused with tumors in this location.

Tumors of the Cervical Enlargement

Tumors of the cervical enlargement may be of any of the cell types previously described. The important point is that they may produce lower motor neuron signs in the upper extremities (atrophy, weakness, decreased reflexes) and upper motor neuron signs in the lower extremities—and therefore may resemble amyotrophic lateral sclerosis or cervical spondylosis.

Tumors of the Lumbosacral Regions

Tumors in the lumbosacral area may readily be confused with the lumbar disc syndrome of lumbar spondylosis. Ependymomas are probably the commonest tumors of the cauda equina. Tumors here may commonly involve the lowermost segments of the spinal cord and the roots of the cauda. Pain in the low back, buttocks, and hamstrings is common. Restricted lesions involving only the conus medullaris (the sacral and coccygeal segments of the cord that occupy vertebral levels L1 and L2) produce only sensory loss in the appropriate dermatomes and no motor deficit. Cauda equina compression produces weakness, atrophy, impairment of deep tendon reflexes in the lower extremities, sensory signs, and sphincter disturbances, usually urinary retention. If the tumor involves the cauda and the lower cord segments, there may be a confusing mixture of lower and upper motor neuron signs.

Spinal tumors may be difficult to distinguish from a variety of other lesions, which must always be considered in the differential diagnosis. These include: *herniated disc, cervical and lumbar spondylosis, multiple sclerosis, spinal cord arteriovenous anomalies, syringomyelia, amyotrophic lateral sclerosis, epidural abscess, pernicious anemia, CNS lues, and arachnoidal cysts.* A few comments about some of these are in order.

Cervical spondylosis classically causes radicular pain, lower motor neuron signs in the upper extremities, and upper motor neuron signs in the lower. Similar motor deficits occur in amyotrophic lateral sclerosis without the sensory abnormalities. Myelography may be required to distinguish them. Arteriovenous anomalies of the spinal cord may cause slowly progressive spinal cord signs or a sudden deficit due to a bleed. Epidural abscesses are uncommon and usually appear after a skin infection or septicemia. They produce evidence of rapid spinal cord compression and thus may be confused with metastases. Not only does syringomyelia cause motor and sensory deficits characteristic of an intramedullary tumor, but myelography may fail to distinguish the pathology, noting only the enlargement of the cord. Indeed, syringomyelia may coexist in almost half the instances with intramedullary tumors of the cervical cord. Multiple sclerosis may infrequently involve the spinal cord without evidence of cranial nerve or brainstem lesions. This occurs particularly in the instance of middle life onset of the disease. The occurrence of a slowly progressive spinal cord lesion in a patient who may have previously had an episode of optic neuritis or diplopia is usually another sign of multiple sclerosis, but this cannot be taken for granted and a second disease thereby overlooked.

Finally, it should be mentioned that progressive spastic paraparesis occurs in a considerable number of individuals in whom no cause is ever found. These patients must at first be considered to have spinal tumors.

The diagnosis of spinal tumors requires a judicious admixture of techniques. Plain x-ray films of the area of suspected involvement may reveal important clues, viz., bony destruction due to metastatic disease, erosion of the pedicles, and widening of one or more neural foramina (neurofibroma). The technique of myelography has evolved and changed since the introduction of the CAT scan and the water-soluble contrast medium metrizamide. Traditional myelography with Pantopaque is still widely applied. There is no standard quantity of Pantopaque which should be used but, rather, enough to visualize the lesion properly and characterize it if possible. This may require that the spinal needle be removed and the patient examined in the supine as well as the prone position. This is particularly important in lesions of the foramen magnum where it is essential to visualize the posterior rim. Adequate visualization of the thoracic portion of the spinal cord is particularly difficult because the contrast tends to run over the dorsal hump into the cervical region without pooling in the thoracic region. The solution to this must depend on use of sufficient contrast to "cover" the suspected area completely. After myelography the Pantopaque should be removed to avoid the rare complication of arachnoiditis.

Metrizamide is best suited for visualization of the lumbosacral region because it permits much better delineation of the nerve roots than does Pantopaque. The amount of the agent which can be used is limited, so levels of the contrast may not be adequate in the thoracic or cervical regions. The combination of metrizamide and CAT scanning of appropriate levels of the cervical cord may provide an effective means of evaluating spinal cord size and displacement, and may even allow visualization of different densities (e.g., a cyst) within the cord itself.

Air myelography may be invaluable in the differential diagnosis of an intramedullary mass lesion because it permits the distinction between solid (noncollapsible) and cystic (syringomyelia) collapsible intramedullary mass lesions.

Angiography is rarely used in the evaluation of spinal cord tumors; it is reserved for those instances in which an angioma is suspected.

Worsening of symptoms and signs after myelography may occur, particularly if the tumor (almost always extramedullary) has blocked the spinal canal, presumably because the reduction of cerebrospinal pressure caudal to the lesion causes the tumor to impact.

Treatment of primary spinal tumors is mainly surgical, although there is some use for radiation therapy in the management of spinal cord astrocytomas. Here again the operating microscope has reduced surgical morbidity by permitting the surgeon to visualize all the vascular attachments of the tumor, thereby helping to prevent ischemia or infarction of part of the cord from surgical injury to tiny blood vessels.

Metastatic tumors of the spine present with symptoms and signs that are similar to those seen with any other spinal tumor, but with a much faster course. Indeed, some patients may progress from an initial symptom to paraplegia in less than 24 hr, probably because the metastatic lesion causes marked edema of adjacent tissues. Back pain is a frequent accompaniment of metastatic spine disease due to adjacent vertebral involvement or to nerve root stretching. The usual story is back pain, weakness or awkwardness of legs, paresthesias or numbness of legs, progressing to severe paraparesis. The development of sphincter signs (e.g., urinary retention or incontinence) denotes severe spinal cord compression and often means that the prognosis for recovery of function is poor despite therapy.

Although there is still some difference of opinion about the best mode of management, there is increasing evidence that surgical decompression of the spinal cord offers little or no advantage over treatment with steroids and radiation. The first step in the management of a patient suspected from the history and physical findings to have spinal cord or cauda equina compression by metastases is to establish the diagnosis if possible. Obviously, the task is easier if the patient is known to have a primary malignancy, but metastases to the spine may be the first sign of a malignancy, previously undiagnosed. The precise location of the metastasis and its extent should, if possible, be determined by roentgenology of the area in question and by myelography. X-ray of the spine may show areas of bony destruction but may also be normal; in any event, myelography assists in localizing the exact site of the lesion, which has often caused a complete block because of epidural compression.

Even as these diagnostic measures are being carried out, the patient should receive steroids, preferably in the form of dexamethasone, 16 mg at once and 24 to 96 mg per each 24 hr thereafter. The steroids act on the metastasis to reduce its bulk and to inhibit its growth, thereby relieving some of the pressure on the cord or cauda equina. Once the lesion has been radiographically localized, further therapy then depends on what is known about the primary lesion. *If the primary lesion is known, it is my belief that radiation therapy directed at the site of the metastasis should be instituted at once, unless it has already been established that the primary carcinoma is radiation-insensitive. In that instance or in the circumstance that a primary lesion cannot be found, surgical decompression and biopsy are indicated.* The commonest cancers which metastasize to the spine are those in the lung, breast, lymphoma, gastrointestinal tract, and prostate. The prognosis varies with each of these and is probably poorest in lung carcinoma and best in lymphoma. Indeed, the response to steroids and irradiation in patients with evidence of spinal spread of a lymphoma is usually quite good; the response of the others is variable. However, that is also true of their response even after surgical decompression, and it must be recalled that the extent of an epidural and bony metastasis may be considerable, so that surgical procedure may be difficult and complicated. In that case radiation therapy to the site of the metastases will have to wait until the surgical wound is healed.

SYRINGOMYELIA

Although not a neoplasm, syringomyelia is a spinal cord and/or medullary lesion that often simulates, and requires differentiation from, a tumor. It is a fluid-filled cavitation of the cord, usually in the central area and most commonly observed in the cervical region, although it occasionally extends into the medulla or caudally into the dorsal and lumbar regions. Pathological studies have not entirely clarified the pathogenesis of the lesion. About 15% of patients are reported to show some type of intramedullary tumor in or near the syrinx, and the lesion is associated with a variety of other conditions, some congenital, such as Arnold-Chiari malformation, basilar impression of the skull, Klippel-Feil syndrome, neurofibromatosis, and myelomeningocele. One theory as to pathogenesis is that congenital obliteration of the foramina of Luschka and Magendie results in an increased cerebrospinal fluid pulse wave impacting into the obex and therefrom into the central canal of the spinal cord, dilating it and causing diverticulae to spread outward from it.

It is an interesting disorder because the clinical picture so exactly reflects the location of the pathology, which interrupts crossing pain and temperature fibers in the spinal cord, sparing the dorsal descending and ascending tracts. As the syrinx enlarges, it compresses the anterior horns of the gray matter of the spinal cord, destroying the motor cells there. The neurological findings, therefore, are segmental loss of pain and temperature (most frequently in the distribution of a cape, because the cervical cord is the most commonly involved location), with preservation of other sensory abnormalities, plus segmental weakness and atrophy of the muscles innervated by the anterior horn cells compressed by the syrinx. Deep tendon reflexes are lost and muscle fasciculations are common. Painless infections, injuries, and burns to the fingers occur because of the anesthesia, and neural arthropathy (Charcot joints) due to denervation of the joints is also seen. Pain in an extremity may also occur and Horner's syndrome may appear because of involvement of the sympathetic cells in the intermediolateral cell column of C-8 and D-1 cord segments. As the syrinx expands, descending and ascending tracts may be involved, so that late in the disease corticospinal tract signs often appear along with sphincter disturbances.

The enlarging syrinx actually becomes a tumor mass in the spinal cord, even though no neoplasm is present. Plain x-rays of the cervical spine or other involved areas may reveal erosion of the pedicles, and myelography demonstrates a widened cord. Air myelography may establish the diagnosis because air may enter the syrinx and outline it, displacing the cerebrospinal fluid. The differential diagnosis includes ependymoma or astrocytoma, both of which are usually solid tumors. An additional diagnostic procedure is to place a needle into the syrinx through the dorsal median raphe under x-ray control and aspirate fluid. The syrinx will usually collapse, whereas a tumor will not.

Syringobulbia occurs if the syrinx begins or extends into the medulla, causing impaired facial sensation, nystagmus, palatal and laryngeal palsies, and atrophy and weakness of part or all of the tongue.

Treatment is rarely satisfactory. Radiation therapy has not been proven to be useful. Decompression of the syrinx usually provides only temporary relief; the fluid recurs. Extensive laminectomy allowing decompression of the expanded cord may be of benefit, but results are unpredictable. Occlusion of the superior end of the spinal central canal at the obex by a piece of muscle has been advocated, but opinion concerning its effectiveness is far from unanimous. Fortunately the syrinx may stop growing spontaneously and, therefore, neurologic abnormalities may not progress beyond a certain point.

SUGGESTED READINGS

Brain Tumors

Types

Abramson N, Raben M, and Cavanaugh PJ: Brain tumors in children: analysis of 136 cases. *Radiology* 112:669, 1974.

Banna M: Craniopharyngioma in adults. *Surg Neurol* 1:202, 1973.

Bramlet D, Giliberti J, and Bender J: Meningeal carcinomatosis: case report, review of the literature. *Neurosci Behav Physiol* 26:287, 1976.

Camins MB, and Mount LA: Primary suprasellar atypical teratoma. *Brain* 97:447, 1974.

Cushing H: *Intracranial Tumors*. Charles C Thomas, Springfield, Ill., 1932.

Cushing H, and Eisenhardt L: *Meningiomas*, Part One. Hafner Publications, New York, 1962.

Cushing H, and Eisenhardt L: *Meningiomas*, Part Two. Hafner Publications, New York, 1962.

Danziger I, Bloch S, and Podlas H: Schwannomas of the central nervous system. *Am J Roentgenol Radium Ther Nucl Med* 125:692, 1975.

Dastor DK, and Lalitho VS: Pathological analysis of intracranial space occupying lesions in 1000 cases including children. 4. Pituitary adenomas, developmental tumours, parasitic and developmental cysts. *J Neurol Sci* 15:397, 1972.

Dohrmann GJ, Farwell JR, and Flannery JT: Glioblastoma multiforme in children. *J Neurosurg* 44:442, 1976.

Fee WE Jr, Epsy CD, and Konrad HR: Trigeminal neuronomas. *Laryngoscope* 85:371, 1975.

Frowein RA: Proceedings: meningiomas of the tentorium. *Acta Neurochir (Wein)* 31:283, 1975.

Hoff JT, and Patterson RH Jr: Craniopharyngiomas in children and adults. *J Neurosurg* 36:299, 1972.

Hooper K: Intracranial tumours in childhood. *Child Brain* 1:136, 1975.

Hoyt WF, Meshel LG, Lessell S, Schatz NJ, and Suckling RD: Malignant optic glioma of adulthood. *Brain* 96:121, 1975.

Jeffreys R: Pathological and haematological aspects of posterior fossa haemangioblastomata. *J Neurol Neurosurg Psychiatry* 38:112, 1975.

Karasick JL, and Mullen ST: A survey of metastatic meningiomas. *J Neurosurg* 40:206, 1974.

Kershing G, and Neumann J: Malignant lymphoma of the brain following renal transplantation. *Acta Neuropathol [Suppl] (Berl)* 6:131, 1975.

Littman P, and Wang CC: Reticulum cell sarcoma of the brain: a review of the literature and a study of 19 cases. *Cancer* 35:1412, 1975.

Magrath IT, Mugerwa J, Bailey I, Olweny C, and Kiryabwire Y: Intracerebral Burkitt's lymphoma: pathology, clinical features and treatment. *Q J Med* 43:489, 1974.

Miller NR: Optic nerve glioma and cerebellar astrocytoma in a patient with Von Recklinghausen's neurofibromatosis. *Am J Ophthalmol* 79:582, 1975.

Nurnberger JI, and Korey SR: *Pituitary Chromophobe Ademomas.* Springer, New York, 1953.

Obrador S, and Blazquez MG: Benign cystic tumours of the cerebellum. *Acta Neurochir (Wein)* 32:55, 1975.

Olson ME, Chernik NL, and Posner JB: Infiltration of the leptomeninges by systemic cancer: a clinical and pathologic study. *Arch Neurol* 30:122, 1974.

Raimondi AJ, and Gutierrez TA: Diagnosis and surgical treatment of choroid plexus papillomas. *Child Brain* 1:81, 1975.

Ransohoff J II: Parasagittal meningiomas. *J Neurosurg* 37:372, 1972.

Rubenstein LJ, Herman MM, Long TF, and Wilbur JR: Disseminated necrotizing leukoencephalopathy: a complication of treated central nervous sytem leukemia and lymphoma. *Cancer* 35:291, 1975.

Russell DS, Rubenstein LJ, and Lumsden EE: *Pathology of Tumors of the Nervous System.* Edward Arnold, London, 1959–1960.

Sansregret A, and Ledoux R: Lesser wing meningiomas: a few unfamiliar differential diagnoses. *Neuroradiology* 2:19, 1971.

Sato O, Tamura A, and Sano K: Brain tumors of early infants. *Child Brain* 1:121, 1975.

Schechter MM, Liebeskind A, and Azar-Kia B: Intracranial chordomas. *Neurology (Minneap)* 8:67, 1974.

Schmidek HM, and Sweet WH: Pathological and clinical aspects of pineal tumors. *Trans Am Neurol Assoc* 99:245, 1974.

Schoenberg BS, Schoenberg DG, Christine BW, and Gomez MR: The epidemiology of primary intracranial neoplasms of childhood: a population study. *Mayo Clin Proc* 51:51, 1976.

Vannucci RC, and Baten M: Cerebral metastatic disease in childhood. *Neurology (Minneap)* 24:981, 1974.

Vincent FM: Intracranial ependymomas: report of a case and literature review. *Minn Med* 58:877, 1975.

Zeller RS, and Chutorian AM: Vascular malformation of the pons in children. *Neurology (Minneap)* 25:776, 1975.

Zimmerman HM, Netsky MG, and Davidoff LM: *Atlas of Tumors of the Nervous System.* Lea & Febiger, Philadelphia, 1956.

Zimmerman HM: Malignant lymphomas of the nervous system. *Acta Neuropathol [Suppl] (Berl)* 6:69, 1975.

Zulch KJ: *Brain Tumors, Their Biology and Pathology.* Springer, New York, 1965.

Symptoms and Signs

Bakay L, and Cares HL: Olfactory meningiomas: report on a series of 25 cases. *Acta Neurochir (Wein)* 26:13, 1972.

Bluestein J, and Seeman MV: Brain tumors presenting as functional psychiatric disturbances. *Can Psychiatr Assoc J* 17 (Suppl 2):SS59, 1972.

Burr IM, Slonim AE, Danish RK, Gadoth N, and Butler IJ: Diencephalic syndrome revisited. *J Pediatr* 88:439, 1976.

Carey JP, Fisher RG, and Pelofsky S: Tentorial meningiomas. *Surg Neurol* 3:41, 1975.

Christiansen CB, and Greisen O: Reversible hearing loss in tumours of the cerebellopontine angle. *J Laryngol* 89:1161, 1975.

Degirolami U, and Schmidek H: Clinicopathological study of 53 tumors of the pineal region. *J Neurosurg* 39:455, 1973.

Derby BM, and Guian RL: Spectrum of symptomatic brainstem metastasis. *J Neurol Neurosurg Psychiatry* 38:888, 1975.

Gregorino FK, Hepler RS, and Stern WE: Loss and recovery of vision with suprasellar meningiomas. *J Neurosurg* 42:69, 1975.

Hussey HH: Editorial: optic neuritis of obscure origin. *JAMA* 230:881, 1974.

Kennedy HB, and Smith RJ: Eye signs in craniopharyngioma. *Br J Ophthalmol* 59:689, 1975.

Klug W: Proceedings: the clinical picture of meningiomas from a neurosurgical point of view. *Acta Neurochir (Wein)* 31:278, 1975.

Levine G, Winkelstein A, and Shadduck RK: CNS involvement as the initial manifestation of acute leukemia. *Cancer* 31:959, 1973.

Little JR, Dale AJ, and Okazak H: Meningeal carcinomatosis—clinical manifestations. *Arch Neurol* 30:122, 1974.

Marton LJ, Heby D, Levin VA, Lubich WP, Crafts DC, and Wilson CB: Presence of central nervous system tumours. *Cancer Res* 36:973, 1976.

Maurice-Williams RS: Mechanisms of production of gait unsteadiness by tumours in the posterior fossa. *J Neurol Neurosurg Psychiatry* 38:143, 1975.

Maurice-Williams RS: Micturition symptoms in frontal tumours. *J Neurol Neurosurg Psychiatry* 37:431, 1975.

Maurice-Williams RS: Multiple crossed false localizing signs in posterior fossa tumour. *J Neurol Neurosurg Psychiatry* 38:1232, 1975.

McNealy DE, et al: Brainstem dysfunction with supratentorial mass lesions. *Arch Neurol* 7:26, 1962.

Mohr PD, Anderson JM, Fletcher P, and Jefferson JM: The diagnostic problem of multiple intracranial tumors—case report of a pituitary chromophobe adenoma and cerebellar haemangioblastoma. *Postgrad Med J* 51:423, 1975.

Negri S, Caraceni T, and De Lorenzi L: Facial myokymia and brainstem tumour. *Eur Neurol* 14:108, 1976.

Pruett RC, and Wepsic JG: Delayed diagnosis of chiasmal compression. *Am J Ophthalmol* 76:229, 1973.

Rovit R, and Fein JM: Pituitary apoplexy: a review and reappraisal. *J Neurosurg* 37:280, 1972.

Rushworth RG: Pituitary apoplexy. *Med J Aust* 1:251, 1971.

Smith KR Jr: Diencephalic syndrome. *Arch Neurol* 29:206, 1973.

Stern WE: Meningiomas in the cranioorbital junction. *J Neurosurg* 38:428, 1973.

Walker AE: Syndromes of the tentorial notch. *J Nerv Ment Dis* 136:118, 1963.

Weir B: The relative significance of factors affecting postoperative survival in astrocytomas, grades 3 and 4. *J Neurosurg* 38:448, 1973.

Diagnosis

Baker HL, Houser OW, Campbell JK, Reese DF, and Holman CB: Computerized tomography of the head. *JAMA* 233:1304, 1975.

Edner G: Proceedings: sterotaxic brain tumor biopsy—5 year experience. *Acta Neurochir (Wein)* 32:258, 1975.

Feizin DS, Welch DM, Siegel BA, and James AE Jr: The efficacy of the brain scan in diagnosis of brainstem gliomas. *Radiology* 116:117, 1975.

Gado M, and Bull JW: The carotid angiogram in suprasellar masses. *Neuroradiology* 2:136, 1971.

Gliday DL, and Ash J: Accuracy of brain scanning in pediatric craniocerebral neoplasms. *Radiology* 117:93, 1975.

Harwood-Nash DC, Fitz CR, and Reilly BJ: Cranial computed tomography in infants and children. *Can Med Assoc J* 113:546, 1975.

Kistler JP, Hochberg FH, Brooks BR, Richardson EP Jr, New PF, and Schner J: Computerized axial tomography: clinicopathologic correlation. *Neurology (Minneap)* 25:201, 1975.

Kolar OJ: Differential diagnostic aspects in malignant lymphomas involving the cerebral nervous system. *Acta Neuropathol [Suppl] (Berl)* 6:181, 1975.

Kramer RA, Poole GJ, Moody OM, and Newton H: Angiography in craniopharyngiomas. *Radiology* 109:99, 1973.

Rowan AJ, Rudolf N De M, and Scott DF: EEG prediction of brain metastases: a controlled study with neuropathological confirmations. *J Neurol Neurosurg Psychiatry* 37:888, 1974.

Symon L, and Kendall B: Proceedings: differential diagnosis of cerebellopontine angle lesions by vertebral angiography. *J Neurol Neurosurg Psychiatry* 38:826, 1975.

Management

Berry HC, Parker RG, and Gerdes AJ: Irradiation of brain metastases. *Acta Radiol Ther (Stockh)* 13:533, 1974.

Brown LJ: Letter: management of cerebral metastases. *JAMA* 235:1552, 1976.

Chen TT, and Mealey J Jr: Effect of corticosteroid on protein and nucleic acid synthesis in human glial tumor cells. *Cancer Press* 33:1721, 1973.

Fewer D, Wilson CB, Boldrey EB, Enot KJ, and Powell MR: The chemotherapy of brain tumors: clinical experience with carmustine (BCNU) and vincristine. *JAMA* 222:549, 1972.

Fields WS, and Sharkey PC: *The Biology and Treatment of Intracranial Tumors.* Charles C Thomas, Springfield, Illinois, 1962.

Garrett MJ, Hughes HJ, and Ryall RD: CCNU in brain tumors. *Clin Radiol* 26:183, 1975.

Gjerris F, Klee JG, and Klinken L: Malignancy grade and long term survival in brain tumours of infancy and childhood. *Acta Neurol Scand* 53:61, 1976.

Glasscock ME, and Hays JW: The translabyrinthine removal of acoustic and other cerebellopontine angle tumors. *Ann Otol Rhinol Laryngol* 82:415, 1973.

Graffman S, Haymaker W, Hozosson R, and Jung B: High energy protons in the postoperative treatment of malignant glioma. *Acta Radiol Ther (Stockh)* 14:443, 1975.

Hazra T, Mullins GM, and Lott S: Management of cerebral metastasis from bronchogenic carcinoma. *Johns Hopkins Med J* 130:377, 1972.

Hendricks GL Jr, Barnes WJ, and Hood HL: Seven year cure of lung cancer with metastasis to the brain. *JAMA* 220:127, 1972.

Jeffreys R: Clinical and surgical aspects of posterior fossa haemangioblastomata. *J Neurol Neurosurg Psychiatry* 38:105, 1975.

Katz E: Late results of radical excision of craniopharyngiomas in children. *J Neurosurg* 42:86, 1975.

Kohler PO, and Ross GT: *Diagnosis and Treatment of Pituitary Tumors.* American Elsevier, New York, 1973.

Lokich JJ: The management of cerebral metastasis. *JAMA* 234:748, 1975.

Lusins J, and Sencer W: Posterior fossa vascular malformations: long term follow-up. *NY State J Med* 76:416, 1976.

Marsa GW, Goffinet DR, Rubinstein LJ, and Bagshaw MA: Megavoltage irradiation in the treatment of gliomas of the brain and spinal cord. *Cancer* 36:1681, 1975.

Miller MR, Iliff WJ, and Green WR: Evaluation and management of gliomas of the anterior visual pathways. *Brain* 97:743, 1974.

Modesti LM, and Feldman RA: Solitary cerebral metastasis from pulmonary cancer: prolonged survival after surgery. *JAMA* 231:1064, 1975.

Newman SJ, and Hansen HH: Proceedings: frequency, diagnosis and treatment of brain metastasis in 247 consecutive patients with bronchogenic carcinoma. *Cancer* 33:492, 1974.

Norrell H, Wilson CB, Slagel DE, and Clark TB: Leukoencephalopathy following the administration of methotrexate into the cerebrospinal fluid in the treatment of primary brain tumors. *Cancer* 33:923, 1974.

Onoyama Y, Abe M, Takahashi M, Yabumoto E, and Sakamoto D: Radiation therapy of brain tumors in children. *Radiology* 115:687, 1975.

Painter MJ, Chutorian AM, and Hilal SK: Cerebrovasculopathy following irradiation in childhood. *Neurology (Minneap)* 25:189, 1975.

Posner JB, and Shapiro WR: Editorial: brain tumor; current status of treatment and its complications. *Arch Neurol* 32:781, 1975.

Rand RW, and Jannella PJ: Microneurosurgery: application of the binocular surgical microscope in brain tumors, intracranial aneurysms, spinal cord disease and nerve reconstruction. *Clin Neurosurg* 15:319, 1968.

Shaffi CM, and Lekias JS: Meningiomas treated and untreated. *Med J Aust* 1:589, 1975.

Shapiro WR, and Young DF: Treatment of malignant glioma: a controlled study of chemotherapy and irradiation. *Arch Neurol* 33:494, 1976.

Stewart I, Millac P, and Sheppard RH: Neurosurgery in the older patient. *Postgrad Med* 51:453, 1975.

Walker MD: Recent advances in treatment for brain tumors. In: *Cancer Chemotherapy.* Year Book Medical Publishers, Chicago, 1975, pp. 251–262.

Walker MD: Diagnosis and treatment of brain tumors. *Pediatr Clin North Am* 23:131, 1976.

Walker MD, Alexander E Jr, et al: Evaluation of BCNU and/or radiotherapy in the treatment of anaplastic gliomas. *J Neurosurg* 49:333, 1978.

Walker MD, and Strike TA: An evaluation of methyl CCNU, BCNU and radiotherapy in the treatment of malignant glioma. *Proc Am Assoc Cancer Res* 17:163, 1976.

Walker MD, and Weiss HD: Chemotherapy in the treatment of malignant brain tumors. *Adv Neurol* 13:149, 1975.

Weinstein JD, Toy FJ, Jaffe ME, and Goldberg HI: The effect of dexamethasone on brain edema in patients with metastatic brain tumors. *Neurology (Minneap)* 23:121, 1973.

Wilson CB: Brain tumors. *N Engl J Med* 300:1469, 1979.

Spinal Cord Tumors

Amer MH, Al-Sarraf M, Baker LH, and Vaitkevicius VK: Malignant melanoma and central nervous system metastases: incidence, diagnosis, treatment and survival. *Cancer* 42:660, 1978.

Dijindjian M, Djindjian R, Houdart R, and Hurth M: Subarachnoid hemorrhage due to intraspinal tumors. *Surg Neurol* 9:223, 1978.

Fearnside MR, and Adams CB: Tumours of the cauda equina. *J Neurol Neurosurg Psychiatry* 41:24, 1978.

Giannotta SL, and Kindt GW: Metastatic spinal cord tumors. *Clin Neurosurg* 25:495, 1978.

Handel S, Grossman R, and Sarwar M: Case report: computed tomography in the diagnosis of spinal cord astrocytoma. *J CAT* 2:226, 1978.

Kawano N, Miyasaka Y, Yada K, Atari H, and Sasaki K: Diffuse cerebrospinal gliomatosis: case report. *J Neurosurg* 49:303, 1978.

Logue V: Angiomas of the spinal cord: review of the pathogenesis, clinical features, and results of surgery. *J Neurol Neurosurg Psychiatry* 42:1, 1979.

Malis LI: Intramedullary spinal cord tumors. *Clin Neurosurg* 25:512, 1978.

Onofrio BM: Intradural extramedullary spinal cord tumors. *Clin Neurosurg* 25:540, 1978.

Stern WE: Localization and diagnosis of spinal cord tumors. *Clin Neurosurg* 25:480, 1978.

Yasudka S, Okazaki H, Daube JR, and MacCarty CS: Foramen magnum tumors: analysis of 57 cases of benign extramedullary tumors. *J Neurosurg* 49:828, 1978.

16

Neurologic Aspects of Medical Diseases

Although many of the disorders discussed in this chapter are described in other sections of this monograph, it is useful to be able to think of the various neurologic complications that may occur in patients with specific types of medical disease. It may be of help to the physician when evaluating a patient with neurologic symptoms or signs to recognize the medical disorders that may produce them.

CARDIOVASCULAR DISEASES

The relationship between cardiovascular and cerebrovascular diseases is well known and was previously described in this volume. It is worth re-emphasizing that hypertension is probably the most important risk factor in the genesis of cerebrovascular disease, particularly cerebral hemorrhage, but that any prior history of heart disease, including myocardial infarction, coronary insufficiency, congestive heart failure, valvular disease, or atrial fibrillation, greatly increase the risk of that patient developing occlusive cerebrovascular disease, either thrombotic or embolic. The multiple cerebral lacunar infarcts that occur in chronic hypertensive disease are sometimes diagnostically confusing, for they may not cause the usual cerebrovascular symptomatology of lateralizing motor or cranial nerve deficits; rather, such patients may present with dementia, gait abnormalities, and movement disorders. The dramatic and often catastrophic symptomatology of hypertensive encephalopathy is another special case in point.

Certain types of syncopal attacks occur specifically in patients with cardiac disease. True vasodepressor syncope has no cardiogenic basis. Although its exact mechanism is not known, it is thought to occur mainly under circumstances of emotional stress or fear and is characterized by a feeling of faintness, a sensation as if the lights were dimming, voices fading, and the environment receding, along with nausea, bradycardia, diaphoresis, and pallor. The patient regains consciousness shortly after assuming the recumbent posture and is not drowsy, even though he may be slightly confused.

Syncope in patients with persistent bradycardia (pulse less than 40) and electrocardiographic (ECG) evidence of conduction defect in the form of an atrioventricular (A-V) block, is called Adams-Stokes syndrome. The onset of unconsciousness is dramatically sudden, with no more than a momentary warning, and may occur whether the patient is upright or supine. It is difficult to understand why these patients have little or no premonitory feeling of faintness, because it is presumed that the loss of consciousness is caused by cardiac asystole and consequent global cerebral ischemia. The faint may occur so rapidly that injury resulting from a fall is not uncommon, particularly since the syncopal attacks may occur several times a day. If the asystole persists, cerebral ischemic damage occurs, with infarctions in the cerebral watershed areas, causing many types of neurologic abnormalities, particularly disturbances of mental function. Brief seizure activity and urinary incontinence during an attack are not rare. Diagnosis depends on the cardiac evidence of severe bradycardia and heart block; the latter may be temporary, and therefore the ECG may show only evidence of myocardial disease. These patients may respond at least temporarily to anticholinergic drugs, particularly atropine, but a cardiac pacemaker may eventually be necessary.

Aortic stenosis also seems to result in syncopal attacks, although the mechanism is not clear. It is due to heart block in some instances. The attack almost invariably occurs immediately after or, less frequently, during exercise; there may be little or no warning, a phenomenon suggesting that some type of reflex mechanism is responsible for the syncope.

Syncope may occur during paroxysmal atrial or ventricular tachycardia, but the patient usually has the warning of palpitation. The mechanism for the syncope is the precipitous drop in cardiac output caused by the tachycardia.

Carotid sinus syncope, although much discussed in the literature, is a rare phenomenon. A hypersensitive carotid sinus is said to be the mechanism for the severe bradycardia, hypotension, and occasionally heart block which occurs when the carotid sinus is massaged in some elderly males. The syncope that occurs is usually preceded by weakness and faintness, although apparently some patients have little or no warning. Atropine is the preferred treatment.

The neurologic complications that follow cardiac arrest depend on the duration of asystole (Fig. 16.1). They vary from mild, temporary confusion—to significant deficits in mental function—to profound movement abnormalities, including myoclonus, choreoathetosis, and cerebellar ataxia—to persistent vegetative state—to brain death. As the neurologic prognosis is often difficult to predict in any given instance, such patients must be treated vigorously with steroids to inhibit brain edema and with bicarbonate to control systemic acidosis.

Cerebrovascular occlusion in young adults should prompt consideration that the cause might be an atrial or ventricular myxoma. Although rare, these tumors are surgically treatable and should therefore be considered. Echocar-

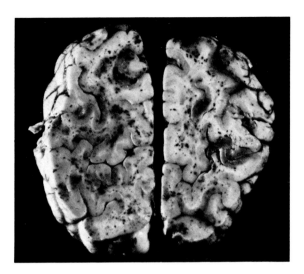

FIG. 16.1. Multiple punctate hemorrhagic infarctions and necrosis in a patient who expired 3 days after open-heart surgery.

diography is a reliable diagnostic tool for this purpose and should be included in the work-up of any young adult with cerebral infarction in whom there is no obvious other cause for the illness. Echocardiography is also used to diagnose mitral valve prolapse, which is reputed by some to cause cerebral embolization, without cardiac symptoms or signs. Mitral valve prolapse associated with cardiac arrhythmias, congestive heart failure, and myxomatous degeneration of the valve is a rare disorder of women.

Ventricular aneurysms which develop following myocardial infarction may be a source of cerebral embolization because clots may form in the adynamic portion of the aneurysm. Diagnosis can often be established by the gated cardiac flow study. Treatment is by surgical excision or anticoagulation.

HEPATOCEREBRAL SYNDROMES

A wide variety of neurologic disorders may appear in patients suffering from liver disease. Some are acute and fulminant, others chronic and progressive. The following description includes those most frequently seen.

Acute Hepatic Encephalopathy

Acute hepatic encephalopathy is usually ushered in by a period of confusion, agitation, and a variety of involuntary movements, the most characteristic of which are asterixis (Chapters 1 and 4) and myoclonus. There is progression to stupor and coma, at which time examination also reveals hyperventilation (respiratory alkalosis), small reactive pupils, bilateral

Babinski signs, and, in deep coma, decortication and decerebration. The oculocephalic reflexes are always intact. Seizures are extremely rare.

Signs of liver disease are usually evident, but there is little correlation between the neurologic deficit and the severity of liver dysfunction. Signs of portocaval shunting are usually evident. The syndrome is often precipitated by gastrointestinal bleeding, sedation, diuresis or paracentesis, infection, or any surgical procedure. The blood ammonia (NH_3) level is usually elevated (> 50 μg%) *but may be normal.* The electroencephalogram (EEG) shows high-voltage 1- to 3-sec waves; these are not specific for hepatic encephalopathy, however, and may also occur in other types of metabolic encephalopathy.

The pathogenesis of acute hepatic encephalopathy is still being debated. Many believe that the increased blood NH_3 interferes with brain metabolism at the level of glutamine synthesis or in reductive amination of α-ketoglutarate. NH_3 originates in the bowel from bacterial decomposition of protein and is usually converted into urea by the liver. In liver disease, particularly with portocaval shunting, it enters the systemic circulation. Some investigators believe that acute hepatic encephalopathy is caused by increased blood levels of short-chain fatty acids (butyric, caproic, valeric), which are elevated in hepatic disease and exert their effects by action on the reticular activating system. Increased blood levels of these fatty acids cause coma in experimental animals. It was recently suggested that aromatic amines, produced in the gut from protein and catabolized by monoamine oxidation in the healthy liver, act as false neurochemical transmitters in the brain, thereby blocking dopaminergic transmission.

Treatment of hepatic coma is directed at reducing the blood ammonia level by clearing the colon with enemas, reducing dietary intake of protein, administering neomycin orally or by nasogastric tube to suppress the organisms which produce increased NH_3 in the bowel, and orally administering lactulose, which acidifies the contents of the colon and further suppresses urease production.

The pathology of hepatocerebral disease is striking and unique. There is a diffuse increase in the number and size of type II (protoplasmic) astrocytes; glycogen inclusions appear in the nuclei of the astrocytes, degenerating nerve cells, and myelin sheaths; and microcavitation occurs in the cortex and basal ganglia.

Aside from acute hepatic encephalopathy, there are other chronic neuropsychiatric syndromes associated with severe hepatic disease. These include the following:

1. *Movement disorders.* These are not infrequent in chronic hepatocerebral disease. Movement disorders usually occur in patients who previously suffered and recovered from acute hepatic encephalopathy. The patients may show cerebellar ataxia, lurching gait, dysarthria, reduced voice volume, tremor, rigidity, and chorea.

2. *Psychosis.* This may appear 2 weeks to several months after surgical portocaval shunt and is characterized by hypomania or paranoid-delusional state.

3. *Spastic paraparesis.* The primary lesion is thought to be in the motor cells of the cortex with secondary demyelinization of the corticospinal tracts.

4. *Dementia.* This may appear along with the movement disorder; it is usually progressive and global.

5. *Brain edema.* In patients with massive acute hepatic necrosis, severe brain edema may cause uncal or cerebellar herniation.

6. *Peripheral neuropathy.* It is difficult to distinguish nutritional neuropathy from that caused by hepatic disease. In both instances, segmental demyelinization occurs.

Encephalopathy and fatty degeneration of the viscera (Reye's syndrome) has received wide scientific and lay publicity during the past few years. It is a disorder of unknown cause, possibly viral, which attacks children or young adolescents. There is a history of upper respiratory infection followed by persistent vomiting, wild delirium, coma, decerebration, severe convulsions, hyperventilation, firmness or enlargement of the liver, positive Babinski signs, elevated serum glutamic oxalic transaminase (SGOT), and hypoglycemia which has a poor response to intravenous glucose. The illness is extremely fulminant and may be fatal within 48 to 72 hr. Pathology includes brainswelling, fatty yellow liver, and fatty degeneration of myocardium and kidneys. Treatment consists of exchange transfusion.

PANCREATIC DISEASE

Although the correlations are not as clearly drawn as in hepatic disorders, there is some evidence that patients with chronic interstitial pancreatitis may show behavioral abnormalities, anxiety, restlessness, dysarthria, and muscular rigidity. Acute pancreatic encephalopathy must be rare, but it is described as being characterized by an acute delirium and the diffuse neurologic changes that occur in acute necrotizing pancreatitis. The consensus is that there are probably several etiologies for acute pancreatic encephalopathy. Disseminated intravascular coagulation has been incriminated, as have dehydration and severe electrolyte abnormalities induced by the pancreatitis. It has also been suggested that the acute necrotizing pancreatitis liberates fat-splitting pancreatic enzymes into the circulation and that these act to destroy brain tissue. Apparently a similar clinical and pathologic picture can be produced in animals by injection of lipase, so one treatment recommended for this condition is injection of pancreatic antienzymes (aprotinin, 200,000 units per day). The other possible causes must be looked for by appropriate laboratory investigation.

MALABSORPTION SYNDROMES

Neurologic complications are present in about 50% of the patients with adult steatorrhea (gluten enteropathy). These include myopathy, peripheral neuropathy, corticospinal tract disease, cerebellar ataxia, and optic atrophy. Tetany and convulsions have been reported, probably secondary to decreased serum calcium and potassium.

Neurologic complications in Whipple's disease are frequent and include Wernicke-Korsakoff psychosis, ophthalmoplegias, dysarthria, and spastic paresis. These are thought to be caused by widespread infiltration of the central nervous system (CNS) with the protein-polysaccharide complex found in these patients.

HEMATOLOGIC DISORDERS

Vitamin B_{12} Deficiency

It is traditional but probably inappropriate to think of pernicious anemia as a hematologic disorder when, in fact, the primary lesion is deficiency of intrinsic factor in gastric cells, with subsequent malabsorption of vitamin B_{12} by the intestinal mucosa. The neurologic complications of B_{12} deficiency are well known, and that they may occur in the absence of significant anemia is also well recognized. Posterolateral sclerosis of the spinal cord is the classic neurologic lesion. This is associated with loss of vibration and position sensibilities in the feet and legs; progressive spastic paraparesis, ageusia, peripheral neuropathy, and defects in mental function have been described and respond to some degree to B_{12} administration.

Porphyria

Acute intermittent and tardive porphyria may produce neurologic abnormalities. Symptoms in the latter may be vague and are often interpreted as psychogenic. Acute intermittent porphyria is characterized by recurrent bouts of abdominal pain, obstipation, progressively ascending peripheral neuropathy, confusion, agitation, hallucinations, and convulsions. Diagnosis is made through increased urinary excretion of porphyrobilinogen and δ-aminolevulinic acid. Treatment consists of high-carbohydrate (500 to 600 g daily) diet. Barbiturates must be avoided.

Platelet Disorders

Neurologic complications may occur in thrombocytopenic purpura due to any cause; the most feared complication is intracerebral or spinal hemorrhage. Disseminated intravascular coagulation (DIC) is a consumptive coagulopathy that may be precipitated by a wide variety of systemic disorders, e.g., trauma, severe infection, carcinoma, and parturition. It is characterized by widespread ecchymoses in the presence of decreased platelets, increased prothrombin and partial thromboplastin time, decreased fibrinogen and increased fibrin split products. The neurologic disturbance may be profound, with convulsive seizures, motor deficits, and coma. The pathology results from the intravascular coagulation rather than hemorrhage, so early treatment with intravenous heparin is essential if these patients are to survive.

Leukemia

Neurologic complications occur rarely in chronic leukemia and frequently in the acute leukemias, particularly during childhood. Meningeal and peripheral nerve infiltration are relatively common. Mixed infiltration and hemorrhagic pictures are seen in the CNS of patients with acute leukemia (Fig. 16.2).

Lymphoma

Hodgkin's disease and lymphosarcoma cause neurologic symptoms and signs by compressing nervous tissue. This is usually due to an epidural mass in the spinal canal and less commonly in the skull; not infrequently there is

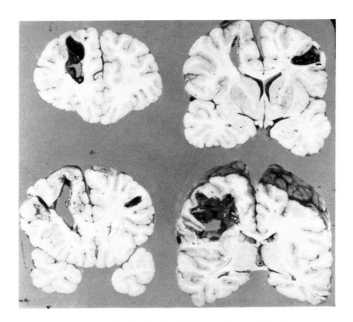

FIG. 16.2. Massive leukemic hemorrhages in brain.

retroperitoneal invasion and compression of peripheral nerves and the lumbosacral plexus. The patient with known lymphoma in whom signs of spinal cord compression (weakness or numbness of legs, urinary urgency, or incontinence) develop requires *immediate* myelography to confirm and localize the lesion. This should be treated by steroids (dexamethasone 24 mg daily) and irradiation to the area of block as soon as possible. Surgical decompression is rarely required.

Multiple Myeloma

Myeloma and other causes of alterations in the serum gammaglobulins produce an unusual and severe form of sensory peripheral neuropathy characterized by involvement of the larger myelinated sensory fibers of the nerves with resultant loss of proprioception, although pain sensibility may be retained. The diagnosis of myeloma should be considered in any patient with this type of neuropathy. Serum protein immunoelectrophoresis is an important diagnostic tool in these patients.

Sarcoidosis

There is no reason other than convenience for considering sarcoidosis under the heading of hematologic disorders. It is actually a systemic granulomatous disease of unknown etiology involving lymph nodes, liver, lungs, spleen, skin, eyes, parotid glands, fingers, and the nervous system. The typical neural involvement is by meningeal invasion and bilateral cranial nerve pathology. The nodules may involve the optic chiasm and nerves, causing optic atrophy and blindness. Bilateral facial nerve involvement is common, but all cranial nerves may be diseased. The cerebrospinal fluid (CSF) shows modest pleocytosis (10 to 50 mm^3; all mononuclear cells), increased protein, and hypoglycorrhachia. CSF gamma-globulin is often elevated.

The neurologic involvement in sarcoidoses may be extreme. There may be damage to the hypothalamus and pituitary (amenorrhea, obesity, altered libido, diabetes insipidus), peripheral neuropathy, or myopathy.

Treatment of sarcoidosis is difficult once there has been evidence of CNS involvement. Steroids must be given as promptly as the diagnosis can be made.

Polycythemia Vera

The usual neurologic complication in polycythemia vera is related to thrombosis of small cerebral vessels with repeated episodes of cerebrovascular insufficiency. Modern management is based on oral or intravenous administration of a single dose of ^{32}P 0.1 m/kg.

The special association of polycythemia with the phacomatosis Hippel-Lindau's syndrome should be mentioned. These patients usually present because of symptoms related to a cerebellar hemangioma, which may have bled or produced cerebellar symptoms by virtue of its presence. Retinal hemangiomatosis is often present.

ENDOCRINE DISORDERS

Pituitary-Hypothalamic Lesions

Lesions of the pituitary and hypothalamus are appropriately considered together because of the close interrelationships of the neural control systems of the hypophysis and hypothalamus. *Lesions of the hypothalamus* such as tumors of the floor of the 3rd ventricle (craniopharyngioma, teratoma, or ectopic pinealoma) or *intrinsic hypothalamic tumors* such as gliomas produce disturbances in visceral function, e.g., changes in appetite and food consumption (an increase or a decrease), diabetes insipidus, disturbed temperature regulation, alteration in sleep patterns (particularly somnolence), apathy, and altered gonadal and menstrual activity. In the infant, tumors of the hypothalamus produce the syndrome known as "failure to thrive."

Pituitary lesions are of two basic types: tumor or infarction. Rapid destruction of the pituitary, particularly infarction of the anterior lobe, occurs rarely during the immediate postpartum period (Sheehan's syndrome) and is probably secondary to hemorrhage or shock or to embolic occlusion of the hypophysial vessels. The syndrome consists of amenorrhea, general and breast atrophy, decreased axillary and pubic hair, hypoglycemia, and evidence of decreased adrenal function. Pituitary dwarfism is due to a deficiency of growth and gonadotropic hormones, and the patient remains a sexually immature dwarf into adult life.

Pituitary tumors produce endocrine as well as neighborhood signs. The neighborhood signs are those of compression of the optic chiasm or optic nerves, or both, as the tumor expands superiorly out of the sella turcica. Visual disturbances in the presence of a pituitary tumor means that the tumor has escaped its diaphragm and extends at least 0.5 cm superiorly. The type of visual disturbance which results is dependent on whether the chiasm is located anteriorly or posteriorly. Although the classic field abnormality is said to be bitemporal hemianopsia because of compression of crossing fibers in the chiasm, unilateral blindness is also frequent because the optic nerve may be compressed. The chiasm is actually squeezed between the superiorly expanding tumor from below and the anterior cerebral and anterior communicating arteries which lie just superior to the chiasm.

Rapidly expanding pituitary tumors may either outgrow their blood supply or cause infarction and necrosis of part of the tumor as the arteries supplying it are compressed, resulting in a syndrome called pituitary apoplexy. This is characterized by dramatically worsening headache, loss of vision, ophthalmoplegia, hypotension, tachycardia, shocklike picture, and coma. These patients require adrenal cortical replacement therapy promptly while being prepared for surgery to decompress the chiasm and extraocular nerves.

Almost all pituitary tumors are composed of several types of cell, with one type predominant. The most common tumor is the chromophobe adenoma (Fig. 16.3), which usually results in deficiency of thyroid stimulating hormone, gonadotropins, and adrenal cortical tropic hormones, with a clinical picture appropriate to these deficiencies. Eosinophilic adenoma produces neighborhood signs similar to those caused by the more common chromophobe and results in giantism if it occurs during childhood or adolescence and acromegaly in adult life. The eosinophilic cells secrete an increased quantity of somatotropin. Acromegalic patients not uncommonly develop a typical picture of myopathy, with proximal muscle weakness so severe they may have difficulty getting about.

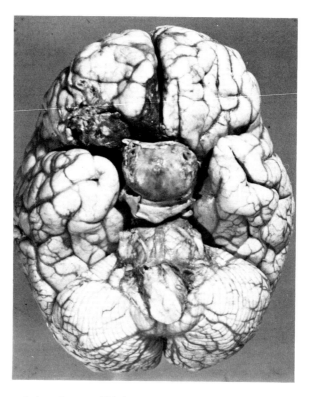

FIG. 16.3. Chromophobe adenoma. This huge cystic mass had resulted in left monocular blindness and right temporal hemianopsia.

The rarest pituitary tumor, which usually does not expand outside the sella turcica, is the basophilic adenoma. This tumor produces the clinical picture of Cushing's syndrome, often in association with adrenal cortical hyperplasia.

Craniopharyngiomas are usually discussed along with pituitary tumors because they frequently cause similar visual disturbances. In fact, they arise from ectodermal rests in the pars tuberalis of the hypophysis. They are cystic masses that are difficult to remove surgically and poorly responsive to radiation therapy. They produce symptoms of hypothalamic origin, e.g., amenorrhea, altered appetite, diabetes insipidus, and impaired libido.

Thyroid Disease

Hypofunction

Congenital thyroid hypofunction results in cretinism with permanently impaired mental function. Myxedema is characterized by a variety of neurologic symptoms and signs, including dizziness, ataxia of gait, somnolence, impaired mental function, carpal tunnel syndrome, and myopathy. The last is usually associated with pseudomyotonia. The CSF protein may be quite elevated, suggesting a brain tumor. The EEG shows a loss of alpha activity and a predominance of low-voltage slow-wave activity with almost no organized pattern. These patients may develop ophthalmoplegia in which any one or several of the extraocular muscles function incompletely. The involved extraocular muscles are fibrotic, and histologic examination reveals them to be infiltrated with round cells and scar tissue. Clinical examination reveals that these contracted muscles cannot be stretched even by forced traction. A similar type of ocular syndrome occurs in hyperthyroidism. Its mechanism is not understood.

Hyperfunction

Although more bizarre neurologic syndromes have been described (e.g., acute thyrotoxic psychosis), the most frequent neurologic abnormalities observed in the hyperthyroid state are myopathy and ophthalmoplegia. As mentioned in other chapters in this monograph, there is an increased incidence of association between thyrotoxicosis and myasthenia gravis and thyrotoxicosis and periodic paralysis.

Parathyroid Disease

The parathyroid glands play a dominant role in the regulation of serum and tissue calcium and phosphorus levels, which are vital to normal neural function in the central and peripheral nervous systems.

Hypoparathyroidism is usually secondary to thyroid surgery, although there is also an idiopathic form and a sex-linked inherited defect termed *pseudohypoparathyroidism* in which the patients are obese, short, and usually mentally defective. The symptoms in all these groups of patients are similar and seem to be related to hypocalcemia. The defect in pseudohypoparathyroidism is failure of parathyroid hormone to increase adenyl cyclase activity. Idiopathic hypoparathyroidism occurs in increased incidence in conjunction with autoimmune disorders.

The decrease in calcium ion results in increased neuronal excitability in the peripheral and central nervous systems. The manifestations in the peripheral nervous system include tingling, acroparesthesia, and laryngeal spasm, usually precipitated by cold. Trousseau's and Chvostek's signs and carpopedal spasms are frequently seen.

Hypocalcemia produces a variety of CNS signs, including convulsions, mental deficiency and dementia, pseudotumor cerebri, intracranial calcifications sometimes associated with extrapyramidal signs, and rarely psychotic behavior. Symmetrical basal ganglia calcifications are an almost certain sign of hypoparathyroidism (Figs. 16.4 and 16.5).

The hyperparathyroid state produces its effect on the nervous system by virtue of increased serum and tissue calcium. Parathyroid adenomas are not uncommonly associated with pancreatic islet cell adenomas and pituitary adenomas. The neurologic picture of hypercalcemia is weakness and diminished pain sensitivity. Myopathy may be present. Patients with chronic hypercalcemic states are easily exhausted, apathetic, and can even be demented or

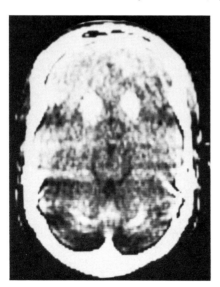 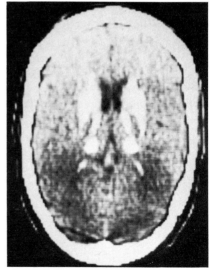

FIGS. 16.4, 16.5. Pseudohypoparathyroidism. There is heavy calcification in the basal ganglia and cerebellar nuclei.

eventually stuporous. Removal of a parathyroid adenoma often results in complete remission of neurologic signs.

COLLAGEN-VASCULAR DISEASES

Some of the collagen-vascular diseases were discussed under the topic of neuromuscular disorders (Chapter 13). The designation collagen-vascular diseases usually applies to systemic lupus erythematosus (SLE), polyarteritis nodosa, systemic sclerosis (scleroderma), dermatomyositis, rheumatoid arthritis and related diseases, and Wegener's granulomatosis. In addition, there are other rare syndromes which are considered by some authorities to be connective tissue disorders. Perhaps the best known of these is *Sjögren's syndrome*, which occurs in association with other connective tissue diseases. There is, in fact, considerable disagreement as to whether these diseases should be grouped together at all, for there is no known common etiologic agent. Some believe that the common unifying factor is a disturbance in immunologic mechanisms. In any case, the common denominator clinically is that they are all multiple-system diseases, causing symptoms related to all the organ systems of the body and usually associated with fever, weight loss, and malaise. The symptoms and signs of these illnesses, including those of the nervous system, are usually caused by degenerative changes in the connective tissue of small blood vessels with resultant ischemic tissue changes.

Collagen-vascular diseases may involve the nervous system in several ways: (1) direct involvement by inflammation or by ischemia secondary to vascular changes; and (2) indirect effects of the disease on other organs, viz., renal disease, which causes uremia or hypertension; cerebral hemorrhage from thrombocytopenia; cerebral emboli from marantic endocarditis; spinal cord compression in rheumatoid arthritis; complications of drug therapy.

Systemic Lupus Erythematosus

Neurologic involvement is frequent in SLE; indeed, it is the second most frequent cause of death in SLE patients, the first being uremia. The disease is five times more frequent in women than men. Neuropsychiatric manifestations occur in about 60% of patients, including confusional states, dementia, and psychotic behavior. Seizures occur in about 25%, and signs of multifocal CNS involvement (e.g., clear-cut stroke syndrome, chorea, and myelopathy) are not rare. In addition, several varieties of peripheral neuropathy may occur, including polyneuropathy which resembles Guillain-Barré syndrome, cranial nerve palsies, and mononeuritis multiplex. Myopathy indistinguishable clinically from other causes may occur.

The CSF is usually abnormal, with mononuclear pleocytosis, increased protein, and increased gamma-globulin. This last feature may serve to confuse the diagnosis with multiple sclerosis, as the neurologic signs of SLE may also be remitting and diffuse, occasionally with minimal systemic symptomatology. Other laboratory data help to confirm the diagnosis of SLE, including elevated erythrocyte sedimentation rate (ESR), anemia, thrombocytopenia, leukopenia, abnormal serum electrophoresis, false-positive serologic tests for syphilis, and of course the presence of the diagnostic LE cells, which may be found in the blood and bone marrow.

Although spontaneous remission of SLE occurs in about 50% of instances, signs of nervous system involvement usually herald a poor prognosis. The best form of treatment is still debated, but adrenocortical steroids are the mainstay.

Polyarteritis Nodosa

Polyarteritis nodosa is an illness of unknown etiology, long thought to be in some way related to a hypersensitization reaction to certain drugs or infections. It is characterized by evidence of inflammation and necrosis in the small arteries and arterioles of all organs. It is the male counterpart of SLE, occurring four to five times more frequently in men. The symptoms and signs are caused by tissue ischemia, infarction, and necrosis secondary to the arterial involvement.

The evidence of neurologic involvement is high, probably more than 80% at some time during the course of the illness. Certain types of neuropathy occur more frequently than others, including polyneuropathy (occasionally of the Guillain-Barré type) and scattered individual peripheral nerve lesions (mononeuropathy multiplex). Spinal cord involvement is seen less frequently. CNS signs are caused by infarction from the arteritis and may therefore be indistinguishable from cerebral infarction due to arteriosclerosis except for the other signs of the disease. Temporal arteritis is considered by some to be a variant of polyarteritis, although it is a much more localized and benign process (see Chapter 2).

There are other unique neurologic syndromes thought by many to have a pathogenesis similar to that of polyarteritis, viz., *Cogan's syndrome* (nonluetic interstitial keratitis with deafness, vertigo, and tinnitus in young adults) and the *painful ophthalmoplegia of Tolosa-Hunt*, characterized by extraocular muscle weakness, optic nerve disease, proptosis, and pain and hypalgesia in the distribution of the first division of the trigeminal nerve.

The prognosis of polyarteritis is similar to that of SLE. About 50% of the patients have significant remissions. Treatment is with adrenocortical steroids.

Systemic Sclerosis

The clinical features of systemic sclerosis are well known. Neurologic complications except for myopathy are infrequent.

Dermatomyositis and Polymyositis

Some authorities do not classify the syndromes dermatomyositis and polymyositis, which affect skin and muscle predominantly, with other collagen vascular diseases. Both entities are discussed in some detail in Chapter 13.

Rheumatoid Arthritis

Rheumatoid arthritis, a protean symptom complex, may occur as a separate entity involving only joints or be associated with a variety of systemic and neurologic symptoms. The syndrome may be blurred by a mixture of features of SLE. The interesting and neurologic complications include the following:

1. *Entrapment neuropathy.* Although carpal tunnel syndrome is the most frequent, any may occur (see Chapter 13).
2. *Atlantoaxial dislocation.* This unique complication of cervical rheumatoid arthritis has been thought to be due to incompetence of the transverse ligament of C_1. Because this ligament holds the anterior arch of C_1 to the odontoid process, incompetence results in anterior dislocation of C_1 on C_2, causing compression of the upper cervical cord or low medulla, or impinging on and obstructing the vertebral arteries resulting in brainstem infarction.
3. *Polymyositis and peripheral neuropathy.* This is rare.
4. *Cryoglobulinemia.* This is associated with increased blood viscosity and cerebral symptoms.
5. *Toxic encephalopathy.* This occurs together with active rheumatoid spondylitis (Still's disease).
6. *Ankylosing spondylitis.* Rarely, this causes arachnoiditis and severe pain in lower extremities due to involvement of the cauda equina.

Wegener's Granulomatosis

Wegener's granulomatosis is a rare disease of unknown etiology; it is thought to be a variant of polyarteritis nodosa and is characterized by vasculitis involving many organs, renal glomerulitis, and necrotizing granulomas of the upper respiratory tract and lungs. The nervous system is involved by contiguous invasion by granulomas from the nose and paranasal sinuses, by brainstem granulomas, or by inflammatory involvement of the vasa nervorum. Cerebral infarction and hemorrhage secondary to vasculitis have been reported. Although these patients are usually treated with steroids, the response of the nervous system lesions is variable.

Sjögren's syndrome (sicca syndrome) occurs in conjunction with several of the other collagen vascular disorders and should therefore probably not be considered a separate entity. It occurs almost exclusively in postmenopausal women and causes dryness of the ocular and oral mucosa and enlargement of the salivary glands. There is an inconsistent association with several neurologic signs, including cranial nerve palsies, myopathy, and peripheral neuropathy.

PULMONARY INSUFFICIENCY

Acute pulmonary insufficiency—as with aspiration, acute pneumonitis, atelectasis, or pneumothorax—produces cerebral symptoms and signs of disturbance of consciousness and seizures, but rarely lateralizing neurologic deficits. The neurologic involvement is due to cerebral hypoxia. If sufficiently prolonged, myocardial instability increases and ventricular tachycardia and cardiac arrest are not uncommon. In chronic pulmonary insufficiency the pathophysiology is more complex, and the neurologic picture may be confusing inasmuch as it develops gradually and may simulate brain tumor. Chronic pulmonary insufficiency due to pulmonary emphysema and fibrosis is often associated with right heart failure. Hypercapnia and hypoxia are present. A fairly typical blood gas picture might reveal $PaCO_2 > 55$ torr, $PaO_2 < 45$ torr, pH < 7.30, and HCO_3^- about 25 mEq/liter. It is believed that the respiratory acidosis in conjunction with hypoxia produces the mischief in the brain. There is an increase in cerebral blood volume owing to dilatation of cerebral vessels, so patients complain of headache and may develop papilledema. The patients are confused, apparently demented, and lethargic to stuporous; they may have extremity tremor, twitching, or myoclonus. CSF pressure is elevated, which may add further to the confusion, but CSF protein is normal. The EEG shows diffuse slow waves and is not further helpful.

It is important to identify respiratory acidosis caused by pulmonary insufficiency because therapy depends on recognizing that the response of the respiratory center to $PaCO_2$ is depressed owing to increased cerebral HCO_3^-; respiration is therefore controlled by the coexisting hypoxia. These patients require close observation. Intubation and elimination of alveolar CO_2 by respiratory assistance is the best method of treatment, keeping in mind that the patient may have to be ventilated artificially for the first several hours after $PaCO_2$ reduction.

RENAL DISEASE

There are three neurologic manifestations of renal failure and uremia:

1. Peripheral motor and sensory neuropathy.
2. Encephalopathy which has no distinctive characteristics. The patients may be irritable, drowsy, mentally cloudy, and, late in the disease, comatose.
3. Generalized myoclonus which causes involuntary asymmetrical jerking movements of muscles and extremities, occasionally terminating in convulsions.

The pathogenesis of these uremic complications is thought to be in some fashion related to the elevation of blood urea nitrogen (BUN), but the correlation between BUN and the severity of the neurologic disturbances is poor. There is no characteristic pathology of uremic encephalopathy.

The treatment of renal failure by dialysis may cause neurologic abnormalities. Dialysis often causes rather severe vascular headaches; and in a small percentage of patients, nausea, vomiting, muscle cramps, restlessness, confusion, convulsions, or any combination of these may occur. This phenomenon is termed the *disequilibrium syndrome* and may appear less than 12 hr or more than 36 hr after dialysis. The mechanism is thought to be due to a temporary increase in brain water.

Dialysis encephalopathy is a more chronic process complicating long-term dialysis. It is characterized by dementia, dysarthria, myoclonic jerks, and convulsions, which may be focal or generalized. The symptoms increase in frequency and may eventually persist. The CSF is normal; and the EEG shows seizure activity, with bursts of slow waves and spikes in various foci. The pathogenesis was formerly attributed to increased cerebral concentration of aluminum, but recent studies failed to confirm this relationship. There are no specific ionic abnormalities in the blood.

Hypoglycemia

Hypoglycemia has long been known to produce severe encephalopathy characterized by confusion, convulsion, and coma. Glucose is an essential substrate of cerebral metabolism which begins to fail as the cellular stores of glucose and glycogen diminish. Fortunately, the brain can survive for a much longer period in the hypoglycemic than the hypoxic state, and complete recovery is possible when blood sugar is restored to normal even though the patient may have been unconscious for more than 1.5 hr. Prolonged hypoglycemia results in irreversible cerebral pathology which is quite similar to that seen in hypoxia. The commonest causes of hypoglycemia are:

1. Overdosage of insulin or oral hypoglycemic agents
2. Islet cell adenoma of the pancreas
3. Hypoglycemia of infants
4. Reye's syndrome
5. Glycogen storage disease (Pompe's disease)

Hyperosmolar and Hypo-osmolar States

Abnormal osmolar states were alluded to in Chapter 11. Hyper- and hypoosmolar states may cause severe encephalopathy, including mental clouding, irritability, muscle twitching, convulsions, and coma. Hyperosmolar encephalopathy may occur with the following:

1. Hyperosmolar aketonic hyperglycemic coma
2. Severe dehydration particularly following diarrhea

Hypo-osmolar states include the following:

1. Inappropriate ADH secretion
2. Water intoxication from any cause
3. Addison's disease

NONMETASTATIC EFFECTS OF CANCER

Approximately 15 to 20% of patients with cancer have serious neurologic complications, the majority of which are caused by metastases, although nonmetastatic neurologic disturbance of the nervous system occurs with considerable frequency as well.

Remote Effects

The term "remote effects" is customarily used to describe a central or peripheral nervous system disorder presumably due to some metabolic or toxic effect of a cancer but not due to organ failure or cancer invasion of the nervous system. Perhaps the best known of these is the myasthenic syndrome, sometimes called Lambert-Eaton syndrome, in which there is extremity and trunk weakness but no involvement of muscles innervated by the cranial nerves. Clinically the illness resembles myasthenia gravis; electrically it appears that the muscle action potential increases with repeated neural stimulation. The syndrome occurs almost exclusively in oat cell carcinoma of the bronchus and is sometimes improved by guanidine, a drug which potentiates the effect of acetylcholine.

Polymyositis and dermatomyositis (previously described) are associated with carcinoma frequently enough that carcinoma should be looked for in such patients, particularly those of middle age or beyond. About 50% of men over age of 50 with polymyositis or dermatomyositis will ultimately be found to have a cancer. Peripheral neuropathy, cerebellar degeneration, myelopathy, and dementia have been described as remote effects of carcinoma.

Infections

The use of immunosuppressive agents in the management of various types of cancer has resulted in increased incidence of infection of the brain and meninges by viral, bacterial, and fungal organisms. Lymphomas, leukemias, and patients who have tumors and have had operations around the head and spine account for over 80% of the infections. Progressive multifocal leukoencephalopathy is an opportunistic viral invasion of the nervous system by a papovavirus in patients with impaired immune mechanisms. It usually occurs late in the course of Hodgkin's disease or chronic leukemia and is characterized by progressive and multifocal neurologic signs, leading to death within a few months. A more acute viral infection by herpes-type inclusion bodies is now seen with increasing frequency as a complication of cancer and its treatment.

The bacteria that most commonly cause infections are *Listeria monocytogenes*, *Pseudomonas*, and *Escherichia coli*. Fungi are the incriminating organisms in 50% of the cases, the most frequent being *Aspergillus* and *Cryptococcus*. These occur with particular frequency in patients with lymphoma.

Treatment depends, of course, on the organism identified. The clinical picture consists of headache, fever, stupor or coma, seizures, and sometimes localizing CNS signs.

Metabolic Encephalopathy

Organ failure, in particular the liver or lung, caused by cancer is the usual cause for encephalopathy. Metabolic encephalopathies due to failure of organ function are usually readily identified and are described in Chapter 11.

Cerebrovascular Disease

A significant complication of cancer and its treatment is cerebrovascular disease. Intracerebral or subdural hemorrhage may occur in patients with thrombocytopenia. This syndrome is probably seen most frequently in acute myelogenous leukemia. Embolic infarction secondary to marantic endocarditis occurs in patients with solid tumors, particularly bronchogenic carcinoma. There is a recent report of intravascular coagulation causing multifocal brain infarctions and diffuse neurologic signs and symptoms. Most were in women with leukemia or lymphoma. These patients rather abruptly develop signs of diffuse brain disease (focal seizures, hemiparesis, delirium, stupor) and eventually show laboratory evidence of coagulation abnormalities, e.g., decreased platelets, increased prothrombin times, and decreased fibrinogen and fibrin-split products. It is important to recognize the nature of this consumption coagulopathy, for early treatment with intravenous heparin may be life-saving.

Syncope

Fainting is a common problem; and although in most instances it has no sinister significance, it is dramatic and frightening, and not infrequently brings the patient to a physician for evaluation, particularly if it is not a solitary episode. Recurrent fainting may point to a serious systemic disorder, and occasionally a syncopal attack must be differentiated from a convulsive seizure.

By definition, syncope is a brief temporary loss of consciousness caused by decreased cerebral perfusion. Recovery is complete, usually soon after the patient assumes the horizontal posture. It is never caused by disease of the brain, but is secondary to any disturbance, usually cardiovascular in origin, which temporarily decreases cerebral perfusion. Obviously, brief cardiac arrest causes syncope; but if the arrest is prolonged for more than a few seconds, the syncopal attack becomes a much more serious event.

Etiologies of syncope are quite varied and are described in more detail below, but the pathophysiology of the final event is a function of the cerebral circulation. The brain requires a constant delivery of oxygen for it has no oxygen stores. It also requires a steady supply of glucose, but glucose and glycogen stores in the brain are sufficient to maintain some function for 60 to 90 min, whereas the effects of oxygen deprivation are felt within a few seconds. Cerebral blood flow (CBF) averages about 700 ml/min, about 12% of the total resting cardiac output; cerebral oxygen consumption is about 60 ml/min, about one-fifth the total oxygen resting consumption of the body. The brain receives 70 to 80 mg glucose per minute, about 75% of the total glucose production of the liver. With this background we can describe the physiologic events which lead to syncope. In many instances there is first a failure of the neurogenic and humoral mechanisms which ordinarily constrict peripheral resistance vessels on assuming the upright posture, causing a drop in systemic and cerebral perfusion pressure. So long as autoregulatory function of the cerebral arteries is retained, CBF remains unchanged because of cerebral vasodilatation. When autoregulation fails (about 60 torr), CBF decreases and oxygen and glucose extraction from cerebral blood are increased to maintain a stable cerebral metabolism. As CBF decreases further, this compensatory mechanism also fails and cerebral oxygen consumption drops, eventually causing failure of the reticular activating system and loss of consciousness.

The symptoms caused by the above sequence of events are fairly typical, but the physician often must rely on an eyewitness's description of the event in order to distinguish syncope from an epileptic attack. Onset of syncope is *usually* (not invariably) not abrupt and, with few exceptions (e.g., the Adams-Stokes syndrome), begins with the patient in the upright position. Patients usually complain of nausea, giddiness, weakness, sweating, pallor, deep breathing, dimness of vision and hearing. Upon losing consciousness the patient usually lies motionless, although mild clonic jerks may occur if the syncope lasts 30 sec or more. Usually the patient regains consciousness rapidly once horizontal and, although weak, is oriented and not confused or drowsy. During unconsciousness, the patient appears pale with slowed pulse and respiration.

Syncope Classification

The two major etiologies of syncope are orthostasis and heart disease, the former benign, the latter potentially serious. Other etiologies exist, but they are of small importance statistically. The classification is as follows:

I. Syncope due to orthostasis.
   A. *Vasodepressor (vasovagal) syncope.* By far the commonest cause of syncope, particularly in young individuals, it may be induced by fright, sight of blood, a threatening situation, etc.
   B. *Defective vasopressor mechanisms.* When a person stands upright, 600 to 1,000 ml blood pools in the visceral and omental veins and the legs. The momentary decrease in circulating blood volume causes vasoconstriction, mediated by baroreceptors in the carotid sinuses and aorta via the autonomic control centers in the hypothalamus and medulla. Continued standing is compensated by humoral mechanisms. Failure of any of these regulatory mechanisms may allow arterial pressure to drop below the initial level necessary for adequate cerebral perfusion. The causes of this type of syncope are:
      1. Drug-induced syncope. Ganglionic blocking agents, diuretics, salt restriction, phenothiazines, tricyclic antidepressants, and L-DOPA are the major ones.
      2. Diseases of the nervous system. These include diabetic neuropathy, peripheral neuropathies of other cause, and primary dysautonomia (Shy-Drager syndrome).
      3. Poor postural adjustment due to disease or age.
      4. Sympathectomy.
      5. Impaired venous return to the heart.
         a. Severe venous insufficiency in the lower extremities.
         b. Tussive syncope. Syncope usually occurs after a prolonged coughing paroxysm, with its associated increased intrathoracic pressure.
         c. Micturition syncope. The usual clinical story is that the patient has ingested some alcohol the previous evening, awakens from sleep, and gets out of a warm bed to void. The syncope occurs without warning at the end of micturition. Recent observations suggest an association with hypokalemia and atrial fibrillation.
         d. Valsalva's maneuver.
II. Syncope due to heart disease.
   A. *Cardiac arrhythmias.*
      1. Adams-Stokes syndrome. Patients usually have a pulse less than 40 and a complete A-V block shown by ECG. The mechanism for the syncope is ventricular arrest. A pacemaker is the usual required therapy.
      2. Tachyarrhythmias. Those responsible for syncope are said to be paroxysmal atrial fibrillation or flutter, ventricular tachycardia and fibrillation.
   B. *Aortic stenosis.* Syncope is associated with exercise.
   C. *Other cardiac causes* include primary pulmonary hypertension,

myocardial infarction, tetralogy of Fallot, dissecting aneurysm, and atrial or ventricular myxoma.

III. Other causes of syncope.
  A. *Hypersensitive carotid sinus.*
  B. *Vagovagal syncope.* This is said to be an esophageal disorder. The swallowing reflex may cause reflex vagal stimulation with bradycardia, decreased cardiac output, and syncope.
  C. *Hyperventilation.*
  D. *Hysterical syncope.*

The differential diagnosis of syncope includes epilepsy, drop attacks, cataplexy, pulseless disease, vestibular disease, herniation of cerebellar tonsils after sneezing or coughing, and rarely hypoglycemia.

The treatment of recurrent syncope is the management of the responsible pathology.

Sleep Disorders

Although neurologists clearly have no monopoly on the management of patients with disturbed sleep patterns, it is equally true that it is reasonable to think of sleep as a function of the CNS, a state of altered consciousness, and therefore that sleep disorders are in some way related to altered function in some part of the CNS. We know remarkably little about the nature of sleep, but that is no more surprising than our lack of understanding of the mechanisms responsible for many other common physiologic functions, e.g., speech, comprehension, memory, abstraction, behavior in general, and countless other simple and complex tasks of the CNS. Of all sleep disorders, only insomnia is truly common and that is probably ubiquitous, affecting everyone on occasion.

We do know a bit about some physiologic events which occur during normal sleep, and that these vary among the stages of sleep, which are defined mainly by altered EEG patterns. The decrease in arterial pressure, pulse, and respiratory rates observed in non-rapid eye movement (non-REM) sleep changes to evidence of autonomic activation during REM sleep. Penile erection occurs regularly in 90-min cycles, particularly during REM sleep, and this phenomenon is utilized in the evaluation of impotence. The absence of penile erection during sleep indicates an organic basis for impotence. Secretion of growth hormone, prolactin, and luteinizing hormones increases during sleep in adolescents, and there is also an increase in the secretion of antidiuretic hormone.

Physiologic sleep is traditionally divided into five EEG stages, according to the observations made by Aserinsky and Kleitman in 1953. During stage 1 the subject's eyes roll slowly and his muscles relax. The EEG shows low-voltage and mixed frequencies. In stage 2 there are 12- to 14-Hz sleep spindles accompanied by high-amplitude complex long-duration waves called K complexes. Stage 3 is characterized by high-voltage 1- to 2-Hz waves, which increase in number during stage 4. REM sleep, or stage 5 sleep, shows an EEG pattern similar to that of stage 1, accompanied by REMs. This usually begins about 70 min after the subject enters stage 1, and the cycle is repeated four to six times a night. During REM sleep brain metabolism (in cats) is generally increased; and in addition to tumescence, dreams appear to occur almost exclusively during REM. It is said that individuals deprived of REM sleep develop behavioral abnormalities, including irritability, impulsivity, acting out, and poor judgment.

The biochemical basis for sleep is not at all understood. Although it is assumed that the reticular activating system is somehow involved in the sleep process, even that is conjectural. Recent studies have claimed that serotonin acting somewhere in the brainstem or hypothalamus is somehow concerned with sleep induction, whereas norepinephrine, synthesized by neurons originating almost exclusively in the locus ceruleus, supresses sleep.

Insomnia

As previously mentioned, insomnia is by far the commonest sleep abnormality. Indeed it may be one of the most frequent complaints (along with constipation) encountered by physicians. Most insomnia is secondary to depression (which does not have to be severe), situational problems, simple worry, or physical discomfort. There is evidence that insomniacs often sleep much more than they claim or believe they do. Management of chronic insomnia is not easy. Many patients become habituated to various types of sedative, the physiologic effects of which are in question. Treatment of depression by pharmacologic means, as with tricyclic antidepressants, may be helpful. The patient must be encouraged to abandon sedatives and allow the sleep-wake cycle to adjust physiologically.

"Jet lag" is an interesting form of insomnia. Susceptible individuals may experience great difficulty in the normalization of the sleep cycle after long air trips, particularly across the international dateline.

Hypersomnia

There are several clinical syndromes characterized by excessive sleep.

Sleep apnea

The term "sleep apnea" has been used only for the past 12 years to describe the mechanism responsible for excessive daytime drowsiness in some patients. As the name implies, the patient become apneic for a brief period during sleep. The apnea is accompanied by hypoxia, which seems to serve as a stimulus to awaken the patient sufficiently to stimulate respiration again.

Continued recurrence of the apneic spells does not permit the patient to go beyond stage 2 sleep and often not beyond stage 1. As a consequence he is sleep-deprived and is drowsy and falls asleep uncontrollably during daylight hours.

The mechanism responsible for the apnea is usually mechanical obstruction of the nasopharynx or larynx following muscle relaxation when the patient begins to fall asleep. Jaw deformities, nasopharyngeal masses, obesity, and short neck have been incriminated. The patients are often short and obese. In this regard, the sleep apnea syndrome is probably what is occurring in pick-wickian syndrome, and it is the hypoxia rather than hypercapnia which is the culprit. Diagnosis is made by history (daytime drowsiness, and recurrent snorting and snoring during sleep) and by observation during sleep. Monitoring the respiration will reveal the apnea, arterial blood will show hypoxia, and the EEG will confirm that the patient does not go beyond stage 2 sleep. Treatment is by tracheostomy, which usually results in a dramatic cure. Persistence of sleep apnea may cause hypertension, systemic and pulmonary, and congestive heart failure.

Narcolepsy

Narcolepsy is probably the most frequent of the hypersomnic disorders. It is a fascinating syndrome characterized by some or all of the following:

1. *Attacks of uncontrollable sleepiness.* These may occur at any time, not only when the patient is sitting quietly, listening to a lecture, or after eating. They may occur while driving or, as in the case of a nurse, at the operating table. The patient is easily awakened and is immediately alert. The usual sleep period is about 15 min if the patient is undisturbed. These episodes may occur several times daily.

2. *Cataplexy.* This is a sudden loss of muscle tone occurring usually during a period of excitement or laughter. The patient's knees buckle, the head falls forward, the arms drop to the side. The patient may actually fall to the ground, but this is rare. The cataplectic periods may last 2 sec to 2 min.

3. *Sleep paralysis.* This is a phenomenon experienced by many normal individuals, particularly on awakening from a dream. It occurs with considerable frequency as a part of the narcoleptic syndrome. The patient may be unable to move either on awakening or while falling asleep. A touch or sharp command by someone may be sufficient to break the spell.

4. *Hallucinations*—visual, auditory, or both—may occur at the beginning of the period of sleep paralysis. These constitute the rarest part of the syndrome.

Some classify somnambulism as a part of the narcoleptic syndrome, but it occurs occasionally in otherwise normal individuals, particularly children who are difficult to arouse.

The etiology and physiologic mechanisms remain a mystery. No distinctive pathology has ever been described. It is known that these patients enter directly into REM sleep during a sleep attack and that the nocturnal sleep pattern varies from normal. The significance of this is not at all clear.

Fortunately, treatment may be quite effective, utilizing methylphenidate HCl (Ritalin) in doses of 10 to 15 mg t.i.d.; the dose may be decreased in amount or discontinued altogether after a symptom-free period of several weeks. Dextroamphetamine (Dexedrine) is also useful.

Klein-Levin syndrome

The Klein-Levin syndrome is a remarkable disorder with bizarre characteristics and no identifiable etiology. The patients are usually young adults or adolescents, more frequently males. Four or five times yearly they retire to their beds and sleep for hours or days at a time, venturing out only to eliminate and eat. They eat excessively during this period, which may last several days to 3 weeks, and appear to be withdrawn, inappropriate, negative, slow to respond, and even incoherent. No neurologic abnormalities can be found, and no evidence of endocrine disorder has been demonstrated. The EEG is normal. There is no effective therapy, nor is there any evidence that the patients wish to be helped during the attacks.

Miscellaneous hypersomnic disorders

Hypersomnia occurs also in various encephalopathies, particularly certain types of viral encephalitis, trypanosomiasis (a protozoal infestation transmitted by mosquito bite in certain areas of Africa), and deep midline (particularly hypothalamic) brain tumors.

Ondine's Curse

Ondine's curse cannot be classified strictly as a sleep disorder, but it is certainly a dramatic event which occurs only during sleep. The name is derived from the curse placed on an unfaithful lover by a river maiden or nymph in Teutonic mythology. The unfortunate victim was forced to stay awake in order to breathe. Cessation of respiration during sleep has been reported in low medullary and high cervical cord lesions and was quite frequent following bilateral cervical tractotomy for intractable pain.

Neurologic Complications of Alcoholism

Some of the neurologic complications of alcoholism were attended to in the discussions of hepatic encephalopathy, peripheral neuropathy, and Wernicke-Korsakoff syndrome, but excessive ingestion of alcohol is so commonplace— not only in the United States but in practically all industrialized societies—

that some comments about some of its other neurologic complications are in order. It is estimated that perhaps 7 to 8% of adults in the United States are alcoholics, i.e., are addicted to alcohol. The number of those who drink substantially is staggering. These figures are even more impressive in many European countries where wine is preferred to water, even by children, particularly in the Scandinavian countries, Iceland, Greenland, and Finland.

There is, of course, no doubt at all that alcohol is a poison which rapidly affects the metabolic activity of practically all tissue cells—gastric, hepatic, hematopoietic, muscle, and neural. These toxic effects on the CNS are readily observed in the ataxia, speech slurring, and impaired mentation and judgment of the intoxicated person; the EEG taken during intoxication shows excessive moderate-voltage slow-wave activity diffusely. It is further known that alcohol acts in a complementary fashion with a wide variety of other supressant drugs; this more than additive effect not infrequently is fatal.

Alcohol withdrawal produces abstinence syndromes in the majority of heavy drinkers. Tremulousness, restlessness, sleeplessness, excessive perspiration, and anorexia appear 8 to 12 hr after the last drink, and some portions of that syndrome may persist for days to weeks. *Alcoholic hallucinosis*, visual and auditory, may appear 24 to 48 hr after withdrawal. Although usually temporary, a small percentage of these patients remain with chronic auditory hallucinosis, often of a paranoid nature.

Withdrawal seizures ("rum fits") may occur within 24 to 36 hr after abstinence begins. The seizures are usually major motor seizures, generalized and single, but several may occur within a 24-hr period. Since alcoholics are notorious for sustaining head injuries, a seizure in the setting of withdrawal must not be viewed cavalierly. It may represent the first sign of a subdural hematoma.

Delirium tremens is the most dangerous complication of alcohol withdrawal, appearing 60 to 72 hr after withdrawal, sometimes when the patient has already had a surgical operation and is presumably recuperating. It is preceded by tremulousness, hallucinations, seizures, illusions, confusion, irritability, insomnia, anorexia, and psychomotor and autonomic overactivity. Approximately 10 to 15% of these patients die, but mortality can be reduced by the judicious use of benzodiazepines or phenothiazines and appropriate fluid and electrolyte (including magnesium) replacement and monitoring. These patients should be in an intensive care unit if possible.

The previously discussed major complications of alcoholism are not reviewed again here. The magnitude of the problem is evident. One recent note has been added which should strike terror in the hearts of even "social" drinkers. Computerized axial tomography (CAT) scanning suggests a correlation between sulcal widening and increased ventricular size and alcohol ingestion, and alcohol ingestion has been demonstrated to produce cortical atrophy and neuronal loss in rats. So much for the two-martini lunch—or supper, for that matter.

SUGGESTED READINGS

Cardiovascular Disorders

Adams CW, et al: Intracardiac myxomas and thrombi. *Am J Cardiol* 7:176, 1961.

Denker SJ and Landahl A: Major mental disturbances in patients surgically treated for mitral stenosis. *Acta Psychiatr Scand* 38:117, 1962.

Derbes VJ, and Kerr A: *Cough Syncope.* Charles C Thomas, Springfield, Ill, 1955.

Engel GL: *Fainting.* Charles C Thomas, Springfield, Ill, 1962.

Hutchinson EC, and Stock JP: The carotid sinus syndrome. *Lancet* 2:445, 1960.

James TN: Observations on cardiovascular involvement in progressive muscular dystrophy. *Am Heart J* 63:48, 1962.

Johannson BW: Adams-Stokes syndrome. *Am J Cardiol* 8:76, 1961.

Jordan RA, et al: Mural thrombosis and arterial embolism in mitral stenosis. *Circulation* 3:363, 1951.

Karp HR, et al: Vasodepressor syncope. *Arch Neurol* 5:106, 1961.

Krinsky CM, and Merritt HH: Neurologic manifestations of subacute bacterial endocarditis. *N Engl J Med* 218:263, 1938.

Silverstein A, and Krieger HP: Neurologic complications of cardiac surgery. *Arch Neurol* 3:601, 1960.

Stephens JW: Neurological sequelae of congenital heart surgery. *Arch Neurol* 7:450, 1962.

Swanson PF: Neurologic disorders in aortic stenosis. *Johns Hopkins Hosp Bull* 103:287, 1958.

Tyler HR, and Clark DC: Incidence of neurologic complications in congenital heart disease. *Arch Neurol* 77:17, 1957.

Hepatic Disorders

Adams RD: Acquired hepatocerebral degeneration. In: *Handbook of Clinical Neurology, Vol 6: Diseases of Basal Ganglia*, pp 279–297. North-Holland, Amsterdam, 1968.

Asao H, and Oji K: *Hepatocerebral Degeneration.* Charles C Thomas, Springfield, Ill, 1968.

Cullity GJ, and Kakulas BA: Encephalopathy and fatty degeneration of the viscera. *Brain* 93:77, 1970.

Fischer JE, and Baldessarini RJ: False neurotransmitters and hepatic failure. *Lancet* 2:75, 1971.

Gibson JB: Encephalopathy after portocaval shunt. *Br Med J* 1:1652, 1963.

Knill-Jones RP, Goodwill CJ, Dayan AD, et al: Peripheral neuropathy in chronic liver disease. *J Neurol Neurosurg Psychiatry* 35:22, 1972.

Parkes JD, Sharpstone P, and Williams R: Levodopa in hepatic coma. *Lancet* 2:1341, 1970.

Read AE, Sherlock S, Laidlaw J, et al: The neuropsychiatric syndromes associated with chronic liver disease and an extensive portal-systemic collateral circulation. *Q J Med* 36:135, 1967.

Reye RDK, Morgan G, Baral J, et al: Encephalopathy and fatty degeneration of the viscera: a disease entity in childhood. *Lancet* 2:749, 1963.

Selby G: Subacute myelo-optic neuropathy in Australia. *Lancet* 1:123, 1972.

Sherlock S: Hepatic coma. *Gastroenterology* 54:754, 1968.

Victor M, Adams RD, and Cole M: The acquired (non-Wilsonian) type of chronic hepatocerebral degeneration. *Medicine (Baltimore)* 44:345, 1965.

Zieve L: Pathogenesis of hepatic coma. *Arch Intern Med* 118:211, 1966.

Malabsorption Disorders

Banerji NK, and Hurwitz LJ: Neurological manifestations in adult steatorrhea. *J Neurol Sci* 14:125, 1971.

Banerji NK, and Hurwitz LJ: Nervous system manifestations after gastric surgery. *Acta Neurol Scand* 47:485, 1971.

Cooke WT, and Smith WT: Neurological disorders associated with adult coeliac disease. *Brain* 89:683, 1966.

Koudouris SD, Stern TN, and Utterback RA: Involvement of central nervous system in Whipple's disease. *Neurology (Minneap)* 13:397, 1963.

Maizel H, Ruffin JM, and Dobbins WO III: Whipple's disease: a review of patients from one hospital and a review of the literature since 1950. *Medicine (Baltimore)* 49:175, 1970.
Smith WT, French JM, Gottsman M, et al: Cerebral complications of Whipple's disease. *Brain* 88:137, 1965.

Parathyroid Disorders

Clunie GJA, Gunn A, and Robson JS: Hyperparathyroid crisis. *Br J Surg* 54:538, 1967.
Dimich A, Bedrossian PB, and Wallach S: Hypoparathyroidism: clinical observations in 34 patients. *Arch Intern Med* 120:449, 1967.
Riddick FA: Primary hyperparathyroidism. *Med Clin North Am* 51:871, 1967.

Hematologic Disorders

Alpers BJ, and Duane W: Intracranial hemorrhage in purpura hemorrhagica. *J Nerv Ment Dis* 78:260, 1933.
Amorosi ES, and Ultmann JE: Thrombotic thrombocytopenic purpura: report of 16 cases and review of the literature. *Medicine (Baltimore)* 45:139, 1966.
Darnley JD: Polyneuropathy in Waldenström's macroglobulinemia. *Neurology (Minneap)* 12:617, 1962.
Fraser TN: Cerebral manifestation of addisonism in pernicious anemia. *Lancet* 2:458, 1960.
Freeman AG, and Heaton JM: The aetiology of retrobulbar neuritis in addisonian pernicious anemia. *Lancet* 280:908, 1961.
Goldberg A: Diagnosis and treatment of the porphyrias. *Proc R Soc Med* 61:193, 1968.
Holmes JM: Cerebral manifestations of vitamin B_{12} deficiency. *Br Med J* 2:1394, 1956.
Kaufman G: Hodgkin's disease involving the central nervous system. *Arch Neurol* 13:555, 1965.
Portnoy BA, and Nerron JC: Neurological manifestations in sickle cell disease. *Ann Intern Med* 76:643, 1972.
Stein JA, and Tschudy DP: Acute intermittent porphyria: a clinical and biochemical study of 46 patients. *Medicine (Baltimore)* 49:1, 1970.
Strachan RW, and Henderson JG: Psychiatric syndromes due to avitaminosis B_{12} with normal blood and marrow. *Q J Med* 34:303, 1965.
Strong RR, and Tovi D: Subdural hematoma complicating anticoagulant therapy. *Br Med J* 11:845, 1962.
Victor M, and Lear AA: Subacute combined degeneration of the spinal cord. *Am J Med* 20:896, 1956.

Pancreatic Disorders

Fras I, Litin EM, and Bartholomew LG: Mental symptoms as an aid in the early diagnosis of carcinoma of the pancreas. *Gastroenterology* 55:191, 1968.
Rothermich NO, and von Haam E: Pancreatic encephalopathy. *J Clin Endocrinol* 1:872, 1941.
Sharf B, and Bental E: Pancreatic encephalopathy. *J Neurol Neurosurg Psychiatry* 34:357, 1971.
Texter EC Jr, Danovitch SH, Kuhl WJ, et al: Physiologic studies of autonomic-nervous system dysfunction accompanying diabetes mellitus. *Am J Dig Dis* 7:530, 1962.

Diabetes

Appenzeller O, and Richardson EP Jr: Sympathetic chain in patients with diabetic and alcoholic polyneuropathy. *Neurology (Minneap)* 16:1205, 1966.
Greenbaum D, Richardson PC, Salmon MV, and Urich H: Pathological observations on six cases of diabetic neuropathy. *Brain* 87:201, 1964.
Greenbaum D: Observations on the homogeneous nature and pathogenesis of diabetic neuropathy. *Brain* 87:215, 1964.
Halmos PB, Nelson JK, and Lowry RC: Hyperosmolar nonketoacidotic coma in diabetics. *Lancet* 1:675, 1966.
Mayne N: the short-term prognosis in diabetic neuropathy. *Diabetes* 17:270, 1968.

Raff MC, and Asbury AK: Ischemic mononeuropathy and mononeuropathy multiplex in diabetes mellitus. *N Engl J Med* 279:17, 1968.

Raff MC, Sangaland V, and Asbury AK: Ischemic mononeuropathy multiplex associated with diabetes mellitus. *Arch Neurol* 18:487, 1968.

Endocrine Disorders

Barttler FC: The parathyroid gland and its relationship to disease of the nervous system. *Proc Assoc Res Nerv Ment Dis* 32:1, 1952.

Fessel W: Myopathy of thyroidism. *Ann Rheum Dis* 27:590, 1968.

Havard CWH: Thyrotoxic myopathy. *Br Med J* 1:440, 1962.

Hed R, Kirstein L, and Lundmark C: Thyrotoxic myopathy. *J Neurol Neurosurg Psychiatry* 21:270, 1958.

Jackman RL, and Jones RE: Hyperthyroidism and periodic paralysis. *Arch Intern Med* 113:657, 1964.

Jefferson A: Symposium on pituitary adenomata. *Arch Neurol* 12:326, 1965.

Jellinek EH, and Kelly RE: Cerebellar syndrome in myxedema. *Lancet* 2:225, 1960.

Logothetis J: Neurologic and muscular manifestations of hyperthyroidism. *Arch Neurol* 5:533, 1961.

Petersen P: Psychiatric disorders in primary hyperparathyroidism. *J Clin Endocrinol* 28:1487, 1968.

Sanders V: Neurologic manifestations of myxedema. *N Engl J Med* 266:547, 599, 1962.

Scholz DA, Haines SF, and Henderson JW: Ophthalmopathy associated with Grave's disease: unusual clinical manifestations and their management. *Arch Intern Med* 112:555, 1963.

Sheehan HL: Postpartum necrosis of anterior pituitary. *J Pathol Bacteriol* 45:189, 1937.

Wright RL: Hemorrhage into pituitary adenomata. *Arch Neurol* 12:326, 1965.

Autonomic System Disorders

Riley CM: Familial dysautonomia. *Adv Pediatr* 9:157, 1957.

Collagen-Vascular and Rheumatoid Disease

Attwood W, and Poser CM: Neurologic complications of Sjögren's syndrome. *Neurology (Minneap)* 11:1034, 1961.

Bleehen SS, Lovelace RE, and Colton RE: Mononeuritis multiplex in polyarteritis nodosa. *Q J Med* 127:193, 1963.

Drachman DA: Neurological complications of Wegener's granulomatosis. *Arch Neurol* 8:45, 1963.

Gordon AL, and Yudell A: Cauda equina lesions associated with rheumatoid spondylitis. *Ann Intern Med* 78:555, 1973.

Hollenhorst RW, et al: Neurologic aspects of temporal arteritis. *Neurology (Minneap)* 10:490, 1960.

Johnson RT, and Richardson EP: The neurological manifestations of systemic lupus erythematosus. *Medicine (Baltimore)* 47:337, 1968.

Kao CC, Messert B, Winkler SS, and Turner JH: Rheumatoid C_1-C_2 dislocation: pathogenesis and treatment reconsidered. *J Neurol Neurosurg Psychiatry* 37:1069, 1974.

Matthews NT, and Chandy J: Painful ophthalmoplegia. *J Neurol Sci* 11:243, 1970.

Matthews WB, and Burne JC: The neurological aspects of dermatomyositis. *J Neurosurg Psychiatry* 16:49, 1953.

O'Connor JF, and Musher DM: Central nervous system involvement in systemic lupus erythematosus: a study of 150 cases. *Arch Neurol* 14:157, 1966.

Rose AL, and Walton JN: Polymyositis: a survey of 89 cases with particular reference to treatment and prognosis. *Brain* 89:747, 1966.

Schmid R, et al: Arteritis in rheumatoid arthritis. *Am J Med* 30:56, 1961.

Smith JL: Cogan's syndrome. *Laryngoscope* 80:121, 1970.

Smith PH, et al: Natural history of rheumatoid cervical luxations. *Ann Rheum Dis* 31:431, 1972.

Tuffonelli DL, and Winkelmann RK: Systemic scleroderma: a clinical study of 727 cases. *Arch Dermatol* 84:359, 1961.

Renal Disorders

Asbury AK, Victor M, and Adams RD: Uremic polyneuropathy. *Arch Neurol* 8:413, 1963.
Locke S, Merrill JP, and Tyler HR: Neurologic complications of acute uremia. *Arch Intern Med* 108:519, 1961.
Mahurkar SD, Dhar SK, Salta R, Meyers L Jr, Smith EC, and Dunea G: Dialysis dementia. *Lancet* 1:1412, 1973.
Raskin NH, and Fishman RA: Neurological disorders in renal failure. *N Engl J Med* 294:143, 204, 1976.
Tyler HR: Neurological complications of dialysis, transplantation, and other forms of treatment in chronic uremia. *Neurology (Minneap)* 15:419, 1965.
Tyler HR: Neurologic disorders in renal failure. *Am J Med* 44:734, 1968.

Sarcoidosis

Jefferson M: Sarcoidosis of the nervous system. *Brain* 80:540, 1957.
Wiederholt WC, and Siekert RG: Neurological manifestations of sarcoidosis. *Neurology (Minneap)* 15:1147, 1965.

Carcinoma

Brain WR, and Norris F: *The Remote Effects of Cancer on the Nervous System.* Grune & Stratton, New York, 1965.
Brain WR, and Wilkinson M: Subacute cerebellar degeneration associated with neoplasms. *Brain* 88:465, 1965.
Chernik NL, et al: Central nervous system infections in patients with cancer. *Medicine (Baltimore)* 52:563, 1973.
Clark E: Peripheral neuropathy associated with multiple myelomatosis. *Neurology (Minneap)* 6:146, 1956.
Croft PB, and Wilkinson M: Incidence of carcinomatous neuromyopathy in patients with various types of carcinoma. *Brain* 88:427, 1965.
Henson RA, Hoffman HL, and Urich H: Encephalomyelitis with carcinoma. *Brain* 88:449, 1965.
Henson RA, Russell DS, and Wilkinson M: Carcinomatous neuropathy and myopathy: a clinical and pathological study. *Brain* 77:82, 1954.
Hutchinson EC, Leonard BJ, Mandoley C, and Yates PO: Neurological complications of the reticuloses. *Brain* 25:1, 1965.
Hyman CB, Bogle JM, Brubaker CA, Williams K, and Hammond D: Central nervous system involvement by leukemia in children. I. Relationship to systemic leukemia and description of clinical and laboratory manifestations. *Blood* 25:1, 1965.
Hyman CB, Bogle JM, Brubaker CA, Williams K, and Hammond D: Central nervous system involvement by leukemia in children. II. Therapy with intrathecal methotrexate. *Blood* 25:13, 1965.
Phair JP, Anderson RE, and Namiki H: The central nervous system in leukemia. *Ann Intern Med* 61:863, 1964.
Posner JB: Neurological complications of systemic cancer. *Med Clin North Am* 55:625, 1971.
Posner JB: Spinal cord compression: a neurological emergency. *Memorial Hosp Clin Bull* 1:65, 1971.
Sperling HJ, Adams RD, and Parker F: Involvement of the nervous system by malignant lymphoma. *Medicine (Baltimore)* 26:285, 1947.
Victor M, Banker BQ, and Adams RD: The neuropathy of multiple myeloma. *Trans Am Neurol Assoc* 80:99, 1955.

Pulmonary Disorders

Austen FK, Carmichael MW, and Adams RD: Neurological manifestations of chronic pulmonary insufficiency. *N Engl J Med* 257:579, 1957.

Syncope

Corbett JJ, Butler AB, and Kaufman B: "Sneeze syncope," basilar invagination and Arnold-Chiari type I malformation. *J Neurol Neurosurg Psychiatry* 39:381, 1976.

Engel GS (ed): *Fainting*. Charles C Thomas, Springfield, Ill, 1962.

Johnson RH: Orthostatic hypotension in neurologic disease. *Cardiology* 61:150, 1976.

Levin B, and Posner JB: Swallow syncope. *Neurology (Minneap)* 22:1086, 1972.

Noble RJ: The patient with syncope. *JAMA* 237:1372, 1976.

Schoenberg BS, Kuglitsch JF, and Karnes WE: Micturition syncope—not a single entity. *JAMA* 229:1631, 1974.

Thulesius O: Pathophysiological classification and diagnosis of orthostatic hypotension. *Cardiology* 61 (Suppl 1):180, 1976.

Sleep Disorders

Dement WC, and Guilleminault CG: Sleep disorders: the state of the art. *Hosp Pract* November:57–70, 1973.

Dement WC, Guilleminault C, and Zarcone V: The pathologies of sleep: a case series approach. In: *The Nervous System*, Vol 2, edited by DB Tower. Raven Press, New York, 1975.

Dement WC, Guilleminault C, Zarcone V, Wilson R, and Carskadon M: The narcolepsy syndrome. In: *Current Diagnosis*, Vol 5, edited by H Conn and R Conn. Saunders, Philadelphia, 1977.

Dement WC, and Kleitman N: Cyclic variations in EEG during sleep and their relation to eye movements, body motility and dreaming. *Electroencephalogr Clin Neurophysiol* 9:673, 1957.

Guilleminault C, Eldridge FL, and Dement WC: Insomina with sleep apnea: a new syndrome. *Science* 181:856, 1973.

Guilleminault C, Tilkian A, and Dement WC: The sleep apnea syndromes. *Annu Rev Med* 27:465, 1976.

Jouvet M: Paradoxical sleep: a study of its nature and mechanism. In: *Sleep Mechanisms*: *Progress in Brain Research*, Vol 20, edited by WA Himwick and JP Schade. Elsevier, Amsterdam, 1965.

Tilkian A, Guilleminault C, Schroeder J, Lehrman K, Simmons B, and Dement WC: Sleep-induced sleep apnea syndrome: prevalence of cardiac arrhythmias and their reversal after tracheostomy. *Am J Med* 63, 1977.

Miscellaneous Disorders

Aita JA: *Neurologic Manifestations of General Diseases*. Charles C Thomas, Springfield, Ill, 1964.

Glaser GH: Metabolic encephalopathy in hepatic, adrenal and pulmonary disorders. *Postgrad Med* 27:611, 1970.

Zavon MR: Treatment of organophosphorus and chlorinated hydrocarbon insecticide intoxication. *Mod Treatm* 4:625, 1967.

Alcoholism

Allsop J, and Turner B: Cerebellar degeneration associated with chronic alcoholism. *J Neurol Sci* 3:238, 1966.

Victor M: Treatment of alcoholic intoxication and the withdrawal syndrome. *Psychosom Med* 28:636, 1966.

Victor M: The pathophysiology of alcoholic epilepsy. *Proc Res Nerv Ment Dis* 46:431, 1968.

Victor M, Adams RD, and Mancall EL: Restricted form of cerebellar cortical degeneration occurring in alcoholic patients. *Arch Neurol* 1:579, 1959.

Subject Index